Psychiatric ethics

Psychiatric ethics

Edited by

SIDNEY BLOCH
Consultant Psychiatrist and Honorary
Clinical Lecturer, University of Oxford

and

PAUL CHODOFF
Clinical Professor of Psychiatry,
George Washington University
Washington DC

OXFORD
OXFORD UNIVERSITY PRESS
NEW YORK MELBOURNE
1981

Oxford University Press, Walton Street, Oxford OX2 6DP

London Glasgow New York Toronto
Delhi Bombay Calcutta Madras Karachi Kuala
Lumpur Singapore Hong Kong Tokyo
Nairobi Dar es Salaam Cape Town
Melbourne Wellington

and associate companies in
Beirut Berlin Ibadan Mexico City

British Library Cataloguing in Publication Data

Psychiatric ethics.
  1. Medical ethics   2. Psychiatry
  I. Bloch, Sidney, 19—   II. Chodoff, Paul
  174'.2   R724
ISBN 0-19-261182-8

Typeset by King's English Typesetters Ltd, Cambridge
Printed in Great Britain by
Butler & Tanner Ltd., Frome and London

Contents

vi   Contents

Contributors

JOHN BANCROFT, M.D., F.R.C.Psych., Research Scientist, MRC Reproductive Biology Unit, Edinburgh.

JEROME BEIGLER, M.D., Clinical Professor of Psychiatry, University of Chicago, and Consultant, Committee on Confidentiality, American Psychiatric Association.

SIDNEY BLOCH, M.B., Ph.D., Consultant Psychiatrist and Honorary Clinical Lecturer, University of Oxford.

PAUL CHODOFF, M.D., Clinical Professor of Psychiatry, George Washington University, Washington DC.

PHILIP GRAHAM, F.R.C.P., F.R.C.Psych., Professor of Child Psychiatry, Institute of Child Health, Hospital for Sick Children, London.

R. M. HARE, F.B.A., White's Professor of Moral Philosophy and Fellow of Corpus Christi College, University of Oxford.

DAVID HEYD, Ph.D., Lecturer in Philosophy, Hebrew University, Jerusalem.

TOKSOZ KARASU, M.D., Director, Department of Psychiatry, Bronx Municipal Hospital Center and Associate Professor of Psychiatry and Vice-Chairman, Albert Einstein College of Medicine, New York.

GERALD KLERMAN, M.D., Professor of Psychiatry, Harvard Medical School, Boston.

LOUIS McGARRY, M.D., Medical Director, Division of Forensic Services, Nassau County Department and Professor of Clinical Psychiatry, State University of New York, Stony Brook.

DAVID MECHANIC, Ph.D., Professor of Social Work, Graduate School of Social Work and Professor of Sociology, Acting Dean, Faculty of Arts and Sciences, Rutgers University, New Brunswick, New Jersey.

HAROLD MERSKEY, M.D., F.R.C.Psych., Professor of Psychiatry, University of Western Ontario, Canada.

ROBERT MICHELS, M.D., Psychiatrist-in-Chief, The New York Hospital and Barklie McKee Henry Professor and Chairman, Department of Psychiatry, Cornell University Medical College, New York.

DAVID MUSTO, M.A., M.D., Professor of Psychiatry (Child Study Center) and History of Medicine, Yale University.

JONAS RAPPEPORT, M.D., Chief Medical Officer, Supreme Bench of Baltimore, Maryland; Clinical Professor of Psychiatry, University of Maryland and Assistant Professor of Psychiatry, Johns Hopkins University, Baltimore.

WALTER REICH, M.D., Research Psychiatrist and Program Director, The Staff College, National Institute of Mental Health, Washington D.C.

GAIL SCHECHTER, M.A., Psychologist, Alcohol, Drug Abuse, and Mental Health Administration, Washington DC.

JOHN WING, M.D., Ph.D., Professor of Social Psychiatry, Institute of Psychiatry and London School of Hygiene, University of London.

1
Introduction

Sidney Bloch and Paul Chodoff

Why a book on psychiatric ethics?

Some psychiatrists might well pose the question: Why is there a need for a book on psychiatric ethics? The profession after all has existed for centuries and during this time its practitioners have managed to care for the mentally ill without becoming unduly preoccupied with moral questions. They might go further and aver that the psychiatrist's prime and sole interest is in his patients: it is inherent in the nature of his work that their optimal welfare is his *raison d'être*. These psychiatrists could buttress their argument by demonstrating the strong links between psychiatry and its parent profession of medicine, which has an even longer tradition of tending the ill along well established and self-evident principles of ethical conduct. Thus, the first principle of the American Medical Association's Principles of Medical Ethics,[†] which originated in 1847, states: 'The principal objective of the medical profession is to render service to humanity with full respect for the dignity of man.'[1] What could be more explicit?

Evidently psychiatrists, along with their medical colleagues, have, throughout the history of their profession, assumed implicitly that they could perform their task without ethical difficulties by serving the best interests of their patients. In the process they have tended by and large to ignore the ethical foundations of their work. One reflection of this state of affairs is the neglect of ethics in the education of psychiatrists; most training programmes have devoted little or no attention to the subject (see Chapter 16). Can there be elements of denial in this process of neglect? This would be partially to be expected: the psychiatrist who had to consider the ethical component of each decision he made would soon be immobilized. Psychiatric practice is characterized by uncertainties and ambiguities which must be kept within bounds.

Thomas Szasz was one of the first psychiatrists to highlight his colleagues' denial: 'Unfortunately these (ethical considerations) are often denied, minimised or merely kept out of focus; for the ideal of the medical profession as well as of the people whom it serves seems to be having a system of medicine (allegedly) free of ethical value'.[2] More

---

[†] The appendix contains codes of medical ethics relevant to psychiatry.

specifically in the case of American psychiatrists, Seymour Halleck has argued that they: 'are still convinced that their professional mandate is simply that of healing a form of illness and that their therapeutic activities do not and should not have political consequences'.[3] Halleck believes that a psychiatrist has a political role whether he is prepared to recognize it or not, and that this role has significant social and ethical implications. We would thoroughly agree with these contentions of both Szasz and Halleck. The contemporary psychiatrist, by virtue of his complex professional role, is required to grapple with a broad range of ethical problems. These problems may be relatively simple and direct and susceptible to easy remedies; most, unfortunately, will be far too complex for ready solution. In some instances the ethical dimension of the problem will be obvious but it will be hidden in others and require careful disentanglement. It is necessary, however, to remember that not every difficulty a psychiatrist faces is an ethical one. Room must be left for mistakes and errors in judgment made in good faith.

Psychiatrists may be relatively blind to ethical aspects of their profession for several reasons. As mentioned above, the ethical quality of a situation which a psychiatrist faces may not be easily apparent. Personal qualities within himself may hamper the psychiatrist's perception (denial has already been mentioned) or he may not have acquired a coherent and integrated set of principles with which to guide his conduct. Possibly the most significant barrier is that the psychiatrist, like other men, is necessarily involved in an internal conflict between forces motivating him towards or away from right behaviour.

Unfortunately a psychiatrist cannot rely on 'dedication to his patients' to lessen the immensity of the ethical problems facing him any more than he can cling to the proposition that psychiatry is basically an objective, scientifically based discipline and therefore unaffected by values. As we hope will become obvious in the chapters that follow, the need for the psychiatrist to make vital moral decisions is pervasive, infiltrating almost every facet of his work. And his task is made more complicated by the fact that most of the ethical problems he faces have not hitherto been adequately dealt with, let alone resolved. Some problems have not even begun to receive systematic study.

The contemporary interest in psychiatric ethics

The situation, however, appears to be changing. In the past two decades interest among psychiatrists (and the medical profession generally) in the ethical foundations of their work has blossomed, perhaps more so than in any other period of psychiatry's history. Psychiatric ethics has within a relatively short period become a most respectable subject. For example, its literature has mushroomed, particularly in the 1970s. Many psychiatric journals contain papers on ethical topics, and the bibliography is growing rapidly. The 1979–80 bibliography of the Hastings Centre (the Institute of Society, Ethics, and the Life Sciences), for example, lists nearly 300 references in the section on behaviour control.[4] The Centre's journal and its British counterpart, the *Journal of Medical Ethics*, regularly publish articles pertinent to mental health. The comprehensive *Encyclopaedia of bioethics*[5] published by the Kennedy Institute of Ethics in 1978, contains many entries relevant to psychiatry. Conferences and workshops on aspects of psychiatric ethics are becoming commonplace. Thus, the Taylor Manor Hospital in the United States devoted a recent annual symposium to 'moral issues in mental health care',[6] while the American Psychiatric Association co-sponsored a conference on the problems of 'psychiatrist as double agent' in 1977.[7] Ethical topics played an important role in the 1977 Congress of the World Psychiatric Association in Hawaii. The congress was also noteworthy for its adoption of a set of ethical guidelines for practising psychiatrists. The Declaration of Hawaii (see Appendix) was the culmination of several years' concern by the Association about questions concerning the ethical conduct of psychiatry among its member societies. The Congress went further by setting up a framework to implement the investigation of ethical conduct among these member societies. Several national psychiatric organizations have also paid increased attention to ethics and have set up special ethics committees. The British Royal College of Psychiatrists, for instance, established an ethics committee in 1974. A comparable committee in the American Psychiatric Association developed a code of ethics to serve as a guide for American psychiatrists in 1973 (see Appendix). Most district branches of the American Psychiatric Association have actively functioning ethics committees.

The absence of specific psychiatric codes until the 1970s was perhaps related to the notion that general medical codes such as the Hippocratic Oath, the Declaration of Geneva, and the American Medical Association's Principles of Medical Ethics were sufficient to cover the needs of the psychiatric profession. But with the growing focus on psychiatric ethics more specifically, has come the recognition that a number of problems are unique to the psychiatrist and therefore deserve specialized attention.

The reasons for the psychiatrist's new interest in ethics

Several factors have contributed to the burgeoning of interest in ethical issues among psychiatrists in the 1960s and 1970s. Among these are:

1. The 'medical consumer movement': recipients of health care have in recent years come to constitute a potent and more or less coherent social force. Perhaps as an example of the sceptical attitude towards authority which is developing as an apparent general cultural trend in the West, the physician no longer compels blind reverence, nor is there unquestioning compliance with his methods. We are now seeing growing demands that the views of the patient and his family be acknowledged and respected. Moore[8] has likened the movement to a 'social egalitarian revolution' in which demands are made that 'The patient be given greater responsibility in determining his or her care and involving less willingness to accept the opinions of professional experts'. There are calls for greater consumer participation in medical policy-making and for the medical establishment's recognition of decent health care as a basic civil right. Consider among other developments the formation of patient's associations, community health councils, and the phenomenal proliferation of self-help groups.[9] Although many of the last have arisen because they provide a forum for mutual support, other motives include the disaffection from conventional health care and the determination of patients with particular disabilities to form pressure lobbies to influence government authorities. The psychiatric patient, too, has thus been instrumental in forcing the psychiatrist to scrutinize more closely his professional activities.

2. It is no coincidence that the increased interest in ethics among psychiatrists has been associated with vehement, repeated attacks on their profession by what might be termed broadly the civil liberties approach to mental illness. This movement has been generated largely by psychiatrists themselves, a minority among their colleagues, but under the vigorous and articulate leadership of Thomas Szasz and Ronald Laing; and by lawyers who, especially in the United States, have come to comprise a relatively large and influential group known as the mental health bar.

Although many psychiatrists would dismiss figures like Szasz and Laing as polemicists, there is no doubt that they have been spurred by their critiques to adopt a more self-searching and questioning attitude to their profession. Szasz was the first to spark off widespread controversy with his publication in 1960 of *The myth of mental illness*[10] and since that time he has mounted a barrage of books and articles insisting that the psychiatrist is nothing more than a modern day inquisitor labelling and classifying behaviour in order to limit peoples' liberties; his role is that of social engineer.[11] Ronald Liefer, another psychiatric activist and a leader of the American 'Radical Psychiatry Movement', has argued vociferously that 'the State has assumed most of the traditional social functions of regulating and controlling human conduct. Because all moral codes are not codified in law, and because the power of the State is limited by a rule of law, the State is unable satisfactorily to control and influence individuals. This requires a new social institution that, under the auspices of an acceptable modern authority, can control and guide conduct without conspicuously violating publicly avowed ideals of freedom and respect for the individual. Psychiatry, in medical disguise, has assumed this historical function.'[12]

R. D. Laing[13], too, has added fuel to the fires with his claims that what has been called mental illness is but an anguished protest against intolerable social pressure, and that psychiatrists, rather than treating it with drugs and confinement, should examine their role in perpetuating it.

Faced with these criticisms both from colleagues and the legal profession psychiatrists have been provoked into considering more than ever before issues such as the criteria for the diagnoses of mental illness, the vague boundaries of their operations, the clash of loyalties to patient and other parties, the paucity of reliable data on the effectiveness of their treatments, the difficulty of assessing and predicting dangerousness, and the like. No reasonable pyschiatrist can avoid wrestling with the arguments proffered by these critics and in this regard the impact of the civil liberties movement has been favourable to the development of a socially responsible ethical sense. However, it is possible that one effect of so intense a legal involvement in psychiatric issues may have been counterproductive. To attempt to specify every aspect of the professional relationship in contractual terms leaves little room for the exercise of individual ethical judgement, and indeed may discourage its exercise. It has been observed that: 'In hell there will be nothing but law and due process will be meticulously observed'.

3. Contributing to both the previous factors for increased interest in psychiatric ethics is the fact that the treatment of the mentally ill has traditionally conjured up the image of manipulator and hapless victim; particularly so in the case of the patient who, because of his disorder, cannot provide informed consent. Controversy about their ethical permissibility has surrounded the use of all psychiatric treatments from physical manipulations of the brain — like psychosurgery and electroconvulsive therapy — to the psychotherapies, especially behaviour modification. In recent years

there has been much questioning of the efficacy of such treatments and their potency and dangers have been emphasized. The most drastic of these, psychosurgery, has been attacked so vigorously in the United States that a National Commission for its investigation was set up under Congressional auspices. The conclusions of the prestigious members of the Commission incidentally were surprisingly moderate.[14] The use of electroconvulsive therapy, too, has been decried, its critics labelling it as hazardous and barbaric under any circumstances. The reaction was so intense that a vociferous patient's advocacy group was responsible for the passage of legislation in the state of California imposing almost impossible barriers before ECT can be used. Furthermore, a body of opinion has held that many, if not most, psychiatric therapies are basically a form of behaviour control in which the patient has little or no say.

As a result of these controversies and criticisms, psychiatrists have had to exercise greater caution in planning treatment for their patients and have had to be more diligent in obtaining informed consent. These developments in the urgency of their efforts to curb ethical abuses may, ironically, be paving the way for new ethical problems, particularly the dilemma in which the psychiatrist is placed when he is not able to hospitalize or treat a severely disturbed patient.

4. The 1977 World Psychiatric Association Congress was momentous not only for the Declaration of Hawaii, but was also an ethical watershed in the annals of international psychiatric politics for another reason: the Soviet practice of labelling normal dissenters as mentally ill and committing them to mental hospitals was condemned by the Association. Furthermore, a commission was formed to monitor political misuse of psychiatry wherever it might occur.[15] At the previous World Congress in 1971 in Mexico City, the Soviet issue had been raised but summarily swept under the carpet. Between Mexico City and Honolulu, many Western psychiatrists had moved from incredulity that such abuse could take place to a conviction that the allegations were well founded. In the process, several national psychiatric organizations reacted with resolutions condemning their Soviet counterparts, and with other interventions aimed at bringing the practices to an end. Human rights organizations like Amnesty International adopted dissenter-patients as 'prisoners of conscience'. The misuse became (and remains) a prominent feature of international psychiatric discussions. Significantly for our purposes here, it provoked psychiatrists throughout the world to consider how readily psychiatry can be abused. (The Soviet case is discussed in detail in Chapter 18.)

5. Ethical aspects of psychiatric practice have been influenced in recent years by other professional disciplines besides the law; these

include sociology, psychology, theology, and philosophy. For instance, after an extended silence, a significant dialogue between psychiatrist and philosopher has developed. New attitudes in the philosopher, particularly the moral philosopher, have certainly been influential. Traditionally, the philosopher may have used a form of language which proved so abstruse as to intimidate even the most eager psychiatrist. Professor Hare, a contributor to this book, recognized this poor communication by his colleagues as long ago as 1952 when he wrote:'in a world in which problems of conduct become everyday more complex and tormenting, there is a great need for an understanding of the language in which these problems are posed and answered.'[16] His *The language of morals* endeavours to clarify the terms and concepts used by moral philosophers. Hare also emphasizes the need for moral philosophy to develop theoretical concepts which have a bearing on daily human activities, on actual concrete cases. Thus: 'The reason why actions are in a peculiar way revelatory of moral principles is that the function of moral principles is to guide conduct' and this includes the activities of a professional group like psychiatrists. Another Oxford philosopher, Mary Warnock, highlights this movement of focus from the abstract to the concrete case in her conclusions to her book on contemporary ethics. She refers particularly to the period since 1960 in which ethics 'has become a practical subject, and therefore more urgent and more interesting'.[17] She points out that a survey of ethics during this period 'would have to show far greater awareness that what people say philosophically may affect what they do in the real world'. Contemporary figures in philosophy have put forward theoretical propositions which have a distinct relevance for day-to-day conduct. A good example is the work of the American moral philosopher John Rawls: a central assumption in his *A theory of justice*[18] is that all morality is social morality. In the present volume, Professor Hare's chapter on the philosophical basis of psychiatric ethics is written in the same spirit as his *The language of morals* and with a particular sensitivity to the interests and needs of the practising psychiatrist.

Ethics: its boundaries in this book

'Ethics' has several connotations and we need now to examine the way in which we use the term in this book.

'Ethics', derived from the Greek adjective *ēthikos*, from *ēthos* meaning 'nature' or 'disposition', is commonly used in one of two ways which we can refer conveniently to as the philosophical and the practical. In the former case, we are concerned with a branch of philosophy, usually termed moral philosophy, whose purpose is the systematic study of human conduct with respect to the rightness and wrongness of actions and to the goodness and badness of the motives and ends of such actions. The moral philosopher attempts to show how value judgements are arrived at. Further, he tackles the question of whether ethical propositions can be proved. He focuses on concepts such as 'good', 'bad', 'right', 'wrong', 'should', 'ought', 'desirable', 'justice', 'duty', 'obligation', and similar evaluative terms. A fundamental premiss of the moral philosopher is that human conduct occurs within a context of values: where a person has a choice of one or another course of action and his activities are not completely prescribed, the inevitable question presents itself as to whether the particular action chosen is right or wrong, good or bad.

In tackling the questions of what constitutes ethical behaviour and how values are derived, he may offer a conceptual model or theory — this is the most general level of ethics. A number of classical models have been proposed.[19] One which has had a profound influence on moral philosophy is the *utilitarian* position of such writers as John Stuart Mill: the emphasis here is on the consequences of acts, on the balance between good and bad consequences, between benefits and harms. A person's action should be chosen so that it produces the best result, by recognizing the needs of all those persons who will be affected by that action. The final consequence would be the greatest-possible total happiness of all concerned. A competing position is the *absolutist*, or *deontological*, with its core thesis that certain acts are intrinsically wrong, regardless of their consequences, and can never be made right, and that moral judgements have universal applicability. An act like the murder of an innocent person or the theft of another person's property, for example, are judged in the absolutist approach to be always totally wrong. Religious morality is commonly of this kind, e.g. God's moral commands are viewed as absolute and must always be obeyed, or the Bible is accepted as the sole guide to moral conduct. We have already mentioned John Rawls[18] whose central thesis is that basic morality consists of those principles chosen by the rational[†] person with the important proviso that his judgements are made behind a 'veil of ignorance' — i.e. he is unaware of the position he would have in a society in which his principles would operate. Self-interest is thus avoided by the determination of moral principles while covered behind the 'veil'.

These theories may be coherent and well argued but a question still remains as to how they apply to concrete, day-to-day situations. In the case of the psychiatrist, like anyone else faced with complex situations, one could argue that every situation he deals with is in one

† Rawls uses 'rational' to mean 'always doing what is in one's own interest'.

way or another unique and that no general principles or guidelines of conduct can possibly apply. Certainly the psychiatrist must, by virtue of the nature of his work, arrive at ethical judgements in terms of real, concrete, and highly specific cases. The snag with an adherence to this 'situational' approach however is its exhausting and infinite quality — the psychiatrist's effort to reach the correct ethical position *vis-à-vis* each one of his patients, their families, colleagues, other fellow professionals, and all the other persons he must work with. Not even the most integrated individual could withstand such an onslaught of continuous decision-making.

Despite the argument of the uniqueness of each case, it seems to us that situations — many of which are discussed in this book — recur regularly in the psychiatrist's work which call for ethical judgements, and these can be studied systematically. In discussing these ethical questions, our contributors have not come up with easy, ready-made solutions and in fact were not expected to do so, although they have in many instances offered their own views, in a tentative manner, about correct ethical conduct in difficult situations. Their chief objective is to describe the problems involved as clearly as they can so that the reader will appreciate their nature and complexity, and as a result, be better qualified to understand how he makes his own ethical judgements. We should emphasize that even the statement of the problem sometimes is fraught with difficulty. Unfortunately the neutrality and lack of bias with which one would want the problems to be presented are not easy to attain; suppositions and assumptions lie behind the identification of the problem and the way in which it is approached.[20] None the less the project, in our opinion, is still worth pursuing.

It is tempting in a book of this kind to offer guidelines for ethical conduct. As we mentioned earlier, efforts in this direction have been made in recent years as witnessed by the formulation of ethical codes. We feel that to succumb to such temptation would be hazardous. Neither the editors nor the contributors could possibly deceive themselves that they are in a position to prescribe immutable ethical guidelines. Ultimately, ethical conduct depends on the individual, and on his peers as a professional group, to use only those attitudes and practices which they generally agree upon as morally appropriate. Guidelines of conduct may be laid down, but they are, unlike laws and regulations, unenforceable; and, furthermore, a code can only be expressed in general terms. The psychiatrist is still left with the personal responsibility of taking ethical decisions in his daily practice which pertain to specific cases.

'Psychiatric ethics' in the context of general ethics

Can 'psychiatric ethics' be regarded as a specific entity, a realm distinct from other aspects of living in which ethical considerations are involved? The argument has been advanced that a separate ethics is unnecessary, not only for the psychiatrist but for the physician in general, since as a reasonable member of society he can readily adopt ethical principles which have been agreed upon by the society as a whole. Thus, the proposition has been advanced by Braceland that: 'the physician [psychiatrist included] *as a citizen* [our italics] must be an ethical man and act in accordance with the accepted standards that apply to all men'.[21] Clouser, in referring to medical ethics, has contended that: 'Medical ethics is simply ethics applied to a particular branch of our lives — roughly the area touched by medicine. And being the same old ethics that has been around for a long time, medical ethics has no special principles or methods or rules. It is the "old ethics" trying to find its way around in new, very puzzling circumstances.'[22]

Both Braceland and Clouser's points seem valid: psychiatric ethics is, in part, the application of more or less universal principles to the moral problems of a particular professional activity. But it would seem to us that this view tends to minimize the uniqueness of these problems as the physician or psychiatrist faces them. In particular, the psychiatrist's domain is characterized by so many issues specific to the nature of his work that ethical considerations and decisions play a greater role for him than for many other professional groups. To illustrate briefly:

1. No other person apart from the psychiatrist faces the task of assessing the state of another's mind with a need to make a judgement whether to deprive a person of his liberty for the sake of his mental health. This is indeed an awesome responsibility.

2. Unlike other physicians for whom this is a relatively rare occurrence, the psychiatrist's problems often involve a balance between individual and social responsibilities. The boundaries of the psychiatrist's work are blurred and ill-defined. He lacks satisfactory guidelines to indicate where his work starts and ends. Thus his attitude may range from limiting 'his field strictly to the suffering patient'[23] to involving himself in 'fundamental social goals'[24]

3. There is, as yet, poor agreement on what constitutes psychiatric disorder (e.g. the debate over whether homosexuality is a diagnosable condition)[25] and the criteria for reaching a diagnosis remain in large measure subjective, sometimes even arbitrary; no tests have been developed to determine objectively the presence or absence of most mental illnesses.

A perusal of the book will make it clear that the psychiatrist contributors are wrestling with problems which they face every day. These problems, of course, differ depending on the area of psychiatry considered, but certain themes are pervasive. These include: how to assess the moral costs and benefits of what they do professionally; how to maintain confidentiality and at the same time be accountable and responsible; how to come to terms with the critics of psychiatry, whether lawyers or those from among their own ranks; how to treat patients effectively while maintaining their confidence and not keeping them in the dark about what is going on; how to define the nebulous parameters of their own work while avoiding hubris or undue timidity; and how to strike a balance between the ethos of contractual equality which is becoming dominant in Western life, and a benevolent paternalism necessary to them as physicians.

As editors we hope that *Psychiatric ethics* will help to illuminate for interested readers in the profession of psychiatry and elsewhere these themes which permeate all areas of psychiatric practice and in which elements of the human, the contingent, and the ambiguous take precedence over purely scientific and clinical considerations.

Finally, we wish to make two general points about the book. First, our selection is by no means exhaustive but we believe the topics included cover the important and common ethical issues facing the psychiatrist. Some readers will obviously have wanted a more extensive account of the ethics involved in behaviour modification, others a separate chapter on distributive justice, and so on. As editors, however, we have had to recognize the need to keep the volume within reasonable bounds. Second, we realize that the subject matter could be 'sliced' in different ways. Thus, for example, some major topics common to various areas of psychiatric practice — such as confidentiality and informed consent — are dealt with in several chapters. After much deliberation we have opted for the present structure which we feel is the most rational for dealing with what is an enormously diverse subject.

References

1. *American Journal of Psychiatry* **130**:1057–64, 1973.
2. Szasz, T.: The myth of mental illness. *American Psychologist* **15**: 113–18, 1960.
3. Halleck, S.: *The politics of therapy*. New York, Science House, 1971 p. 13.
4. *Bibliography 1979–1980,* Institute of Society, Ethics, and Life Sciences, Hastings, New York.
5. Reich, W. (ed.): *Encyclopaedia of bioethics*. New York, Free Press, 1978.
6. Ayd, F. J. (ed.): *Medical, moral and legal issues in mental health care*. Baltimore, Williams and Wilkins, 1974.
7. *In the service of the state: the psychiatrist as double agent*. Special Supplement, Institute of Society, Ethics, and the Life Sciences, April 1978.

8. MOORE, R. A.: Ethics in the practice of psychiatry — origins, functions, models and enforcement. *American Journal of Psychiatry* **135**: 157–63, 1978.
9. ROBINSON, D. and HENRY, S.: *Self-help and health. Mutual aid for modern problems.* London, Martin Robertson, 1977.
10. SZASZ, T.: *The myth of mental illness.* New York, Harper and Row, 1961.
11. SZASZ, T.: *Law, liberty and psychiatry.* New York, Macmillan, 1963.
12. LIEFER, R.: The medical model as ideology. *International Journal of Psychiatry* **9**:13–21, 1970.
13. LAING, R. D.: *The divided self.* Harmondsworth, Penguin, 1965.
14. US National Commission for the Protection of Subjects of Biomedical and Behavioural Research Involving Psychosurgery — Report and Recommendations. US Department of Health, Education, and Welfare Publication No. (OS) 77–0001 and (OS) 77–0002, March 1977.
15. BLOCH, S.: The political misuse of Soviet psychiatry: Honolulu and beyond. *Australian and New Zealand Journal of Psychiatry* **14**:109–14, 1980.
16. HARE, R. H.: *The language of morals.* Oxford, Oxford University Press, 1952.
17. WARNOCK, M.: *Ethics since 1900.* Oxford, Oxford University Press, 1978.
18. RAWLS, J.: *A theory of justice.* Cambridge, Mass., Harvard University Press, 1971.
19. FOOT, P. (ed.): *Theories of ethics.* Oxford, Oxford University Press, 1967.
20. MONTEFIORE, A. (ed.): *Neutrality and impartiality.* Cambridge, Cambridge University Press, 1975.
21. BRACELAND, F. J.: Historical perspectives of the ethical practice of psychiatry. *American Journal of Psychiatry* **126**:230–7, 1969.
22. CLOUSER, K. D.: Medical ethics: some uses, abuses and limitations. *New England Journal of Medicine* **293**:384–7, 1973.
23. BUSSE, E. W.: APA's role in influencing the evolution of a health care delivery system. *American Journal of Psychiatry* **126**:739–44, 1969.
24. WAGGONER, R.: Cultural dissonance and psychiatry. *American Journal of Psychiatry* **127**:1–8, 1970.
25. See for example: A symposium: Should homosexuality be in the APA nomenclature? *American Journal of Psychiatry* **130**:1207–16, 1973.

2
A historical perspective
David Musto

THREE factors underlie the ethical questions which at all times have preoccupied those delegated to help the mentally ill: the role of the therapist, the nature of mental disease, and the cultural, religious, and even political environment in which the patient and therapist coexist. In the last decade or so these factors and the formal study of psychiatric ethics have been explicitly analysed and have become almost a new subspecialty. Before the mid-twentieth-century, however, few such formal studies existed. This lack of attention is understandable since the profession of psychiatry developed as a medical specialty only recently, and since for much of the last century the codes discussed and adopted for general medicine appeared to have served psychiatry well. The dramatic changes in the scope of psychiatry since the Second World War however, have brought into sharp focus ethical issues peculiar to psychiatry.

The governing factors listed above have varied widely in Western medical tradition since Hippocrates. What we call issues in psychiatric ethics during that time must represent the imposition of categories familiar to us, such as informed consent and 'right to be treated', on to a historical record for which these terms are not entirely appropriate. In reviewing the past we will be looking for ethical concepts deemed pertinent by medical or other cultural authorities when the behaviour of a person was judged to be grossly abnormal and to require treatment or limitation of freedom. Social control in a broad sense could be justified as the theme for a study of psychiatric ethics, but in this brief survey the subject will be studied in the traditional medical context. The realization that ethical issues transcend medicine — and therefore psychiatry — constitutes a fundamental change in outlook which has marked the recent rise of interest. Restriction of the subject to the context of the history of medicine is a concession to space, not a judgment on its proper boundaries. A convenient starting point is the Greco-Roman period.

† The writing of this chapter was supported in part by a Research Scientist Development Award, National Institute on Drug Abuse.
I am indebted to Catherine D. Wilder for aid in preparing this chapter.

Greco-Roman period

It would be an error to consider the Hippocratic Oath as representing Greek or Roman medical practice. The tradition of Hippocratic thinking was akin to Pythagoreanism, a school of thought with strict moral precepts whose tenets more resembled later Christian principles than the flexible mores of Hellenistic practices, which, for example, condoned abortion and suicide[1]. The oath does include, however, some of the earliest affirmations of confidentiality and the primacy of the patient's health:

> Whatever houses I may visit, I will come for the benefit of the sick, remaining free of all intentional injustice, of all mischief and in particular of sexual relations with both female and male persons, be they free or slaves.
> What I may see or hear in the course of the treatment or even outside of the treatment in regard to the life of the men, which on no account one must spread abroad, I will keep to myself holding such things shameful to be spoken about.[2]

Insanity is not mentioned in the oath. In the Greek world there appears to have been little legal provision for the insane, although Roman law did provide for trusteeship of an incompetent's property and other restrictions of his rights. Mental illness as well as drunkenness were conditions that could decrease a defendant's criminal responsibility, although such decisions appear to have been made by judges without the advice of a physician or other expert on mental illness.[3]

Treatment of the insane in the ancient Western world ranged from such harsh methods described by Celsus (first century of the Christian era) as purgation, bleeding, beatings, and cold baths to the milder policies advocated by Soranus (first and second centuries) which are similar to the moral therapy espoused, although rarely practised, in the early nineteenth century: esteem for the patient, relative freedom of movement, and kind treatment.

Just as a range of restraints on freedom can be identified in these early approaches to mental illness, so the causes advanced for insanity extended from divine intervention to organic or natural factors. When ethical issues are drawn from this period, the vague edges of the definition of insanity and various responses to it make firm statements about these issues difficult. Clearly, for those who were treated medically, evidence suggests that harshness of treatment or limitations of freedom were the prerogative of the physician and that the patient and his family had little to say about either. Furthermore, the major determinant in form of therapy depended on the custodian's faith in a particular school of medicine or, perhaps, in a lack of faith in any medical treatment and, instead, a dependence on religious intervention.

The marks of insanity were simple: strange, violent, suicidal, or homicidal behaviour which did not have a likely explanation from the observer's point of view. Bizarre explanations from the patient would only confirm the judgment of the family or other authorities. Treatment might be painful or harmful, but the physician administered it with a clear conscience because his theory of medicine required certain courses of action. In these instances, ethical problems may exist for us but did not for the confident physician or the patient's faithful custodian, or, perhaps, even for the patient himself. The random manner in which those considered insane received care continued for centuries until more formal and elaborate systems evolved, first with hospitals and, much later and very recently, with the varieties of care possible when a large mental health profession exists.

Middle Ages and Renaissance

The Middle Ages brought no medical advance to the insane; rather, the major influence on attitudes toward the mentally ill emanated from religion. For example, the Prophet Mahomet revealed that the insane are the beloved of God and especially chosen by him to declare the truth. This attitude, taken with the founding of hospitals in the Moslem world and the establishment of an enlightened medical profession, suggests that Islam was disposed towards humane care of the ill. Because of the Prophet's statement, the status of the patient was elevated to at least the same level as the therapist, a rare event in the history of psychiatry.[4]

Jewish tradition, as stated in the Talmud, portrayed the insane as victims of a disease, not of possession.[5] Christian religious orders provided humane though limited treatment for the deranged, but outside the monasteries Europeans had diminishing resources for care as the Roman Empire was gradually eroded. The ensuing anarchy apparently was responsible for an increase in jailings, beatings, and torture among the insane. Compounding their misfortune, schisms among Christians led to an increase in the maltreatment of patients by equating deviant opinions with demonic possession and heresy.[6] Among competing religious factions little concern was shown for the rights of heretics whom we would now consider sane, and certainly no more concern was shown for those whose disordered fantasies and opinions were thought the product of heresy. Yet it would be unfair and misleading to suggest that European Christian attitudes toward the insane were characterized by a belief in demonic possession which had to be rooted out by the most severe methods. Toward the end of the Middle Ages, hospitals for the mentally ill were founded, humane physicians and caretakers did exist, and their numbers were to multiply in the sixteenth and seventeenth centuries.[7]

At the same time, legal care for the insane seems to have been in some specific instances balanced and thoughtful. This is the conclusion of Richard Neugebauer,[8] who studied judicial records regarding 'natural fools' and those judged *non compos mentis* in England from the thirteenth to the seventeenth centuries; these records do not support the accepted belief that the era was cruel and dominated by demonological explanations of mental retardation and disorder. There was a growing pattern of reasonable distinctions between congenital and temporary conditions, protection of property and interests of those judged incompetent, and a disinclination to be punitive or cruel.

In monastic hospitals the insane received good care, in keeping with the dictum of St Benedict that 'care of the sick is to be placed above and before every other duty'.[9] With suppression of the monastic orders in Protestant countries and confiscation of their property, care of patients suffered. Still, even taking into account the existence of a few hospitals and of legal protection, the Middle Ages offered only a random and unpredictable response to insanity. The ethical context in which decisions were taken was the religious tradition of the locality. This could mean emphasis on charity and understanding, or it could justify severe measures if demonic possession were suspected. It is probably reasonable to generalize that during this time a person with bizarre behaviour and beliefs was seldom classified as a 'patient,' and moreover, that no broad consensus existed for what we think of as humane treatment. The low level of institutional and public health care for all health or social problems meant that the overall quality of care for the mentally ill would be as low as that for other illnesses such as leprosy and communicable diseases.

Seventeenth Century to the French Revolution

The two centuries preceding the French Revolution were a period of increased hospital building but no significant improvement in the care of the mentally ill. The traditional religious view of mental illness was progressively balanced by advances in anatomy and physiology which suggested that it was the product of organic change. Humane treatment, however, seems to have been related more to culturally inspired responses than to organic explanations of disordered behaviour or beliefs. An assumption that a lesion in the brain or other part of the body caused mental illness brought contrasting treatment. Powerful and destructive therapies were justified on grounds that they were required for the correction of specific lesions while milder treatments were advocated because of the belief that strenuous applications would impair the natural capacity of the body or mind to heal the lesion and restore health.

Mild treatment, though, appears to have been rare in the great hospitals that were built before the French Revolution, with the exception of those administered by religious orders. The rise of the sciences stimulated new explanations for the body's functions; mechanical, physical, and chemical theories challenged the Galenic tradition of four humours whose balance brought health. New theories fostered new regimens: strong medicines and bleeding, purgation, and blistering competed with methods such as isolation, beatings, and instilling fear. Faith in theory continued to outweigh empirical considerations based on the actual effects of the patient's treatment. In general, eighteenth-century therapists considered their task difficult and in need of rough procedures.

The French Revolution and, to a lesser degree, the American Revolution, were movements for political equality which gave a new importance to the individual in terms of his rights in the secular order. This importance rivalled the religious tradition of immortality and equality before God. In the late eighteenth century, particularly in France, mental illness was considered the result of a wrongly ordered society: the patient was the victim of an exploitative social environment. The attitude that placed blame on society exonerated the ill person; it also suggested that care could take a social form and promoted optimism for outcome — at least in the heyday of the Revolution.

Philippe Pinel, so often honoured for removing the chains from patients, was not totally original in his efforts, but he did adopt and promote more humane attitudes than his predecessors. The basis for his action in the 1790s was faith in the Revolution and one of its corollaries — the expectation that an improved society would result in fewer patients and great improvement in those already interned. He did not abolish authority over his patients — in fact, he was quite firm — but he believed that communication with them in as egalitarian a manner as possible was in keeping with the spirit of the French Republic and also beneficial to their health. Pinel was confident that few restraints were necessary if patients were treated with fundamental regard to their individuality and self-respect.[10]

In contrast, George III of Great Britain, who suffered a relapse of his mental condition in 1788, received traditional rugged care and close restraint because his physicians were determined he should receive the best care that their theories commanded: wild behaviour required a strong antidote. Even the king could not escape what we would today consider cruel treatment. Whatever anxiety the physicians felt about the king's response to their care, their consciences were untroubled. Pinel was equally at ease when he moved in the direction of more benign treatments. In both instances the physician had virtually absolute control over his patient.

Benjamin Rush, the father of American psychiatry, introduced improvements for patients under his care at the Pennsylvania Hospital in Philadelphia. As usual in the movement toward less confining treatments, reformers faced the problem of the hyperactive and threatening patient. Rush, whose own son was long a patient at the hospital, devised restraints like the 'tranquillizer chair', which prevented movement that could cause further damage to the patient while reducing blood flow to the brain — required by his theory of insanity. His goal was to ensure that necessary restraint and treatment created no unintended or undesirable effects.[11]

The nineteenth century

In the nineteenth century, ethical formulations for the medical profession were promulgated in many countries. In 1803, for example, Dr Thomas Percival published a formal statement on medical ethics. Percival's immediate goal was the establishment of a code of ethics and etiquette for the Manchester Infirmary in order to reduce controversy among the attending physicians. His comments, however, on mental patients in asylums such as existed on the Infirmary grounds, reveal the conflict between humane care and the need to preserve order. His attitude is not far different from that of Pinel or Rush when he writes:

The law justifies the *beating of a lunatic, in such manner as the circumstances may require*. But it has been before remarked that a physician, who attends an asylum for insanity, is under an obligation of honour as well as of humanity to secure to the unhappy sufferers, committed to his charge, all the tenderness and indulgence compatible with steady and effectual government. And the strait waistcoat, with other improvements in modern practice, now preclude the necessity of coercion by corporal punishment [Percival's italics].[12]

Although he wished to be kind, he believed the physician with special knowledge of the insane could take action which to young and uninformed physicians might appear harsh. 'Certain cases of *mania*', he wrote, 'seem to require a *boldness* of *practice* which a young physician of sensibility may feel a reluctance to adopt.' When this occurs, the novice 'must not yield to timidity, but fortify his mind by the councils of his more experienced brethren of the faculty'. Yet Percival could not let his advice admit of too severe an interpretation, for he warned that 'it is more consonant to probity to err on the side of caution than of temerity.'[13] Repeatedly, these advocates of humane care faced the problem of keeping order in hospitals and regulating the admission of patients. Percival strongly favoured strict inspection of asylums for proper care and for assurance that no one was admitted without a certificate signed by a physician, surgeon, or apothecary. He emphasized the provision for writs of *habeas corpus* and other legal protection of hospital inmates. Here then are two aspects of care of the insane in which ethical problems arise: whether detention is justified, and whether care given during detention is as humane as possible.

Often the adoption of ethical codes in the nineteenth century was related to the advent of professionalism, whereby standards were set for members of a professional organization who were distinguished from physicians or laymen outside the organization. Medical etiquette was a prominent feature of these ethical codes. Procedures for consultation, details about fees, and relations with fellow physicians were regulated by the codes. Through statutory laws and third-party payment procedures, society later would begin to control aspects of practice that physicians had first governed through internal professional standards. But in the last century, especially in the United States, professionalism was not a concern of the state and jurisdictions had few or no licensing powers. So many schools of medical practice existed that the need to distinguish among them became a matter of pride for their adherents as well as a source of economic advantage. Thus, physicians established a variety of medical associations each of which set codes of conduct and standards.

When the American Medical Association was founded in 1847, its members adopted a code of ethics based on Percival's work.[14] The American Medical Association did not become a powerful medical organization until the twentieth century, but its code of ethics is representative of mid-nineteenth-century concerns about proper clinical practice. The first section stresses the physician's high moral obligation, the need for secrecy, the requirement that a physician see a patient through to the end of his illness — whether to cure or to death — balancing hope with realistic warnings to the family. There followed a long section, entirely missing from Percival, entitled 'Obligations of Patients to Their Physicians'. The patient should choose a properly trained physician, provide all relevant information, follow the regimen prescribed, and after recovery 'entertain a just and enduring sense of the value of the services rendered him by his physician'.[15] Later sections of the code detail courtesies of physicians to one another and the qualifications of a regular physician. The title of the last chapter is 'Of the Duties of the Profession to the Public, and the Obligations of the Public to the Profession'. The relationship of physicians to coroners, guidelines for dispensing free service, and the need to educate the public regarding quackery are stated but, unlike

Percival's work, there is no discussion of medical practice within hospitals, and the only reference to insane asylums is in a list of various institutions in which medical authorities must have an interest, such as hospitals, schools, and prisons.

In 1849, two years after adoption of the American Medical Association code, Worthington Hooker, a Connecticut physician, published what is increasingly recognized as a pioneer study of medical ethics in the United States, *Physician and patient; or, a practical view of the mutual duties, relations and interests of the medical profession and the community*.[16] The titles of the chapters, 'Skill in Medicine', 'Popular Errors', 'Quackery', 'Good and Bad Practice', 'Influence of Hope in the Treatment of Disease', 'Truth in Our Intercourse with the Sick', and 'Moral Influence of Physicians' reflect his ethical concerns. Two chapters, 'Mutual Influence of Mind and Body in Disease', and 'Insanity', particularly merit our attention. Hooker, like Percival, advocated removal of the mentally ill to a retreat and reliance upon a 'regimen, or the regulation of their occupations and amusements, bodily and mental, and very little indeed upon medicine'.[17] Hooker deplored the practice, which he admitted was widespread, of intentionally deceiving the insane, or any other patient. He recommended early treatment and that its costs should be shared by the town and state of the patient's residence. On the subject of how best to determine whether a person is insane, Hooker approved of the French system, in which a committee of experts made the decision after an examination conducted over several days. He regretted that, in his experience, police and prison authorities too often had the final decision and, in some instances, regarded the advice of physicians as interference. 'Such having been the opinion and practices of our courts of justice', Hooker reflected, 'it is not strange that the rights of the insane have often been trampled on'.[18] In the matter of who might commit an insane person to institutional care, he noted that in Connecticut and Massachusetts it was the civil authorities, not physicians, who made the decision. Even worse, these authorities often committed someone only after he had performed some dangerous act. 'With such defects in the provision of the law', Hooker concluded, 'it is no wonder that the community is occasionally shocked with outrageous, even fatal acts by insane persons, who through neglect have been permitted to go at large'.[19] In keeping with his desire for early treatment in cases of insanity, he suggested that those suspected of being insane be examined by a 'standing commission of lunacy . . . composed of physicians who are properly qualified'.[20]

Today we witness a trend in direct opposition to a pattern whereby physicians, and particularly psychiatrists, in the United States were given wide latitude regarding commitment to mental institutions. Dr Hooker had sought to introduce expertise into decisions regarding insanity and this is by and large what occured in the century after this advocacy. He saw application of knowledge by professionals as increasing the rights of the committed and reducing the error during commitment procedures. It is worth noting that he did not favour waiting until an overt, dangerous act had been committed before acting on behalf of the community and the patient. He was unaware of the present-day argument that cultural bias might distort professional judgement or that reserving entirely to medical practitioners the decision about confinement might abridge legal protection for the patient.

For several generations thereafter few issues other than the justi-fication for commitment and the humaneness of care were raised regarding psychiatric patients. Such currently significant concerns as the ethics of behaviour control can be dissected away from the practices and concerns of 1800, but only with difficulty. The rights of the committed patient were few and the primitive state of what we might call the psychiatric profession of the time meant that treatment consisted chiefly in admission to a hospital and residence there until reversion to a normal state, improvement, withdrawal by relatives, or death. The chief question for those who worried about the quality of care was how to conduct a paternalistic relationship kindly, effec-tively, and efficiently. Personal attention to a patient was expensive and required great devotion on the part of individual caretakers and hospital authorities. Attempts to make contact with patients through close, kind supervision, mutual respect, and a wholesome environ-ment — 'moral therapy' — could not survive waves of pessimism about the curability of mental illness, the overloading of caretakers with patients and the degradation of hospitals to the status of human warehouses. These conditions obtained in the mid-nineteenth-century in many countries. Attention to ethical questions suffered as the possibility of substantial reform declined.[21]

Superintendents of American institutions for the insane, who formed an organization in 1844 (later to become the American Psychiatric Association), argued especially for the right to make most decisions about their patients, from commitment to the way the hospital was organized. This body, antedating the American Medical Association, testifies to the special role these physicians had assumed within the profession. Increasingly isolated from medical practice in general, the superintendents saw themselves as experts in a field too often neglected financially, misunderstood by the community, and requiring extraordinary powers of insight and judgement. Harassed by patients' complaints of maltreatment and wrongful commitment, the superintendents were more concerned to protect themselves from legal encroachment than they were about the veracity of these accounts. To the extent that an asylum attempted moral management, to use a term of Pinel's and a goal of the English reformers William and Samuel Tuke at the York Retreat, an uplifting and healthy environment was created for the patient.[22] One could hardly find fault with trying to improve the conditions of patients, the authorities believed, and if better conditions did not exist, the cause lay in inadequate financial support from governments, not with the managers of the asylums. Worry over behaviour modification did not exist, nor did the experts wonder whether they were guided by cultural bias in designing a healthy mental environment. In fact, American psychiatrists of the time commonly found the origin of illness in disobedience or ignorance of what would now be called New England Protestant principles of conduct.[23]

An occasional dramatic error in commitment became a popular cause, stimulating the creation of new laws and procedures. Particularly noteworthy was the case of Mrs E. P. W. Packard. She was committed in 1860 by her husband, a clergyman, to an Illinois institution on the grounds that she held dangerous religious beliefs. Her husband was a strict fundamentalist and feared that his wife would poison the minds of their children with liberal ideas. After several years, Mrs Packard was freed by the trustees, but her troubles were not over. Her husband imprisoned her in her own home and sought to have her recommitted. Finally, in 1864, a trial was held at which she was declared sane. She then embarked on a campaign to make commitment for the expression of opinions an impossibility, 'no matter how absurd these opinions may appear to others'.[24] Events like Mrs Packard's wrongful detention seemed to give credibility to claims against the hospital superintendents, although the latter vowed that such miscarriages were extremely rare. As one anonymous writer in the *American Journal of Insanity* explained:

There can be no clashing or division of interest between the public and the institutions. They are one and the same, and no officer of any public institution can have any possible object in receiving or retaining any sane person in an asylum.[25]

While the psychiatric profession and mental hospitals in the United States were becoming established and stimulating a body of law and precedent regarding the care of the ill, increased experimentation with new procedures and operations raised other ethical questions within the profession and among the laity. Prominent among the questioners were those severe critics of nineteenth-century medicine, the anti-vivisectionists.[26] Three instances of what we today might consider abuses of research in Ohio, Maryland, and Ontario led to harsh criticism from physicians in North America and Great Britain. It is noteworthy that the condemnation came first and strongest from peers, illustrating the alertness of professional self-regulation. One other preliminary comment might be made: these experiments were not representative of contemporary treatment. On the other hand, one should be aware that the high-minded aspirations of asylum superintendents did not necessarily reflect, in fact probably did not reflect, the reality of day-to-day existence in mental hospitals. Published reports and admonitions are not good guides to the routine practice of psychiatry.

The Ohio experiment was published in the eminent *American Journal of Medical Science* in 1874. Dr Roberts Bartholow studied the effect of electrically stimulating the exposed surface of a patient's brain through her ulcerated skull. A few days later the patient died but Dr Bartholow denied that the experiment was related to her death.[27] However, the *British Medical Journal* criticized Bartholow's procedure and his conclusions.[28] The editor was reaffirming Claude Bernard's comment in his *Introduction to the study of experimental medicine:*

It is our duty and our right to perform an experiment on man whenever it can save his life, cure him or gain him some personal benefit. The principle of medical and surgical morality, therefore, consists in never performing on man an experiment which might be harmful to him to any extent, even though the result might be highly advantageous to science, that is, to the health of others.[29]

In a reply, [30] Dr Bartholow tried to justify his actions but acknowledged that the procedure was injurious to the brain, and he stated that he would not repeat such an experiment.

Reports such as that of Dr Bartholow became a refrain in the antivivisectionist literature as examples of experimenters meddling with the bodies of poor patients while observing great caution toward fee-paying patients. The antivivisectionists saw a similarity between charity patients and laboratory animals: they opposed experiments on both and sought to arouse the public through dramatic reports.[31]

In 1897, Dr George Rohé, superintendent of a Maryland hospital for the insane, reported on his research of operating on female pelvic organs in order to relieve insanity. He based this treatment on such diagnoses as hysteroepilepsy melancholia, puerperal insanity, and mania, and claimed a recovery rate of about one-third.[32] Similar operations were reported by Dr A. T. Hobbs of the Asylum for the Insane at London, Ontario.[33]

Reproaches against Drs Rohé and Hobbs appeared in the same issue of the *British Medical Journal* which had published their papers. Dr James Russell argued that there was no scientific basis for the widespread belief that gynaecological problems lay at the root of

insanity in many women.[34] 'The relation of gynaecology to psychiatry
has been pretty thoroughly discussed in late years, and the general
consensus of opinion gathered from alienists and neurologists alike is
that . . . to extol it as a great curative method in the treatment of
insanity is nothing short of absurdity.'[35] The procedures closely
approached criminality since the women could not understand their
possible consequences. Dr Russell even queried 120 physicians in
Great Britain and in America and found, as presumably he had
suspected, that few believed female organs were associated with
insanity or that any operation on them would be beneficial. The
operations did not meet the test of conformity with current standards
of medical practice.

Dr Rohé's reply to Dr Russell's severe and sarcastic criticism was
very weak; he had been misunderstood and reasserted his claim for a
cure of insanity. Dr Hobbs, 'in reply, repudiated the idea that he ever
approved of operative interference unless there was actual disease'.[36]
Although reports of the infamous operations had achieved publication, they did not seem to represent the practice of a substantial
fraction of the profession on either side of the Atlantic. Of course, if
the experimenters had not published, their questionable accomplish-
ments might have passed unnoticed.

In looking back over the nineteenth century — keeping in mind
that we are considering, rather narrowly, antecedents to the modern
psychiatric profession — we see that the growth of mental hospitals
and the increase in their inmates, the decline in most instances of
'moral therapy', and a deterioration in the relations between physicians and patients were all evidence of an atmosphere of pessimism
about the ultimate cure of mental illness. This pessimism, in spite of
advances in understanding syphilis, alcoholism, and other specific
causes of mental illness, overshadowed ethical concerns and caused
them to appear unimportant. A further consequence was that patients
who displayed bizarre behaviour were relegated by some caretakers to
a less than fully human status. Even reformers like Benjamin Rush
described such patients as animal-like and fit for being 'broken' like
wild animals.[37] In the twentieth century and especially since the
Second World War there have been powerful changes in most of these
perceptions as new concepts and sensitivities about the activities of
psychiatrists have arisen.

The twentieth century

In this century, hospital psychiatry burgeoned, with some institutions
housing as many as ten thousand patients. At the same time
psychiatry and other mental health professions were evolving and

manifesting new optimism about therapy and the future of their disciplines. This optimism, in the face of the hundreds of thousands of patients with poor prognoses and receiving inadequate care, was based on developments in biological research and psychodynamic and social psychiatry.

Biological research moved from one success to another in medicine, reducing communicable diseases, curbing syphilis, improving surgical procedures, and ameliorating chronic diseases such as diabetes and congestive heart failure. But enthusiastic extension of this research to the field of psychiatry created ethical concerns about, for example, the introduction of prefrontal lobotomy for certain diagnoses. Other treatments for schizophrenia: electro-convulsive therapy, removal of segments of the intestine to cure 'autointoxication', and similar questionable operations were encouraged by two features of institutional care: the need to control highly disturbed patients and repeated frustration in attempts to find a cure for the psychoses. Confidence in a new therapy was created paradoxically not only by difficulty in finding any cure but also by the belief, common in the history of medicine and science, that a line of investigation or theory successful in one area is the likely key to solving a problem in another area.

In the application of these new treatments in the early twentieth century, paternalism was still evident. The physician decided whether to pursue an innovation and on whom to apply it; he would meet few institutional or professional obstacles. Rejection of such a paternalistic attitude is a major theme in contemporary psychiatric ethics, and is dealt with in many of the other chapters in this book. These objections are applicable not only to the rise in biological research and the use of drugs, surgery, and electroshock therapy but also to other aspects of psychiatry in the twentieth century.

The increasing importance of psychodynamic psychiatry has paralleled the one in biological research. Here too, ethical issues have arisen quickly and much more explicitly than in previous centuries. Psychoanalytic psychology, particularly the work of Freud, has raised the study of ethical issues to a new level of sophistication by pointing out the many motivations which may underlie the setting and enforcement of standards for others.

In both social and biological psychiatry a central goal has been to establish norms for behaviour as well as to correct deviance. In recent years, however, the public has become suspicious of the authority of a professional élite and the standards which they have promulgated. The accuracy of expert opinion is less an issue now than the prior issue of whether experts have any right to prescribe norms of behaviour or to modify behaviour without the full consent and understanding of the patient. This attitude contrasts with the enthusiasm following the Second World War in the United States when government psychiatrists looked forward to the full adoption of public health methods by their specialty. Early intervention would follow the pattern of testing for tuberculosis and then treating the incipient illness. The problems that unilateral psychiatric intervention would present in everyday life — at least from our outlook today — reveal the great changes that have taken place in just a few decades among psychiatrists and in their attitude toward their public responsibilities.

The public health model applied to psychiatry appeared to some to be the fulfilment of a great goal — the provision of expert knowledge and treatment of mental illness for everyone, not only for those who could afford a private psychiatrist or who were forced to enter a great warehouse for mental incompetents. Here we note a profound change in the history of psychiatry: transformation of the profession from a passive role — accepting those brought to it — to an active role, seeking ways in which psychiatrists might help everyone in a community. In the United States, efforts to increase the number of psychiatrists, and the establishment of a nationwide network of community mental health centres in the 1960s, had this new role for psychiatry in mind. Certainly there is an association between the expansion of psychiatry into new fields and the current rise in ethical concerns about the psychiatrist's proper role.

While noting the hopeful expectations and the positive therapeutic results, we cannot overlook the damage done by psychiatrists to some patients who have been excessively treated by electroshock therapy, drugs, or surgery. Some patients have been committed without adequate reason, or any reason, and kept in institutions for many years although fit for discharge to their families or to the community. Personal catastrophes occasionally resulting from misguided psychiatric interventions have elicited new legal formulations restricting the powers of psychiatrists. Awareness of ethical issues, however, has not been limited to medicine or psychiatry.

Some of the most severe critics of psychiatry recently have arisen from within its own ranks. In his early writings the British psychiatrist R. D. Laing,[38] questioned the pathological nature of schizophrenia, suggesting that it could be a 'normal' reaction to modern life and a positive experience. Other psychiatrists have followed this line of reasoning and opposed medication or customary restrictions on the behaviour of those diagnosed as schizophrenic.

Dr Laing appears a member of the old guard compared to Thomas Szasz. Dr Szasz questions the existence of mental illness across the board and argues that to restrict the actions of patients is unethical. For example, should a person be severely depressed and wish to take his life, Dr Szasz would oppose restraining him by force and imposing psychiatric hospitalization and treatment. Szasz is not, it should be emphasized, opposed to intervention but only on terms acceptable to the patient. He takes issue with coercion in the name of help, and sees psychiatrists who so impose their 'help' as policemen and jailers, mental hospitals that confine such persons as prisons, and the insanity defence as a mechanism whereby offenders try to avoid responsibility for their acts and the courts evade their duty to punish.[39,40] In an atmosphere of suspicion about authority, and with the existence of real abuses in psychiatry and a strong activist movement in the profession, such strident criticisms from within psychiatry have had an influence greater than has been possible at any time in the past.

An interesting discussion of recent historical trends in the ethics of psychiatry has come not from a member of the psychiatric profession but from a philosopher, William J. Winslade.[41] Professor Winslade has analysed medical, philosophical, and social components of approaches to mental illness since 1870. In ethical terms, he sees a conflict today between utilitarian thinking, characterized by cost-effective treatment often relying on behavioural control by drugs, and values advocating individually tailored, possibly long-term and expensive care.

The tragic abuse of medicine during the Second World War was an important factor in rekindling the profession's interest in ethics and led, first, to the Code of Nuremberg — rules for medical research — which were subsequently incorporated into the Declaration of Helsinki (see Appendix). In 1948, the World Medical Association promulgated the Declaration of Geneva and, a year later, the International Code of Medical Ethics, which was designed to be a model for national medical codes. These two texts are modern restatements of the Hippocratic Oath. There has also been growing awareness of abuses in psychiatry which contributed to the adoption in 1977 of the Declaration of Hawaii by the World Psychiatric Association. This is the first code of ethics specifically designed for psychiatrists.[42] This text is a response both to the misuse of psychiatric diagnosis and treatment in order to silence political dissidents in the USSR (see Chapter 18) and to the less dramatic but pervasive role of psychiatry in its aggressive public health and paternalistic stances in the West. To cite a few of the Declaration's statements, it calls for disclosure of diagnosis and discussion of alternative therapies with the patient, requires that detained patients have an avenue of appeal, and calls for the use of patient consent to any treatment, with third-party consent in cases of patient incapacity.

Some national psychiatric associations have formulated their own ethical codes. The American Psychiatric Association, for example, adopted the Principles of Medical Ethics of the American Medical Association, and produced a text, the *Principles of medical ethics with annotations especially applicable to psychiatry* in 1973.[43,44] The most relevant sections of this text concern the appropriate conduct of the psychiatrist in regard to contractual relationships in situations where he works closely with other mental health and medical colleagues; in contexts such as examinations for employment, security, and legal purposes in which the right to confidentiality must be waived; and in circumstances where the psychiatrist may feel called to draw on his knowledge in speaking out about social issues. The American Psychiatric Association text, unlike the Declaration of Hawaii, does not advocate an essentially egalitarian relationship between therapist and patient; its emphasis — demonstrating its direct descent from Hippocratic tenets — is rather on the need for the psychiatrist to merit and maintain the trust of patients and other professionals alike.

Thus, in a short period thoughtful laymen and members of the psychiatric profession have moved from an almost uncritical enthusiasm for the benefits of psychiatry in the three decades since the Second World War to a more judicious attitude about what psychiatrists say they can do and what they actually can accomplish. Psychiatry is in an era of unprecedented professional development, yet finds itself in crisis in its relations with patients and the public. In this quandary the welfare of the profession depends on sound analysis of ethical questions. Clearly, attempts to remove all authority from psychiatrists would be unhelpful to the profession and those it is able to assist. On the other hand, it is unlikely that countries like the United States or Britain will ever permit the control over the destinies of others which psychiatrists once held. We are at a peak of conflict over the role of psychiatry in modern society, and its resolution will in all likelihood long define the profession.

References

1. EDELSTEIN, L.: The Hippocratic Oath, text translation and interpretation. *Ancient medicine.* Ed. Temkin, O. and Temkin, C. L. Baltimore, The Johns Hopkins Press, 1967, pp. 17–18.
2 *Ibid.,* p. 6.
3 ROSEN G.: *Madness in society: chapters in the historical sociology of mental illness.* Chicago, University of Chicago Press, 1968, pp. 125–8.
4. MORA, G.: History of psychiatry, in *Comprehensive textbook of psychiatry.* Ed. Freedman, A. M. and Kaplan, H. I. Baltimore, Williams and Wilkins, 1967, p. 12.
5. *Ibid.,* p. 5.
6. ACKERKNECHT, E. H.: *A short history of psychiatry.* Trans. Wolff, S. New York, Hafner, 1968, p. 17.
7. MORA, G.: History of psychiatry, in *Comprehensive textbook of psychiatry.* Ed.

Freedman, A. M. and Kaplan, H. I. Baltimore, Williams and Wilkins, 1967, pp. 16–17.

8. NEUGEBAUER, R.: Treatment of the mentally ill in medieval and early modern England: a reappraisal. *Journal for the History of Behavioural Science* **14**:158–69, 1978.

9. ELLENBERGER, H. F.: Psychiatry from ancient to modern times, in *American Handbook of Psychiatry*, 2nd edn, Vol 1. Ed. Arieti, S. New York, Basic Books, 1974, p. 14.

10. HUNTER, R., MACALPINE, I.: *Three hundred years of psychiatry 1535–1860: a history presented in selected English texts*. London, Oxford University Press, 1963, pp. 602–10.

11. DAIN, N.: Concepts of insanity in the United States, 1789–1865. New Brunswick, N. J., Rutgers University Press, 1964, pp. 18–19, 23.

12. PERCIVAL T.: *Medical ethics (1803)*. Ed. Leake, C. D. and Huntington, N. Y. Robert E. Krieger 1975, p. 126.

13. *Ibid.*, p. 89.

14. Code of medical ethics adopted by the National Medical Convention in Philadelphia, June, 1847, in Hooker, W.L.: *Physician and patient; or, a practical view of the mutual duties, relations and interests of the medical profession and the community (1849)*. New York: Arno Press, 1972, pp. 440–53.

15. *Ibid.*, p. 444.

16. HOOKER, W. L.: *Physician and patient; or, a practical view of the mutual duties, relations and interests of the medical profession and the community (1849)*. New York: Arno Press, 1972.

17. *Ibid.*, p. 334.

18. *Ibid.*, p. 340.

19. *Ibid.*, p. 342.

20. *Ibid.*, p. 342.

21. Musto D.: Therapeutic intervention and social forces: Historical perspectives, in *American Handbook of Psychiatry*, vol. 5. Ed. S. Arieti. New York, Basic Books, 1975, pp. 34–42.

22. HUNTER, R. and MACALPINE, I.: *Three hundred years of psychiatry 1535–1860. A history presented in selected English texts*. London, Oxford University Press, 1963, pp. 602–10, 684–90.

23. GROB, G. N.: *Mental institutions in America: social policy to 1875*. New York, The Free Press, 1973, pp. 160–1.

24. PACKARD, Mrs. E. P. W.: *Marital power exemplified in Mrs. Packard's trial, and self-defence from the charge of insanity; or three years' imprisonment for religious belief, by the arbitrary will of a husband, with an appeal to the Government to so change the laws as to protect the rights of married women*. Hartford, 1866, p. 55.

25. *American Journal of Insanity* **29**: 302, 1872.

26. HARVEY, J.: Human experimentation in the nineteenth century. Unpublished manuscript. Harvard University, 1977. (I am indebted to Ms. Harvey for calling my attention to this reference to psychosurgery.)

27. BARTHOLOW, R.: Experimental investigations into the functions of the human brain. *American Journal of Medical Science* **67**:305–13, 1874.

28. *British Medical Journal* **i**: 687, 1874.

29. BERNARD, C.: *An introduction to the study of experimental medicine (1865)*. Trans. Greene, H. C. New York, Henry Schuman, 1949, p. 101.

30. BARTHOLOW, R.: Experiments on the functions of the human brain. *British Medical Journal* **i**:727, 1874.

31. FRENCH, R. D.: *Antivivesection and medical science in Victorian society*. Princeton, Princeton University Press, 1975.

32. Rohé, G. E.: The etiological relation of pelvic disease in women to insanity. *British Medical Journal* **ii**: 766–9, 1897.
33. Hobbs, A. T.: Surgical gynaecology in insanity. *British Medical Journal* **ii**: 769–70.
34. Russell, J.: The after-effects of surgical procedure on the generative organs of females for the relief of insanity. *British Medical Journal* **ii**:770–7, 1897.
35. *Ibid.*, p. 770.
36. *Ibid.*, p. 774.
37. Deutsch, A.: *The mentally ill in America* (1938). New York, Columbia University Press, 1949.
38. Laing R. D.: *The divided self* (1960). Baltimore, Penguin, 1971.
39. Szasz, T. S.: *The myth of mental illness: foundations of a theory of personal conduct* (1961). New York, Harper and Row, 1974.
40. Szasz, T. S.: *The manufacture of madness: a comparative study of the inquisition and the mental health movement.* New York, Harper and Row, 1970.
41. Winslade, W. J.: Ethics and ethos in psychiatry: historical patterns and conceptual changes. Unpublished paper presented at the American College of Psychiatrists, Annual Meeting, San Antonio, Texas, 6 Feb. 1980.
42. Blomquist, C. D. D.: From the Oath of Hippocrates to the Declaration of Hawaii: *Ethics in Science and Medicine* **4**: 139–49, 1977.
43. Moore, R. A.: Ethics in the practice of psychiatry — origins, functions, models, and enforcement. *American Journal of Psychiatry* **135**: 157–63, 1978.
44. The Principles of Medical Ethics with annotations especially applicable to psychiatry. *American Journal of Psychiatry* **130**: 1057–64, 1973.

3

The philosophical basis of psychiatric ethics

Richard Hare

THE editors are plainly right when they say in their introduction that 'the contemporary psychiatrist . . . is required to grapple with a broad range of ethical problems'. Some of these problems afflict other branches of medicine equally; some are, for the reasons the editors give, peculiarly pressing for the psychiatrist. On the relations in general between moral philosophy and medical ethics I have already published a paper, 'Medical Ethics: Can the Moral Philosopher Help?',[1] and this will absolve me from repeating here all the arguments for the method of thinking I there advocate. I will, however, outline the method itself, before I go on to apply it to the problems besetting psychiatrists.

In that paper I drew a contrast between two supposedly incompatible views about the right way to settle moral questions, which I dubbed the 'utilitarian' view and the 'absolutist' view. I then showed how the two views could in fact be combined into a single viable account by carefully distinguishing between two different levels of moral thinking: first, that at which we are faced with particular pressing moral problems without much time for reflection about them; and secondly, that at which we think out, in general, what our attitudes to these problems ought to be. I said that the absolutist approach was most suited to the first kind of thinking, the utilitarian to the second.

But before I explain why this should be so, I must first outline the two approaches. Readers of the huge literature that is accumulating on medical ethics will easily recognize the two kinds of view that I have in mind. We have first those who tend to speak in terms of people's rights and the corresponding duties of other people towards them — rights and duties which are thought of as in some sense absolute. This stance is often adopted by writers on, for example, abortion. They will accordingly claim, depending on which side they take in the dispute, either that the woman concerned, or that the foetus, has certain inalienable rights which there is an absolute duty to respect. It is one of the defects of this approach that it tells us very little about how to decide *what* rights people have, or, if incompatible rights are claimed, which ought to be preserved and which over-ridden.

Though 'absolutist' is a convenient name for this approach, we must be careful not to confuse this use of the term with that in which it is the opposite of 'relativist'; the controversy between absolutists in this second sense and relativists has no bearing on our present topic.

The second, utilitarian, approach is the one attributed by the editors to those who 'assumed implicitly that they could perform their task without ethical difficulties by serving the best interests of their patients', and that 'inherent in the nature of the work is the psychiatrist's prime and sole interest in his patients; their optimal welfare is his *raison d'être*'. But before we assimilate this view to utilitarianism an important qualification has to be made which, as we shall see, introduces a difficulty. A true utilitarian would, it might be said, not consider the interests of his patients solely, or even pre-eminently. For the interests of all are of equal weight for the utilitarian, and he is forbidden by his doctrine to give extra weight to those of some particular person who stands in some special relation-ship to him. To this question we shall return. However, in many, perhaps most, cases the interests of the patient are so paramount, and the interests of others so negligible or so equally balanced, that a utilitarian would without much hesitation make his decision solely by reference to the patient's interests. But to avoid this complication let us simply say that a utilitarian is one who thinks that when faced with a moral decision he ought to act in whichever way is best for the interests of those affected.

Here too we have to be careful in using this term. The name 'utilitarian' is used by philosophers for adherents of a wide variety of doctrines, and in common parlance has got attached to others which are not utilitarian at all in any strict sense. So it must not be assumed that any argument that has ever been brought against any view that has been called utilitarian can be brought against the view we are considering.

It is evident that psychiatrists, like most of us, think from time to time in both these ways. But it is also evident that cases can and frequently do arise in which the two methods will yield different results. For example, in a case involving treatment against the wishes of the patient, a psychiatrist might well think that the treatment was clearly in the patient's best interest and in that of everybody else concerned and yet think that he had no right to impose it if the patient did not want it. To this question too we shall return.

Because of these apparent conflicts between the approaches, philo-sophers and others have suggested various more or less clumsy ways of combining them so as to avoid the conflicts. One way would be to say that the duty to do the best for the patient and others (the so-called duty of beneficence) is one duty among many, and that, as in all cases of conflicts between duties, we have to 'weigh' the relative urgency or importance of the duties in the particular case; in some cases we may decide that the duty of beneficence is the more weighty, in others the duty to respect some right. This way out is utterly unhelpful, relying as it does on a weighing process of which no explanation whatever is given.

Another equally unhelpful suggestion is that the duties in question, including that of beneficence, might be placed once for all in an order of priority, sometimes called 'lexical ordering' (from the practice of lexicographers of putting first all the words beginning with 'a', whatever other letters they contain, and then those beginning with 'b', and so on). So we should, for example, fulfil duty *a* in all cases in which it existed, whatever other duties might also be present, and so on. This suggestion is unhelpful for at least two reasons. The first is that, as before, no account is given of why the duties should have this order of priority rather than some other. The second is more subtle: will it not be the case that on some occasions duty *a* ought to have priority, on others duty *b*? In terms of the same example as before, ought we not sometimes to treat the patient against his will if the harm to which he will otherwise come is very great, but in others respect his right to refuse treatment? No lexical ordering of the duties could allow us to say this, and yet we might often want to say it. Nevertheless the idea of lexical ordering has been quite popular.

These suggestions are handicapped by their failure to distinguish between the different levels of moral thinking. It is indeed hard to see how any one-level account could solve the problem of moral conflicts; for if conflicts arise at one level, they cannot be resolved without ascending to a higher level. That we have a duty to serve the interests of the patient, and that we have a duty to respect his rights, can both perhaps be ascertained by consulting our intuitions at the bottom level. But if we ask which duty or which intuition ought to carry the day, we need some means other than intuition, some higher kind of thinking (let us call it 'critical moral thinking') to settle the question between them. And this kind of thinking has also to be brought to bear when we are asking what intuitions we ought to cultivate, or what our duties at the bottom level are (our *prima facie* duties, as philosophers call them).

An illustration of the difference between the levels, and of its relation to that between the utilitarian and absolutist approaches, may help. A simple case is that of our duty to speak the truth. A common example in the philosophical literature, which goes back to Kant, is this: a madman is seeking out a supposed enemy to murder him, and I know where the proposed victim is; do I, if I cannot get away with evasions, tell the truth to the madman? Most of us, as well as the duty to speak the truth, acknowledge a duty to preserve innocent people from murderers, and here the duties are in conflict. An absolutist will have to resolve the conflict by calling one of the duties absolute and assigning some weaker status to the other. Let us suppose that, as some absolutists have, he calls the duty to speak the truth absolute and therefore requires us to sacrifice the life of the victim to it. A utilitarian, by contrast, is likely to say that neither duty is absolute; what we have to do is to decide what would be for the best in the particular case. In this case it will presumably do most good to all concerned, considering their interests impartially, if I tell a lie. But then it is objected that the utilitarian is making a solemn duty, that of truthfulness, of no account; he simply maximizes utility, and might as well not acknowledge any other duties.

The dispute is easily resolved once we distinguish between the two levels of moral thinking. At the intuitive level, we have these intuitions about duties, and it is a good thing that we do. A wise utilitarian, bringing up his children, would see to it that they developed a conscience which gave them a bad time if they told lies. He would do this because people with such a disposition are much more likely to do, on the whole, what is best than somebody who does cost–benefit analyses on particular occasions; he will not have enough time or information to do them properly, and will probably cook the results to suit his own convenience. Firm moral dispositions have a great utility. So the utilitarian can let the absolutist operate at the intuitive level in much the way that he proposes. But when conflicts arise, or when the question is asked, *what* intuitions we ought to have, or *what* duties we ought to acknowledge, or what would be the *content* of a sound moral education, then intuitive thinking is powerless; for if intuitions conflict or are called into question, it is no use appealing to intuitions to resolve the difficulty, since they will be equally questionable.

A utilitarian can therefore let the absolutists have their say about the intuitive level of thinking and ask them in return to keep their fingers out of the critical level at which intuitions themselves are being appraised. That the method to be used at the critical level has to dispense with the appeal to intuitions seems on the face of it clear; that there is no other method than the utilitarian which can achieve this is more controversial, though I myself know of no other. But it is at any rate clear that *if* the utilitarian is given the monopoly of the critical level, he can readily explain what happens at the intuitive level; we form, in ourselves, and others, for good utilitarian reasons, sound intuitions prescribing duties, and the disposition to feel bad if we go against them; the content of these intuitions is to be selected according to the good or bad consequences of our acquiring them; when they conflict in a particular case, we have to apply utilitarian reasoning and do the best we can in the circumstances; but when the case is clear and there is no conflict, we are likely to do the best by sticking to the intuitions.

This is not the place to give a full account of these two levels of moral thinking, the intuitive and the critical. For our present purposes it will be enough to characterize them briefly. The intuitive level, with its *prima facie* duties and principles, is the main locus of everyday moral decisions for the psychiatrist as for everybody else. Most of us, when we face a moral question, decide it on the basis of dispositions, habits of thought, moral intuitions (it makes little difference what we call them) which we have absorbed during our earlier upbringing and follow without reflection.

It is sometimes suggested that this is a bad thing, and that we ought to be more reflective in our moral thought even about these everyday decisions. It is easy to see that this is not so, however. One of the qualities we look for in a good man is a readiness to do the right thing without hesitation. A man would not, for example, have the virtue of dependability if, when the time came to fulfil some undertaking he had made, he first had to spend some time thinking about whether he ought, after all, to fulfil it. Not only do we seldom have time for such thought (especially if we are doctors); but, if we do engage in it, it is frighteningly easy to deceive ourselves into thinking that the case is a peculiar one in which our ordinary moral principles give the wrong answer, when in fact we would do better to stick to them. Our ingrained moral principles are therefore not merely time-saving rules of thumb, but necessary safeguards against special pleading. On the whole we are more likely to err by abandoning one of these principles than by observing it; for the information necessary in order to be sure that this is a case where the principle gives the wrong answer is seldom available.

Most of us get these sound general principles in the course of our normal upbringing and acquire what is called a conscience, which makes us very uncomfortable if we break them; and this too is a good thing. However, those philosophers are mistaken who think that these moral feelings which we have are by themselves certificates of correctness in the moral judgments which they prompt. For the upbringing which led to our having them might have been misguided; if a Southerner in the old days felt bad about being friendly with blacks, because he had been brought up to believe in keeping one's distance from them, we should not regard that as a proof that he had a duty to keep his distance, but rather condemn his upbringing. In the medical and other professions the *prima facie* principles which apply specially to their members have been to some extent made articulate, if not in codes of conduct, at least in the consistent practice of disciplinary bodies like the General Medical Council in Britain and the medical licensing authorities of each State in the US. But even more obviously in this case, it is possible to ask whether the particular practices which at any one time have this official blessing are the right ones.

That is one reason why the intuitive level of moral thinking is not self-sufficient. Another is that the *prima facie* principles, to be of much use, have to be fairly simple and general, or they could not become second nature, as they have to. This has the consequence that cases can easily arise in which the principles conflict and thus yield no determinate answer. It is good for doctors to strive always to save life, and to strive always to relieve pain; but what if the only way to relieve pain is to kill? Or what if we can save one life only by destroying another? Such cases are the main fuel of controversy in medical ethics.

For these reasons a full account of moral thinking will include an account of the critical as well as of the intuitive level. The critical level is that at which we select the principles to be used at the intuitive level, and adjudicate between them in cases where they conflict. But how is this to be managed, and how do we know when to engage in critical moral thinking? For, as we implied above, it is sometimes even dangerous to do so.

To answer the first question I should have to survey almost the whole of moral philosophy. Good brief general introductions to ethical method are to be found in the opening chapters of P. Singer, *Practical ethics*[2] and J. C. B. Glover, *Causing death and saving lives.*[3] My own *Moral thinking: its levels, method and point*[4] will provide a full-scale account. All I can do here is to state my own view briefly, recognizing that other moral philosphers might not share it. My view is based on an analsyis of the moral concepts of words, such as 'ought' and 'wrong', in order to determine clearly, first their meanings; and then, as part of these, their logical properties; and thus, as a consequence of their logical properties, the rules for arguing about questions formulated in terms of these concepts. This is really the only sound basis for an account of moral reasoning. I am perhaps unusual among moral philosophers in insisting that at the critical level no appeal should be allowed to moral intuitions. Such appeals are bound to be viciously circular; for if intuitions are in dispute, no appeal to intuitions could settle the dispute. To this one exception can be made; some of our intuitions are not moral but linguistic or logical, and can be shared by people with the most diverse moral views. Logical intuitions are acquired when we learn our language, not as part of our moral upbringing; they are expressed, not in moral judgments (e.g. that it would be morally wrong to force the patient to submit to treatment), but in statements of logic (e.g. that to say such and such would be to contradict oneself). The failure to distinguish between these two kinds of intuition is one of the main sources of confusion in moral philosophy.

It seems to me that it can be established on the basis of logical intuitions alone that whenever we make a moral judgement of the typical or central sort we are prescribing that something be done in all cases of a certain (perhaps minutely specified) kind, i.e. prescribing universally for a given *type* of case. We cannot consistently claim that some particular individual has some duty, but that some other individual, however like the first in his character, circumstances, etc., might not have it. The thesis that moral judgements represent universal prescriptions can be made the basis of an account of moral reasoning which supports most of our common moral convictions (though it would be quite wrong to quote this fact in support of the account itself — for how are we to know that the moral convictions, implanted in us by our upbringing, are the ones we ought to have?). An example (which is all there is space for) will perhaps help to make clear how this can be done. We most of us accept the principle that it is wrong in general to confine people against their will. If 'wrong' expresses a negative universal prescription, or universal prohibition, this is easy to explain. For then in saying that it is wrong to do this, we are prescribing that it never be done. And the reason why we are ready to prescribe this is that we imagine ourselves in various circumstances in which other people might wish to confine us against our will, and unhesitatingly prescribe that they should not. There are some complications in the logic here which would need to be gone into in a full treatment; but it is not difficult to see intuitively that one who is prepared to prohibit involuntary confinement in all hypothetical cases in which he would be the victim will be prepared to assent to a general prohibition.

The same kind of reasoning can be used to establish exceptions to the general principle. In some cases the patient, if not confined, is likely to kill some other person. If we put ourself in the place of this other person, we find ourself ready to prescribe that the patient *should* be confined. It is a question of balancing the interests of the two parties; presuming that the interest of one in not being killed is greater than that of the other in being at liberty, we shall, if we put ourselves in the places of both in turn and respect their interests impartially, allow the confinement of the patient because this would promote the greater interest of the other person. So by this means we can build up a set of universal principles, each with the necessary exceptions written into it, to cover all contingencies.

At least, we could do this if we had complete information,

superhuman powers of thought, and infinite time at our disposal. Since we are not so gifted, we have to do the best we can to arrive at the conclusions to which such a gifted being would come. That, ideed, is why it is necessary to separate moral thinking into two levels. By doing the best critical thinking of which we are capable, when we have the leisure for it, we may be able to get for ourselves a set of fairly simple, general, *prima facie* principles for use at the intuitive level, whose prescriptions for particular cases will approximate to those which would be given a being who had those superhuman powers. This is really the best that in our human circumstances we can do.

In practical terms, what this means is that psychiatrists should, when they have the time, think about the ethics of their profession and try to decide what principles and practice would, on the whole, be for the best for those affected by their actions. In this thinking, they should consider a wide variety of particular cases and think what ought to be done in them, for the greatest good of those affected. And then they should select those principles and practices whose general acceptance would yield the closest approximation to the actions which would be done if all cases were subjected to the same leisured scrutiny. It is important to notice that cases have to be weighted for the likelihood of their occurring. In deciding whether people ought to wear seat belts when driving, we should be more moved by the huge majority of cases in which this increases the chances of survival than by the small minority where this is not the case.

I have not had the opportunity of reading all of the contributions to this volume; but from the introduction and from those which I have seen it appears that the method I have explained corresponds in general to that adopted by the contributors. I wish now to go through some of the topics mentioned by the editors at the end of their introduction, and ask how this method might be applied to them. We shall, I hope, see that the distinction between the intuitive level of thinking, at which an absolutist stance is appropriate, and the critical level, at which we should rather think in a utilitarian way, enables us to find a path through the philosophical difficulties, and at least pinpoint the empirical, factual questions which we should have to answer in order to solve the practical ones.

I will start with a problem which illustrates especially well the value of the separation of levels: the problem of the medical man's peculiar duty to his *own* patient. As we saw, it is natural for a psychiatrist to regard himself as owing a special duty to his own patient, to safeguard his welfare — a duty which ought to override any duties he may have to the public at large. If, for example, he has as a patient somebody who he knows will be a great deal of trouble to anybody who is so unwise as to employ him, has he any duty to reveal the fact when asked for a medical certificate? Here, as before, it is obviously no use treating the duty of confidentiality to the patient and the duty of candour to the employer as duties on the same level but ranked in order of priority; for it may depend on the case which duty should have precedence. If the patient is an airline pilot and his condition will cause him to lose control of the plane, we may think the public interest paramount; if he is a bank clerk and is merely going to turn up late to work from time to time, we may think that his condition should be concealed.

Dr Rappeport, in his excellent contribution (see Chapter 14), has many good examples of this kind of conflict between duty to one's patient and other duties. It looks at first as if a utilitarian, who is required to treat everybody's equal interests as of equal weight, can find no room in his system for special duties or loyalties to people standing in special relationships to oneself (e.g. that of patient). And indeed this has been often made the basis of objections to utilitarianism. But the two-level account makes it easy to overcome them. At the critical level of moral thinking we are bound to be impartial between the interests of all those affected by actions. So at this level, we shall have to give no special edge to our own patients, but simply ask, in each case we consider, what action would produce the best results for all those affected, treated impartially. A superhuman intelligence, given complete information, might be able to provide specifications, in this way, for all cases that could possibly occur. But if this gifted person were asked to draw up some simple ethical principles for the conduct of psychiatrists, which they ought to cultivate as second nature, it is obvious that he would not give them the single principle 'In every case, do what would be in the best interests of all considered impartially'; for mortal psychiatrists are seldom going to know what this is. It is much more likely that the principle to do the best one can for one's own patients will figure among the principles he recommends. Why? Because if psychiatrists absorb this principle as second nature it is much more likely that the interests of all, even considered impartially, will be served than if psychiatrists think they have to do an impartial utilitarian calculation in every case. This is because the relationship between a psychiatrist and his patient, based on mutual trust and confidentiality, has itself immense utility, and the destruction of this relationship is likely, except in extreme and rare instances, to do much more harm than good. So we have the paradoxical result that a utilitarian critical thinker would recommend, on utilitarian grounds, the cultivation of practices which are not themselves overtly utilitarian, but appeal to such notions as the patient's right to confidentiality.

However, this right to confidentiality is not the only right which

will be entrenched in the principles of a good psychiatrist. There will
be other rights there too, including the right of the public to be
protected. All these rights are important; yet they will sometimes
conflict. A one-level account of moral thinking based on rights is
powerless to deal with such conflicts. The two rights, of the patient to
confidentiality and of the public to protection, exist; but if that is all
we say, we can say nothing about cases where one of these rights has
to be overridden. In such cases, the psychiatrist will have to do some
critical thinking; and it may have different outcomes according to the
severity of the impact on the various parties' interests.

Next, let us take the right to liberty. As we saw, some sort of
prohibition, in general, of forcible deprivation of liberty is likely to be
part of the moral armoury of nearly everybody, because liberty is
something we all value highly. For this reason, the good psychiatrist
will be extremely averse to confining anybody unless there is a very
strong reason. But sometimes there will be. The right of the public to
protection comes in here too. So here too we have the same picture: a
superhumanly well-informed critical thinker who had considered all
possible cases on utilitarian lines might be able to arrive at the right
answer in all of them without saying anything about rights; but if he
were asked to draw up a set of principles to be imbibed by mortal
psychiatrists, which would lead them in the course of their practices to
the nearest approximation to his ideal solutions, he would certainly
place high on the list of such principles that which protects people's
right to liberty. For to confine people against their will does them,
normally, such enormous harm that any psychiatrist who makes light
of this principle will be a public menace.

Two particular cases of this kind of problem require special
consideration. The first is that of when a psychiatrist may justifiably
confine somebody for *his own* good (e.g. to prevent suicide). It is the
case that *in general* people who kill themselves are not acting in their
own best interests (as is shown by the later thoughts of most of those
who have been prevented). However, it may be that some people do
the best for themselves (for example some who face miserable senility
and have no close friends or kin). So here too the right to liberty has to
be balanced against a duty to preserve the patient from great harm to
himself. Both are very important and will be recognized as such by
good psychiatrists; and this recognition can be justified on utilitarian
grounds at the critical level. But at the intuitive level a psychiatrist
will do well to respect *both* these principles without thinking in a
utilitarian way at all — until they conflict; and then he will have,
perhaps at the cost of a great deal of mental anguish, to think critically
and ask what, in these particular circumstances, is for the best.

The other problem is that which arises when the patient is

incapable of judging for himself what is in his own interest. This may be because he is a young child, or because he suffers from some mental disability. Our ideal critical thinker would no doubt, in some of the cases he reviewed, come to the conclusion that the best interests of such people would be served if they were treated without their consent. These would be cases in which the patient is unable to grasp the facts of his own case, and in particular facts about the prognoses with and without the treatment. The psychiatrist may be better able to make such prognoses. But it is terribly easy to stray across the boundary between prognosis, on which perhaps he can claim authority, and judgements of value about possible future states of the patient, on which he cannot. Suppose that the patient, if subjected to brain surgery, will become placid and contented, but lose all his artistic flair; but that if he is not, he will remain an artist of genius, which is what he wants to be, but suffer miserably from recurrent depression and perhaps in the end kill himself after enriching the world with some outstanding masterpieces. An exceptionally gifted psychiatrist might be better able than the patient to predict that these would be the respective outcomes of treatment and of no treatment; but that would not give him the authority to override the patient's preference for the second outcome over the first.

Looked at in terms of our two levels, the picture becomes clearer. At the intuitive level, the patient's right to decide for himself what sort of person he wants to be will seem very important; and we can justify at the critical level the entrenchment of this right by pointing out that in the vast majority of cases patients *are* the best judges of what will in the end suit them, and also that psychiatrists are very subject to the temptation to impose their authority beyond its proper limits, i.e. to stray over the boundary above mentioned. On the other hand we can also justify at the critical level the entrenchment of the duty to preserve patients from the consequences of their inability to grasp what their own future states are likely to be. In most cases there will be no conflict between these principles; but where there is, they can be resolved only by an ascent to the critical level in the particular case. However, there is danger in a too ready ascent; for it is easy to persuade oneself that there is a serious conflict between the principles, when what is really happening is a conflict between the patient's right to liberty and our own propensity to meddle.

We may next consider a group of problems about consent, which are closely related to the problem we have just been considering. One of the rights on which great emphasis is properly laid is the right not to be treated without one's own informed consent. The justification, at the critical level, for the emphasis on this right is the same as before, that patients are on the whole the best judges of their own interests, and their interests are normally much more severely affected than anybody else's; so the ideal outcome from the utilitarian point of view is much more likely to be realized if this right is normally allowed to 'trump' any considerations of utility which might *seem* strong in particular cases (the 'trump' metaphor comes from R. M. Dworkin, *Taking rights seriously*[5]). But if we wish to entrench the right in this way, we have the difficulty on our hands of saying what counts as informed consent. Can people who have neither practised psychiatry, nor actually been in the state which they will get into if not treated, ever be *fully* informed about what they are letting themselves in for? If they are really pretty mad, could they not make crazy choices even if they did grasp the alternative prognoses? And would not this make their refusal of consent not fully informed? These are familiar problems. What our critical thinker will try to do is to find some principles for deciding what criteria of informed consent, if absorbed into the practice of psychiatrists, are likely to lead them in the majority of cases to do what is for the best.

An especially difficult subclass of these problems afflicts psychiatrists who have to deal with patients who are already confined in a mental institution or in prison. In either case the psychiatrist may be in a position to force treatment on patients (for example aversion therapy or psychotropic drugs); and it has sometimes been thought that this presents an ideal opportunity to do good to the patient (and also serve the public interest) against the patient's will. 'Force' need not mean 'physical force'. If the psychiatrist says to the patient that he is likely to get out much earlier if he submits to the treatment, this is not force in Aristotle's strict sense (*Nicomachean ethics* 1110 a 1) of 'that of which the origin is outside [a man], being such that in it the person who acts, or [to be more exact] is acted upon, contributes nothing'; but it is certainly duress, which Aristotle treats of in the next few sentences; the patient is faced with alternatives such that he is highly likely to do what the psychiatrist wants. It has therefore been denied that people in confinement can give meaningful consent, and it has been held, accordingly, that it is always illegitimate to use such treatments on them. But this doctrine too could lead to less than optimum results if it caused offenders to languish in prison who might, if given suitable drugs, be safely allowed out.

This could be a consequence of the failure to distinguish between our two levels, and a resulting rigidity in the application of the principle guaranteeing the right to freedom of choice to be treated or not treated. The principle is immensely important as a safeguard against abuses; if psychiatrists can break it without a qualm, they are not to be trusted with prisoners or even with patients confined in institutions. But in order to determine the limits of the principle, what is needed is not a lot of casuistry about the precise meaning of 'consent', but a set of practical rules whose general adoption will lead to the best decisions being made on the whole.

One such rule would be to insist on the separation of decisions about confinement or release from decisions about treatment. In the case of prisoners, decisions to confine would be left to judges, and decisions to release to the civil authorities; decisions about treatment would be the province of the psychiatrist, who, therefore, could only say to the prisoner that he might be able to improve his condition enough to enable the authorities to release him, and not that he (the psychiatrist) would release him if he successfully underwent treatment. Certainly any mixing up of the roles of judge and doctor is likely to have bad consequences; for a decision on medical treatment requires careful observation over a period of an individual patient, which courts cannot undertake; whereas the sentence of a court aims at consistency and fairness between different offenders, and, subject to this, at the protection of the public, and the psychiatrist has neither the experience nor the expertise nor even the habits of mind required for this judicial role. Sound critical thinking would be likely to insist on such a separation of roles, and thus prevent many abuses. But whether this is so or not, the general point stands: *what* rights ought to be enshrined in *what* rules should be decided in the light of the consequences of making those the rules rather than some others.

Lastly, we may consider a related problem: how are we to decide which conditions are mental diseases and which are merely deviations from the currently accepted social or political norms? This is the problem raised by the political abuse of psychiatry in Russia. For example, is homosexuality a disease; and if it is, is 'revisionism'? Where do we draw the line? The term 'disease' is above all a ticket giving entry to what has been called 'the sick role'. It is an evaluative term, implying that the person with the disease ought, other things being equal, to be treated in order to remove it. If we classify homosexuality, or 'revisionism', as a disease, what we are doing is subscribing to such an evaluation. So it is no use hoping by mere conceptual analysis to settle the question of whether homosexuality is a disease. We shall call it one if we approve of the treatment of homosexuals to remove their homosexuality (if this is possible); and the same with 'revisionism'. The crucial decision, then, is whether to approve of this. And it should depend on whether the approval, and therefore practice, of treatment to remove homosexuality will on the whole be for the best for the homosexuals and others. Confining ourselves for the moment to voluntary treatment, it would seem that sound critical thinking might arrive at the following principle: if the patient wants not to be a homosexual and asks for treatment because he wants to have sexual relations with the opposite sex, he should be given what he wants; on the other hand, if he wants not to be a homosexual only because of the social stigmas and legal penalties attached to homosexuality, it might be better, if we could, to remove the stigmas and penalties. The reason why critical thinking would arrive at this conclusion is that in the first case the interests of the patient and others are advanced by 'cure', whereas in the second they would be better advanced by the removal of the need for it. If the situation is thus clarified, it becomes less important whether we call the condition a disease or something else.

But if *compulsory* treatment for homosexuality or 'revisionism' comes into question, the right to liberty again becomes of the first importance. Since having things done to one against one's will is something that nobody wants (this is a tautology), it is in itself an evil; it can only be justified by large countervailing gains (e.g. as above, the protection of the public from dangerous mental patients). It is hard to see what these gains could be in the two cases we are now considering. In both of them the general good would be much better advanced by removing the political institutions which make 'revisionism' something that the authorities feel impelled to suppress, or by removing the habits of thought which make people want to persecute homosexuals. It will be better all round for everybody if this comes about.

Though I have not had the space to deal with all the topics raised even in the Introduction, I have perhaps done enough to indicate in general how such problems are to be handled. In all cases what we have to do is to find a set of sound principles whose general acceptance and firm implantation in the habits of thought of psychiatrists will lead them to do what is best for their patients and others. In the general run of their professional life, they need not think like utilitarians; they can cleave to principles expressed in terms of rights and duties and may, if they do this, achieve better the aims that an omniscient utilitarian would prescribe than if they themselves did any utilitarian calculations. But if that is all they do, their thought is still defective; for, first of all, it is a matter for thought what these principles should be; and second, we have to know what to do when they conflict in a particular case. And thought about both these questions will be best directed if it has as a target the good of those affected by the application of the principles.

References

1   Hare, R. M.: Medical ethics: can the moral philosopher help?, in *Philosophical medical ethics: its nature and significance*. Ed. Spicker, S. F. and Engelhard, H. T. Jr. Boston, Reidel, 1977, p. 49.

2   SINGER, P: *Practical ethics*. Cambridge, Cambridge University Press, 1979.
3   GLOVER, J. C. B: *Causing death and saving lives*. London, Penguin, 1977.
4   HARE, R. M: *Moral thinking: its levels, method, and point*. (To be published.)
5   DWORKIN, R. M: *Taking rights seriously*. Cambridge, Mass., Harvard University Press, 1977, p.xv.

4
The social dimension

David Mechanic

PSYCHIATRISTS, or any other mental health professionals, are influenced in their activity and judgment by the sociocultural context, by their personal and social biography, by the ideology implicit in their professional training, by the state of perspective, theory, and scientific understanding in their discipline, and by the economic and organizational constraints of the setting in which they practise. The practice of psychiatry involves competing roles. Although psychiatrists may select themselves into certain roles and not others, it is common for them to have multiple professional roles with different social and ethical requirements but with no clear demarcation among them. Much of professional practice has an important social control function, and mental health practitioners are in part political actors. While the foregoing characterizes all physicians and not only psychiatrists, the conflicts in psychiatry are more sharply drawn and the boundaries of appropriate activity somewhat more hazy.

Although the roles psychiatrists play are numerous, they can be separated roughly into three spheres of action: as scientist, clinician, and bureaucrat. While these activities overlap, it is useful to separate them and examine their varying aspects and the ethical dilemmas they pose.

The psychiatrist as scientist and as clinician assumes entirely different stances. As Freidson[1] has noted in his distinction between these two world views, the goal of the clinician is action and not knowledge. He believes in what he is doing, and this is functional for both doctor and patient. The sceptical detachment of the scientist would only discourage the patient and erode the suggestive powers of the therapeutic encounter. While the scientist seeks to develop a coherent theory, the clinician is a pragmatist, depending heavily on his own subjective experience and trial and error in situations of uncertainty. While the scientist seeks to determine regularity of behaviour in relation to abstract principles, the clinician is more subjective and suspicious of the abstract. The responsibility of clinical work makes it difficult to suspend action, to remain detached, and to lack faith that one is helping patients.

† The writing of this chapter was supported in part by a grant from the Robert Wood Johnson Foundation.

The differences between the objectives of science and clinical practice suggest different ways of proceeding in the two roles. The researcher in psychiatry, for example, must be concerned with precise and reliable diagnosis. Only through clear distinctions among varying clinical entities can knowledge about the aetiology, course, and effective treatment be acquired.[2] Although efforts in making finer distinctions or in identifying new conditions may be uncertain and yield no benefit for the patient, they may serve the development of scientific inquiry and understanding. Such a diagnostic orientation used in a clinical context, however, may be of little use or even be dysfunctional. The labelling of questionable conditions may induce anxiety in the patient, may stigmatize, and may divert the clinician from taking constructive therapeutic action.

The professionalization of psychiatry in the nineteenth century and the growing assumption that mental disorders were biological in origin and required organic intervention undermined the useful activity of social reformers who devoted attention to the social context of treatment.[3] If mental disease was an unfolding of a biological propensity, why worry about the social environment? The irony, of course, was that the new conception had little to offer patients and undermined helpful intervention.

Psychiatrists, in their capacity as physicians, have a social role that extends beyond their technical knowledge. Although the scope of their activity may be influenced by their conception of the psychiatrist's role, they have limited control in defining the types of patient who seek their help. Moreover, they have a social responsibility to do what they can to help patients who suffer and seek assistance and thus cannot simply be constrained by the state of established knowledge. In short, the psychiatrist as clinician works in part on the basis of scientific knowledge and practical experience and in part on the basis of his social judgment of what is appropriate to his profession. As problems he faces become more uncertain and he is less able to resolve them through existing psychiatric knowledge, the psychiatrist's social biography and values have a larger impact on his decisions.

Because psychiatry deals with deviance in behaviour, its conceptions run parallel to society's conceptions of social behaviour, personal worth, and morality. These conceptions can be viewed from competing vantage points, and are therefore amenable to different professional approaches. In the absence of clear evidence about aetiology or treatment, disturbance can be seen as biological in nature, as a failure in development, as a moral crisis, or as a result of socioeconomic and other social factors. Remedies may correspondingly be seen in terms of biological restoration, moral realignment, social conditioning, or societal change. Although all of these elements may be present in the same situation, the one that the psychiatrist emphasizes has both moral and practical implications. There is no completely neutral stance: diagnostic and therapeutic judgments have political and social connotations.[4]

The psychiatrist as double agent

In this context it is of great importance whom the psychiatrist represents. To the extent that he acts exclusively as the patient's representative and in the patient's interest as far as this can be known, the situation is relatively simple. The patient suffers and seeks assistance, and the role of the psychiatrist is to do whatever possible to define the available treatment options and to proceed in a manner on which they agree. Such intervention may be at a biological, psychological, or social level, or within a medical, psychodynamic, or educational model. The definition of the endeavour, however, is in terms of the patient's interests and needs. In practice, failure to define options is common, and the psychiatrist's values and ideology may intervene resulting in deviation from the ideal. Indeed, the psychiatrist may not be conscious of his own ideology because it is so entrenched in his own world view. Or he may act against the patient's wishes because he assumes greater knowledge of what the patient's interests are. Despite the complexity, the approach is distinctive in that action taken is for the sake of the patient and no other.

The notion that the psychiatrist's responsibility is to the patient and no other is a value, like other ethical aspects of practice such as confidentiality, which arises from a commitment to the individual as compared to the collective. But it is not universally shared.

In the People's Republic of China, for example, psychiatric practice is a public function with primary commitment to the interests of the State and not of the individual.[5] Clinical practice takes place openly in consultation with family members and with commune leaders. The way the patient is handled is a public issue, and information concerning his problems and management is shared with commune officials, work supervisors, and the like. While the basic content of psychiatry is primarily biological, the social effects of psychiatric advice are recognized. Professional practice cannot be divorced from the existing form of social organization in which it occurs.

In Western societies, psychiatrists may work as agents of individual patients or as agents of organizations such as the family, the school, industry, the court, and the armed services.[6] While under some circumstances psychiatrists may retain an autonomous role in which they act as an agent for patients, in other circumstances their organizational auspices may make such a role uncertain and susceptible to encroachment.[7] Treatment involving couples or parents and children, for example, inevitably entails a clash of wills and interests, and the therapist is forced to take sides, even if only in the most subtle ways. Although the treatment may involve sufficient common interest among the parties to sustain the encounter, the therapist still walks a difficult line. While he may regard himself as playing an autonomous role, it may become especially tenuous as the power of the employing institution intrudes on his relationship with his patients (this is obviously less of a problem in private clinical practice).

While psychiatrists work for organizations other than the patient, they have, by definition, a split loyalty. Although conflict of loyalty may not be a major issue in routine practice, it may at any time become problematic. This is the case whenever the organization and the patient have competing needs or interests. The most dramatic examples of this form of bureaucratic psychiatry occur in totalitarian countries where psychiatrists are State bureaucrats and may perform social control functions for the State, or in the military, in all countries, in which psychiatrists serve as agents of their employer. Similar pressure exists, however, whenever the psychiatrist represents an organization such as the court, prison, school, or industry. In all but the most crass cases, the psychiatrist's position as double agent is sufficiently ambiguous for him to experience a sense of neutrality and believe himself to be participating in the public interest. But it is this comforting feeling of impartiality that is dangerous because it diverts attention from the dilemma in resolving conflict between involved parties. The use of psychiatry to discredit political dissenters, for example, is reasonably obvious, even if disputed. It is the more subtle social influence on the psychiatrist's role that is more difficult to bring into the open.

A major practical issue is how to develop safeguards to protect clients in situations where the psychiatrist is well intentioned and views his role as impartial but is in fact influenced by conflicting expectations. The problem is in no way unique to psychiatry. Comparable problems occur in industrial medicine, in the determination of disability, and in many other activities involving general physicians. If psychiatry is different, it is primarily because the social control aspects of psychiatric practice are far-reaching, particularly in situations involving the patient's freedom: clinical assessment affecting involuntary hospitalization, parole of prisoners, release of soldiers from military service, criminal responsibility, and the like.

When the psychiatrist represents an organization with which a client is in conflict, the possibility that the latter may be betrayed is real, however well-intentioned the psychiatrist. However, the social system of organizations like mental hospitals, prisons, courts and schools brings the psychiatrist into continuing informal association with administrators, with whom he often comes to share a certain common perspective. Conditions are thus ripe for an exchange of information that can harm the interests of the client, who may have communicated with the psychiatrist on the assumption that the material divulged would be used solely in the client's self-interest. Whether the client actually believes this, or even considers the issue, is not crucial. What is important is the fact that the psychiatrist functioning in a bureaucratic role can potentially harm the client's interests without the latter's awareness. The client can be drawn into a situation in which he unknowingly participates in his own betrayal.

Response to this ethical dilemma varies among psychiatrists, ranging from an assertion that they can function impartially in a bureaucratic setting to the position that a double agent's role is a violation of the ethical basis of the discipline. While the former position denies reality, the latter escapes from it. Since society insists that psychiatrists perform such bureaucratic responsibilities and many do so, constructive approaches to the problem are necessary. One position is that organizations should separate therapeutic from bureaucratic practice: those with bureaucratic power over clients, and who do not serve solely as their agents, should not pose as therapists. While these non-therapists may incidentally provide a service that is perceived as therapeutic, there should be no confusion in the social definition of the psychiatrist's role. This separation provides some protection, but it does not insure against abuse for reasons suggested earlier. In any case, with the scarcity of resources for psychiatric services in most organizatios, it is unlikely that a clear-cut separation of psychiatric functions will be implemented.

Some commentators maintain that a psychiatrist performing a role involving conflicting loyalty should warn the patient of the risk in providing confidential information and even of the danger of being assessed by a psychiatrist who is not the patient's agent. While in principle this seems fair, in reality it is unlikely to occur or will be performed only in a formal or perfunctory way. People are resistant to a requirement that makes it difficult to perform their functions, and such an external requirement of 'informed consent' is difficult to implement in an effective way. But perhaps the requirement itself may alert psychiatrists to the conflicting functions of their role, and help them to avoid serious unethical practice. While regulation may have an impact, more important is an awareness among psychiatrists themselves of the gravity of the issue and the extent to which they, as a profession, are prepared to impose sanctions on colleagues who obviously abuse their role. But education, without organizational reinforcement that encourages ethical practice and protects the helping aspect of the psychiatrist's function, is destined to fail.

In noting possible solutions to the problem of the psychiatrist as double agent, I have avoided purposely the many ambiguities and subtleties that actually arise in psychiatric practice. The work of the psychiatrist is interwoven with social values, and it is to an examination of some of this source of influence that we now turn.

Social influences on psychiatric judgement

In most instances of psychiatric judgement, there are no reliable independent tests to confirm or contest them. While psychiatric diagnosis focuses on disordered thought and functioning and not on deviant behaviour *per se*[8], a judgement about disorder is inevitably tied to the social context, and to the clinician's understanding of it — based not only on clinical experience but also on normal life experience. Most lay persons can recognize the bizarre symptoms associated with psychosis; it is the borderline areas that are more at issue, and at these borders it becomes more difficult to disentangle subculture, illness behaviour and psychopathology. The further the patient's subculture is from the psychiatrist's first hand experience, the greater the likelihood that inappropriate contextual norms will be applied. To the extent that the patient comes to the therapist voluntarily and seeks relief from his suffering, the lack of precision in making such contextual judgments is less of a concern than when the psychiatrist acts on behalf of some other interest. Even in the former case, however, the prestige of the therapist reinforces his considerable personal power in the encounter with the patient. It may also reinforce an alternative view of the nature of the patient's problem.

The absence of tests to establish diagnosis independent of the therapist's contextual judgment makes it relatively easy for critics to insist that psychiatrists label patients on the basis of social, ethical, or legal norms and not on clearly established evidence of psychopathology.[9,10] Although the criticism cannot really speak to the scientific validity of applying a disease model to the patient's suffering or deviant behaviour,[2,11] it applies to the role of psychiatrist as clinician or bureaucrat in dealing with social problems and psychological disorder. The psychiatrist who mediates conflict between husband and wife, between parent and child, between employer and employee, and between citizens and official agencies inevitably must mix social judgment with assessment of psychopathology. When the psychiatrist acts as an agent to excuse failure at work, to obtain special preference for housing or other benefits, to obtain disability payment, to excuse deviant behaviour, or in a wide variety of other areas, he typically parades social judgments and personal decisions as psychiatric assessment. Thus it is essential to understand the social orientation and world view of psychiatrists.

Personal and social biography

Psychiatrists have undertaken various selective screenings in their careers: entry into medical school, into psychiatric training, and into particular types of psychiatric work such as psychotherapy, hospital practice, or administration. This process involves not only academic performance and interests but also social background, values, ideology, and aspirations. Various studies show that physicians who specialize in psychiatry differ from their colleagues in other specialities such as surgery or family practice in terms of social background, attitudes, and political orientation,[12,13] Moreover, in their classic book *Social class and mental illness*, Hollingshead and Redlich[14] reviewed the dramatically different social biographies of psychiatrists with an analytic–psychological orientation in New Haven as compared with those who were more directive in their approach and depended more on physical treatments. While there has been an obvious convergence in therapeutic practice, with many psychiatrists using a combination of psychotherapy and drugs, there continues to be a distinctive selection process of mental health professionals into the field of psychotherapy.

Psychiatrists engaged in private psychotherapy, at least in the United States, are both distinctive and relatively homogeneous in their social characteristics. Henry, Sims, and Spray,[15] for example, note in their study of psychotherapists that:

Careers terminating in the private practice of psychotherapy are populated, to a very large extent, by practitioners of highly similar cultural and social backgrounds. They come from a highly circumscribed sector of the social world, representing a special combination of social marginality in ethnic, religious, political, and social-class terms.

Moreover, psychotherapists coming from psychiatry, clinical psychology, and social work are more similar in social background and clinical orientation than psychiatrists who are medically inclined.[16] Those who become therapists, regardless of profession, have a comparable work style, share many viewpoints, and have strikingly similar developmental experiences.

The implications of these similarities are very suggestive. Certainly it is reasonable to assume that therapists who are upwardly mobile, socially marginal, nonreligious, divorced, politically liberal, and so forth, will see social and moral issues differently than more conventional persons and will make quite different judgments. Because the therapist's personality is an important aspect of his treatment, and because psychotherapy is largely a process of influence,[17] the encounter inevitably involves the transmission of values. The therapist may wish to minimize his personal bias, but cannot help but convey what he stands for. To the extent that this is explicit to the patient, it is less of a problem than when masked behind a professional mystique.

Greenley, Kepecs, and Henry [18] provide data collected in 1973 from psychiatrists practising in Chicago, some of whom were also studied in a 1962 survey.[16] These data indicated that, at least in Chicago, a Freudian-analytic approach and private practice continued to be strongly dominant. Although more psychiatrists reported having an eclectic orientation, the enthusiasm of the early 1960s for social and community psychiatry had receded markedly.

There is evidence from this survey that social characteristics of both psychiatrists and their patients are becoming more like those of the general population, although large differences still exist. The growth of psychodynamic treatment in the United States can be viewed as a social movement, developing first among particular practitioners — many of them urban, middle-class, and Jewish — and patients facing certain existential dilemmas.[19] These patients had social inclinations and characteristics similar to those of the therapists. As the movement grew, and therapy became more widely accepted in the culture, one would have expected that it would become more heterogenous in geographic distribution and in the features of both therapists and patients. The indications are that such heterogeneity has developed, and Greenley, Kepecs, and Henry's[18] Chicago data illustrate this trend. Comparing cohorts of psychiatrists who completed training in different periods from before 1960 to the time of the survey, they observed steep declines in the proportion with immigrant fathers, of Jewish faith, and from an urban background. Psychiatrists questioned in 1973 as compared with the 1966 cohort reported more women, blacks, Catholics, and poor people as patients, and somewhat fewer Jewish patients.

The Chicago study, as well as other experience, indicates that psychiatric practice is becoming more varied and complex.[20] This should allow greater opportunity for a patient to select a therapist who has an orientation and perspective closer to his own. It should also promote a healthy diversity within psychiatry itself with regard to the relationship between mental health concerns and values.

The sociocultural context

The sociocultural context in which young psychiatrists develop and mature and within which they practice dramatically influences their views of the world and their professional activity. This is obvious historically as different eras with associated cultural contexts have provided different view of the nature of man, the boundaries of deviance, and the pattern of social and psychiatric intervention.[21] In the European context, for example, psychiatry has remained closer to general medical practice than in the United States where dynamic forms of therapy have been regarded by young psychiatrists as more prestigious than the treatment of severely disturbed or chronic patients. Since the Second World War the psychodynamic school has dominated psychiatric training programmes and influenced markedly the psychiatrist's perception of his role and the practice of his craft. Why the United States and not Europe was the most fertile ground for psychoanalytic ideas is open to many interpretations, and is beyond the scope of this chapter.

The close relationship between psychiatry and its sociocultural context is well illustrated in the United States of the 1960s. During this period there was great ferment in American society, characterized by social activism and an ideology that social problems could effectively be attacked through government intervention. This ideology had a broad sweep and also came to encompass conceptions of the social causes of, and remedies for, mental illness. Psychiatrists caught up in the ethos of the time began making grandiose claims for the potential of community psychiatry. Such advocacy was not based on improvement of programmes for chronic mental patients who were increasingly being returned to the community, but in a claim for special social expertise. In the words of one advocate, 'The psychiatrist must truly be a political personage in the best sense of the word. He must play a role in *controlling* the environment which man has created.'[22]

A major component of the new ideology was the notion that psychiatry could engage in the primary prevention of mental illness. Caplan, [23] for example, maintained that a program of primary prevention involved: identification of harmful influences, encouragement of environmental forces that support individuals in counteracting these influences, and promotion of resistance in the population to future illness. His programme — under the guise of psychiatric expertise was simply a form of social and political action. As Caplan saw it:

The mental health specialist offers consultation to legislators and administrators and collaborates with other citizens in influencing government agencies to change laws and regulations. Social action includes efforts to modify general attitudes and behaviour of community members by communication through the educational system, the mass media, and through interaction between professional and lay committees [p. 56].

Caplan cites the area of welfare legislation as one that psychiatrists ought to be involved in:

In some states, the regulation of these grants [Aid to Dependent Children] in the case of children of unmarried mothers is currently being modified to dissuade the mothers from further illegitimate pregnancies. Mental health specialist are being consulted to help the legislators and welfare authorities improve the moral atmosphere in the homes where children are being brought up and to influence their mothers to marry and provide them with stable fathers [p. 59].

Clearly Caplan wished psychiatrists to become involved in matters of morality and values about which there are many different views. Caplan[24] also saw psychiatrists extending their focus to problems of personnel section, placement, and promotion:

If he accedes to these requests, he will find that he is using his clinical skills and his knowledge of personality and human relations and needs not only to deal with persons suspected of mental disorder, but also to predict the fitness of healthy persons to deal effectively with particular situations without endangering their mental health. He will also be exercising some influence upon the nature of the population in the organization, and hopefully he will be reducing the risk of mental disorder by excluding vulnerable candidates and by preventing the fitting of round pegs into square holes [p. 6]

Caplan[23] even went as far as to speculate that a psychiatrist might 'exercise surveillance over key people in the community and ... intervene in those cases where he identifies disturbed relationships in order to offer treatment or recommend dismissal' [p. 79]. However, he rejected this role not because of lack of ability or knowledge on the part of psychiatrists but because it would be a distasteful role for them and be associated with political and social complications. That some psychiatrists do not find this role distasteful is evidenced by the more than one thousand American psychiatrists who responded to an obviously biased poll by *Fact* magazine in 1964 attempting to discredit Barry Goldwater's psychological fitness to run for the presidency of the United States. A lawsuit resulted in a jury decision that Goldwater had been libelled.

Some of the concepts implicit in preventive psychiatry are unfortunate not only because they are grandiose, naive, and an obvious projection of political values, but also because they continue to divert attention from making remedial efforts which are more consistent with existing knowledge and expertise. For example, adequate antenatal and postnatal care, still not fully available to the poor, is important in preventing mental retardation, prematurity, brain damage, and many other problems. Family planning services and facilities for the family with a handicapped child are often difficult to find. The system of service in the community for chronic mental patients is at best fragmentary. By what values do we divert attention from these needs to pursue illusory goals? The greatest weakness of preventive psychiatry in the 1960s was substitution of vague ideals for tangible action and a failure to specify clearly how psychiatric expertise could lead to the laudable goals that were advocated.

Here again it is essential from an ethical perspective to differentiate between different psychiatric roles. From the point of view of psychiatrist as researcher, it is fully appropriate to examine the value of interventions. Caplan,[23] for example, maintained that various crises and transitional periods (e.g. entering school, having a child, undergoing surgery, moving to a new environment) pose severe stresses that may burden a person's capacity to cope, and entail a high risk of social breakdown. He asserted that during these periods the person had a heightened wish for help and was more responsive to it. Thus he argued that community psychiatrists should identify situations in which people feel vulnerable, provide supportive help to them, and teach new coping techniques. According to his theory, social breakdown could be prevented either by intervening directly in the life of a person and his family during a period of crisis or by working through other professionals, such as doctors, nurses, teachers, and administrators, who naturally would come into contact with the person facing the crisis. Among the contexts Caplan suggested for such crisis intervention were antenatal clinics, surgical wards, divorce courts, and colleges. The basic hypothesis, legitimate and worth detailed inquiry, is that it is possible to give people anticipatory guidance and 'emotional inoculation' to help them cope with threatening events.

When the psychiatric role moves from researcher to clinician, crisis intervention theory involves major ethical dilemmas. First, although aspects of the theory are promising, it is based on a vague conceptualization that environmental trauma and the lack of coping ability cause mental illness. The evidence for this conception is incomplete and far from secure. Second, although such efforts may be laudable, the literature on evaluation attests that crisis intervention often may not only fail to achieve desired objectives, but also may make matters worse.[25] Third, there is little evidence that the type of troubleshooting advocated by preventive psychiatrists, although perhaps valuable in reducing distress, has any impact on the occurrence of mental illness or is directed at those who are likely to become ill if untreated. Despite these ethical concerns, the psychiatrist could justifiably engage in preventive programmes with interested community groups provided that he understands the limitations and elects to participate voluntarily. In this sense, his intervention may be viewed in the same way as any other uncertain therapy, with possible positive and adverse effects that must be balanced.

Preventive psychiatry is on shaky ground when a psychiatrist in a bureaucratic position provides services to people who neither seek nor desire his assistance. Imposition of such intervention in schools, divorce courts, welfare agencies, and the like, buttressed by the coercive authority of the organization, is a serious intrusion of privacy and a violation of the rights of a person to lead his life without interference. Even if the theory were powerful and its effectiveness demonstrated, involuntary application of preventive psychiatry would raise a profound ethical problem.

As the optimism of the late 1960s receded, preventive psychiatry lost much of its lustre, although it remains one of many streams of psychiatric activity. Psychiatry in the 1970s, at least in the United States, has turned to an interest in the biological basis of behaviour and more particularly neurophysiology and genetics. Although psychodynamic views are highly prevalent, the field of practice has become more heterogeneous than ever before, and training centres increasingly have focused on biological research and a more rigorous approach to psychiatric diagnosis. This will, of course, affect the viewpoint and practice of psychiatrists in the future. While these changes result in part from advances in research in biological psychiatry and epidemiology, they also reflect changing conceptions in society at large about the potential for social reform. Each generation of psychiatrists is likely to retain in part the social conceptions and values characteristic of its 'historical life cycle'.

Constraints of practice settings

Professional practice is influenced by the social context of practice organization and the manner in which payment for services is made. Because influence of the employer on the psychiatrist's decision-making is widely recognized and has already been discussed, I focus now on some factors affecting practice that are less well appreciated. In the United States, a considerable section of the psychiatric profession works privately, contracting with patients to provide service on a fee-for-service basis. Although the service may be paid for in whole or in part by an insurance company, there is an implicit contract between psychiatrist and patient. Treatment is typically arranged in time units of 45 to 50 minutes as often as every day or several times a week. Services of this kind are purchased to a disproportionate extent by the affluent or those with insurance cover. The therapists view themselves as responsible to their patients and not to some abstract notion of overall need in the community. The form of payment in this situation — the fee for service per session — presumably creates an incentive on the part of the psychiatrist to offer long-term therapy beyond the point that intervention would be cost-effective.

An alternative model of psychiatric work is found in institutions like health maintenance organizations, community mental health centres, and the British National Health Service, where the psychiatrist theoretically serves a defined population. Because his services are often insufficient to the need and limited by economic factors, decisions must be made as to who need specialized psychiatric services most and to what extent. Typically, this rationing is in part specified in the contract between patients and the institution. For example, there may be a limit on the number of visits over a specific period. Rationing also occurs in that a formal referral is usually necessary from a general practitioner to the consulting psychiatrist. Commonly, long-term therapy for a small number of patients cannot be offered since it would be at the expense of others needing services. The results are shorter consultations, short-term psychotherapy, or drug treatment. Although psychiatrists with a preference for these forms of treatment may be drawn to public-type organizations, there is little question that organizational arrangements help shape the scope and character of psychiatric services.

Similar types of constraints operate in psychiatric hospital practice and in community care. What can be done for a patient depends on the personnel and resources available and the number of other patients requiring help. Frequently, services are stretched thinly or are inadequate to meet the demand. While it is usual to bemoan insufficient financing, it is likely that economic constraints will never allow psychiatrists to provide all possible services to all patients in need. Although there are no easy solutions to the ethical dilemma posed by the need to ration, the psychiatric profession has an obligation to evaluate its methods and approaches in relation to their benefits and costs, in order that the resources available can be applied in the most efficacious way. For example, a prudent society cannot provide public support for psychoanalysis or other long-term psychotherapy in the absence of evidence that these approaches are more beneficial than less costly alternatives.

A note on the care of chronically impaired patients

Deinstitutionalization and community mental health care are as much a social ideology as were earlier conceptions of the care of the mentally ill. The ideology consists of a belief that it is desirable that individuals, to the greatest extent possible, live independently, assume responsibility, and show a desire to adjust to community living. The involuntary hospitalization of patients, in particular, constitutes a violation of cherished beliefs about individual rights. The abuses associated with involuntary commitment have become widely known and have made it more difficult to justify civil commitment. Perhaps less widely appreciated are the pressures, sometimes approaching abuses in their own right, placed on patients and their families to return the patient to the community even if he is unfit to manage, and the tendency to refuse hospital refuge to some highly impaired patients.

The extent to which the community should allow this refuge, and at what point, is very much tied to economic factors and the social ethos. The extent to which coercive therapies should be used to stimulate and maintain 'appropriate functioning' does not easily yeild to a consensus. Practices vary a great deal from one context to another depending on the values and commitments of professionals working with such patients. With the development of aversive techniques of control, 'token economies', and other forms of behaviour modification, profound questions are raised about the limits of coercion and treatment. Other chapters of this volume explore these issues.

Conclusion

Every aspect of psychiatric conceptualization, research, and practice is shaped by social assumptions and ideology. Concepts of deviance, the boundaries between mental disorders and other types of problem, modes of intervention, and selection of clients all vary as a function of time, place, character of the social structure, and dominant social perspective. The biographies of psychiatrists and their practices are culturally shaped, and the economic system poses alternative opportunities and constraints. Because psychiatrists work with models of man which have broad ethical implications for every aspect of their craft, there is no way of escaping the fact that psychiatric practice is as much a moral as a medical endeavour.

References

1. FREIDSON, E: *Profession of medicine: a study of the social structure of applied knowledge.* New York: Dodd, Mead, 1970.
2. MECHANIC, D: *Medical sociology,* 2nd edn. New York: The Free Press, 1978.
3. GROB, G. N: *The State and the mentally ill: a history of Worcester State Hospital in Massachusetts, 1830–1920.* Chapel Hill: University of North Carolina Press, 1966.
4. HALLECK, S. L: *The politics of therapy.* New York: Science House, 1971.
5. KLEINMAN, A. AND MECHANIC, D: Some observations of mental illness and its treatment in the People's Republic of China. *Journal of Nervous and Mental Diseases* **167**:267–74, 1979.
6. SZASZ, T. S: *Ideology and insanity: essays on the psychiatric dehumanization of man.* New York: Doubleday Anchor, 1970.
7. HALLECK, S. L. and MILLER, M. H: The psychiatric consultation: questionable social precedents of some current practices. *American Journal of Psychiatry* **120**:164–9, 1963.
8. LEWIS, A: Health as a social concept. *British Journal of Sociology* **4**:109–24, 1953.
9. SZASZ, T. S: The myth of mental illness. *American Psychologist* **15**:113–18, 1960.
10. ROSENHAN D. L: On being sane in insane places. *Science, New York* **179**:250–8, 1973.
11. SPITZER, R. L: More on pseudoscience in science and the case for psychiatric diagnosis. *Archives of General Psychiatry* **33**:459–70, 1976.
12. CHRISTIE, R. and GEIS, F. L: *Studies in Machiavellianism.* New York: Academic Press, 1970.
13. COLOMBOTOS, J., KIRCHNER, C., and MILLMAN, M: Physicians view national health insurance: a national study. *Medical Care* **13**:369–96, 1975.
14. HOLLINGSHEAD, A. B and REDLICH, F. C: *Social class and mental illness: a community study.* New York: John Wiley, 1958.
15. HENRY, W. E., SIMS, J. H., and SPRAY, S. L: *Public and private lives of psychotherapists.* San Francisco: Jossey-Bass, 1973, p. 3.
16. HENRY W. E., SIMS, J. H., and SPRAY, S. L: *The fifth profession: becoming a psychotherapist.* San Francisco: Jossey-Bass, 1971.
17. FRANK, J: *Persuasion and healing: a comparative study of psychotherapy.* New York: Schocken, 1974.
18. GREENLEY, J. R., KEPECS, J. G., and HENRY, W. H: A comparison of psychiatric practice in Chicago in 1962 and 1973. Unpublished manuscript, Department of Psychiatry, University of Wisconsin, Madison, 1979.
19. MECHANIC, D: Sociocultural and social-psychological factors affecting personal responses to psychological disorder. *Journal of Health and Social Behaviour* **16**:393–404, 1975.
20. REDLICH, F. and KELLERT, S. R: Trends in American mental health. *American Journal of Psychiatry* **135**: 22–8, 1978.
21. FOUCAULT, M: *Madness and civilization: a history of insanity in the age of reason.* New York: Pantheon Books, 1965.
22. DUHL, L. J., (ed.): *The urban condition: people and policy in the metropolis.* New York: Basic Books, 1963, p. 73.
23. CAPLAN, G: *Principles of preventive psychiatry.* New York: Basic Books, 1964.
24. CAPLAN, G: Community psychiatry — introduction and overview, in *Concepts of community psychiatry: a framework for training.* Ed. Goldston, S. E. Washington, DC: Government Printing Office, 1965, pp. 3–18.
25. ROBINS, L. N: Longitudinal methods in the study of normal and pathological development, in *Psychiatrie der Gegenwart*, Vol. I, 2nd edn. Ed. Kisker KP *et al.* Heidelberg: Springer-Verlag, 1979, pp. 627–84.

5
Psychiatric diagnosis as an ethical problem
Walter Reich

SOMETHING — a set of powers, an institution, or a technology — is an ethical problem when its product — an act, a system, or a technique — is capable of good or harm. The only other requirement is the mediation of human will: for the act, the system, or the technique to pose an ethical problem, it must be carried out, supervised, or participated in by persons who at some point possess, or believe themselves to possess, knowledge of their actions and the freedom to carry them out. Accidents of nature do not pose ethical problems, even if they cause harm, because they are not under human control. Should they come under such control — for example, through the creation of a technology, such as amniocentesis or accurate earthquake prediction — then what was once an accident becomes, through human mediation, preventable or predictable, and what was once ethically neutral becomes ethically charged. If a human intervention, in some form, can, through its exercise or restraint, result in good or harm, then that intervention is, by its very nature, an ethical problem.

In psychiatry, powers, institutions, and technologies exist that, through their acts, systems, and techniques, have the potential for good as well as harm. And, as the profession's practitioners, psychiatrists believe themselves both to know their field and have the freedom to act within it. Clearly, the field, as well as those who work in it, satisfy the criteria for ethical concern.

Ever since psychiatry emerged as a separate discipline, it has been criticized for ethical abuses in every sphere of its activity. Probably its ability summarily to cancel a person's freedom through its power to commit has been the subject of most such criticism: psychiatrists have been accused of hospitalizing against their will persons who have not required it — indeed, persons who have not even been mentally ill. Other aspects of the profession have also been found ethically lacking. Thus, the institutions providing psychiatric services have often been seen as debasing; and the technologies of electroconvulsive therapy,

† The opinions expressed here are those of Dr Reich and do not necessarily reflect those of the National Institute of Mental Health.

behaviour modification, medication, psychosurgery, and even psychotherapy have raised vexing and abiding issues regarding the control of behaviour.

But, in an important sense, all of these criticisms have missed the mark — or, to be more precise, have not gone deep enough. For, underlying all of its activities — underlying all of its powers, institutions and technologies — has been one sustaining psychiatric act: diagnosis. It is the prerogative to diagnose that enables the psychiatrist to commit, that delineates the populations subjected to his care, and that sets in motion the methods he will use for treatment. And it is this prerogative therefore, that, should provoke the most fundamental and the most serious ethical consideration.

Of course, the ethical problem of diagnosis — assuming that diagnosis is itself, at least in theory, a valid endeavour — has to do with its capacity for misuse. If enough is really known about mental disorders to be able to categorize them, and if such categorization does indeed represent a scientifically based or at least pragmatically useful professional activity, then the ethical concern must be the actual or potential misapplication of diagnostic categories to persons who do not deserve or require them — a misapplication that unnecessarily places those persons at risk to the harmful effects of psychiatric diagnosis. These effects include not only the loss of personal freedom and the subjection to noxious psychiatric environments and treatments, but also the possibility of life-long labelling[1-3] as well as a variety of legal and social disadvantages ranging from declarations of non-responsibility in family and financial affairs to, under the most extreme circumstance, the deprivation of life.[4]

Now, in general, misdiagnoses can be said to originate in two ways. The first way is purposeful: the psychiatrist applies a standard psychiatric diagnosis to a person for whom he knows it to be inappropriate in order to achieve some end that is not, by common definition, medical. That end may vary from instance to instance. For example, the psychiatrist may be under direct and obvious pressure from a family to hospitalize a troublesome relative, or from political authorities to hospitalize a troublesome dissident. On the other hand, the psychiatrist may also misdiagnose at the person's own request. For example, a diagnosis resulting in hospitalization may be a protection against a worse fate, such as jail in the case of a criminal offender, the military draft in the case of a war resister, or the birth of an unwanted child in the case of a woman seeking an abortion in a place where abortions are available only to those who can show medical need. In both types of case, whether the misdiagnosis is wanted or unwanted by its recipient, harm results. In the first type, the harm is obviously to the person. In the second type, it is to the integrity of the profession. One's main concern should certainly be for the first type; but the second, largely overlooked as a sort of victimless crime, also requires attention.

But though purposeful misdiagnoses should be a serious concern, it is the other kind — misdiagnoses that result not from the wilful misapplication of psychiatric categories but from other, primarily non-purposeful causes — that deserve the greatest scrutiny. They deserve it because most misdiagnoses belong in this category. And they deserve it, too, because misdiagnoses of the other type, the purposeful, are in general clear and easily understood as unethical, while those that are non-purposeful are much more subtle and insidious, much more a part of the fabric of the field itself, and much more difficult to identify and stop.

To be sure, there is a sense in which it could be argued that this other category of misdiagnosis does not constitute a true ethical problem: after all, if a misdiagnosis is not purposefully carried out, then it does not involve knowledge or free will on the part of the psychiatrist, and is beyond his control. But that is not quite the case. The mere fact that something is not completely purposeful does not mean that it is completely non-purposeful. This category involves, in the main, non-medical needs, pressures, and compromises that affect the diagnostic process, but that enter the psychiatrist's awareness to only a partial degree. The fact that the psychiatrist allows himself, for his own comfort, to ignore this awareness, or his responsibility to strengthen it, raises this category of misdiagnosis to the highest level of ethical concern.

Non-purposeful misdiagnoses can be traced to at least three sources. And it will be to these sources that the remainder of this discussion will be devoted.

The inherent limitations of the diagnostic process

Certainly the simplest source of misdiagnoses lies in the vulnerability of the diagnostic process to error. Over the years, it has been shown that the process can have a poor or questionable reliability;[5-7] may be subject to inconsistency and change;[8] often suffers from bias;[8-12] tends to rely on subjective criteria†; and tends to result in diagnoses of health rather than illness because, as Scheff has observed, physicians as a group feel that a 'type 2 error' (accepting a hypothesis that is false) is less dangerous than a 'type 1 error' (rejecting a hypothesis that is true).[2]

All of these inherent limitations have been well described in the

†With regard to schizophrenia, such subjective criteria include: 'understandability'; [13-15] 'peculiar behaviour';[16] 'the feel of the case';[17] the 'praecox feeling';[18] and 'bizarre thinking'.[19]

psychiatric literature and they raise ethical questions only to the degree that they are ignored. In the absence of objective, physical criteria, psychiatric diagnosis is, even in its most informed expression, only a finely tuned and intelligent art; and it is the responsibility of the diagnosing psychiatrist to remember its limitations with humility and to maintain a willingness to review his decisions and to admit his fallibility. At best, the psychiatrist is no better than his tools; and he must acknowledge their limitations as only the starting-points of his own.

The power of diagnostic theory to shape psychiatric vision

But vulnerable as the diagnostic process in psychiatry is to its own limitations, likely as those limitations may be to lead the psychiatrist to a misdiagnosis, and hard as he must try to guard against them, psychiatric diagnosis has yet other vulnerabilities that are even more subtle, more pervasive, and more difficult to recognize, and that, therefore, demand even greater vigilance. Again, the danger is misdiagnosis — non-purposeful but still damaging — and the ethical problem is the degree to which the psychiatrist can allow himself to ignore the forces and circumstances that lead to, and make use of, such disdiagnosis.

In the main, diagnosis is a social act. It takes place in a social context. The psychiatrist observes behaviour and judges it against a social — often local — norm. Nor is this necessarily inappropriate. Psychiatric illnesses, particularly those characterized by psychosis, often affect people in ways that lead them to ignore social norms and to traverse generally accepted verbal and behavioural boundaries; and such trespasses may, in fact, be the most sensitive and early indicators of illness. To be sure, the social basis of diagnosis is itself a problem, since the psychiatrist must know precisely where the social boundaries should be drawn and which trespasses are the result not of illness but of some other cause, such as, for example, social activism, or artistic style, or mere eccentricity, or, for that matter, rearing in another culture. But psychiatrists are, in the main, aware of these problems, at least dimly, having been apprised of them during training or, failing that, in the course of their practice.

Another basis for diagnostic judgement, however — one that shapes the diagnostic vision of the psychiatrist no less powerfully than the social one, but that is, nevertheless, generally unrecognized — is the diagnostic theory itself. In most countries, psychiatrists are guided by one or more theories of mental illness; and often those theories are associated with diagnostic systems that are their functional and practical expression. And, depending on the specificity of the system to which he subscribes, the ways in which a psychiatrist assesses a person's behaviour, draws conclusions about it, weighs the variance between the person and the social norm — indeed, *sees* the person — may be heavily influenced by the assumptions underlying the system and the approach that system takes to recognizing and identifying mental illness. The system, after all, delineates categories of illness and identifies the criteria by which behaviours and the people who exhibit them deserve to be placed in those categories; and every time such a placement is made, the categories, as well as the system itself, are reified. To the psychiatrist who accepts the system as real, this occasions no concern: the reality of the system has merely found a correspondence in the reality of the patient's illness. To one who finds the categories mistaken, however, or the criteria too narrowly or too broadly defined, such reification may be simply self-deceptive and false, and may result in misdiagnoses that are as systematic as only a system can cause.

In many countries, this danger is relatively small. The competition of theories is so great and the impact of systems so circumscribed or diluted that, while errors may result, their scale is necessarily limited. In the United States at the present time, for example, contrasting theories, such as those stressing psychological causation and those stressing the biological basis of mental illness, exist in such active competition, and without official sanction or encouragement from governmental or professional bodies, that the diagnostic system that is in use, even if it is itself codified and official, can hardly represent a unified approach to mental illness, and is unlikely to impose on the psychiatrist a rigid vision of psychiatric reality — a vision that the psychiatrist in turn adopts and that strictly moulds his own sense of the nature, meaning, and limits of psychopathology.

In some countries, however — one, at least — the danger of such an imposition is not only great but, indeed, has already expressed itself. In that country, psychiatrists have adopted an understanding of mental illness on the basis of the theoretical teachings of a dominant school; have accepted, whole, an approach to diagnosis in accordance with the rules of that school's formal and elaborate system; and have come to see — really see people as naturally and precisely falling into the categories that make up that system. That country is the Soviet Union, and its experience has much to teach about the ways in which an official diagnostic system can shape psychiatric vision and skew diagnostic practice, ensnaring people who elsewhere would be considered mentally well in the broad net that defines them irrevocably, as mentally ill. The Soviet experience is important because it exemplifies, in pure and extreme form, a trend that is only now developing in other countries; because its effects can be documented in multiple ways; and because it demonstrates, with grim clarity, how a system that appears to have only scientific origins and professional goals can, simply by virtue of its own nature as a systematic psychiatric technology, result in significant human harm.

What has happened in the Soviet Union has been the development during the past two decades of a diagnostic system that is by now standard in Moscow and nearly so in the rest of the country. That system was developed during the 1960s by Andrei V. Snezhnevsky, the founder of what has come to be called the Moscow School of psychiatry and the head of the Institute of Psychiatry of the USSR Academy of Medical Sciences, the central psychiatric research centre in that country. During the 1940s and 1950s, Snezhnevsky worked at and then became chairman of the Department of Psychiatry of the Central Postgraduate Medical Institute, to which the most talented academic psychiatrists in the country came to obtain their advanced degrees. Upon his ascension to the directorship of the Institute of Psychiatry in 1962, he dedicated the institute and its resources to the problem of schizophrenia, which was the focus of his central theory and of his diagnostic approach. Over the next decade, he and his staff continued to refine the system, doing clinical research designed to elaborate its details. By the early 1970s, many of his former students and trainees were in charge of the nation's academic psychiatric centres; the journal he edited, the *Korsakov Journal of Neuropathology and Psychiatry*, was the only psychiatric periodical in the USSR, and regularly carried news of his school's research and of the fine points of its diagnostic system; and the pattern of psychiatric teaching and research in centres far from Moscow felt the effect of his guidance and views, exerted through his role as an influential member of review committees for government ministries responsible for the approval of research and training grants. By the middle and late 1970s, the hegemony of the Moscow School was almost complete: it was, clearly, the dominant force in Soviet psychiatry, and its system the standard Soviet approach to mental illness.

The system itself focuses on schizophrenia; but because its definition of schizophrenia is so extraordinarily broad, it takes in vast sectors of psychopathology — sectors that, grouped together, encompass almost the whole of mental illness.

The theory behind the system is based on the assumption that schizophrenia has three different forms; that these forms vary from each other not so much in their symptoms, as traditionally has been assumed in the West since Kraepelin, but in their course; and that a particular schizophrenic's course form may be identified on the basis of a retrospective analysis of the development of his or her illness.[20-23]

COURSE FORMS

	Continuous		Periodic	Shift-like		
Life course of the illness						
Subtypes	Sluggish (mild)	Paranoid (moderate)	Malignant (severe)	Mild	Moderate	Severe
Some characteristics	Neurotic; self-consciousness; introspectiveness; obsessive doubts; conflicts with parental and other authorities; 'reformism'	Paranoid; delusions; hallucinations; 'parasitic life style'	Early onset; unremitting; overwhelming	Acute attacks; fluctuations in mood; confusion	Neurotic, with affective colouring; social contentiousness; philosophical concerns; self-absorption	Acute paranoid	Catatonia; delusions; prominent mood changes

A schematic rendering of the characteristics distinguishing the three course forms is presented in Table 5.1. The continuous form is characterized by the development of symptoms early in life, usually by late adolescence or early adulthood, with a general worsening as life progresses. Patients falling into this category do not, as a rule, improve. The second course form, the periodic, is characterized by periods of acute illness, interspersed with periods of remission during which the patient regains his health. The shift-like form is a mixture of the other two. As in the periodic form, there are acute attacks; but each attack leaves the patient more ill than he was prior to that attack, so that, overall, as in the continuous form, there is a general worsening of the illness during the course of the patient's life.

What is so unique — and, in the end, so problematic — about this system is the fact that two of the course forms have subtypes ranging from mild to severe, and that in those two, the continuous and the shift-like, the mild subtypes are characterized by symptoms that are not psychotic. In almost all countries, psychiatrists would probably agree that persons who satisfy the Moscow School's criteria for the moderate and severe subtypes of each of these course forms really are, by their criteria as well, schizophrenic. But they would probably disagree about the Moscow School's criteria for the mild subtypes, and would judge the persons who satisfy them to be not schizophrenic but, rather, neurotic, suffering from a character (personality) disorder, or even mentally well. Table 5.1 notes the characteristics attributed by the Moscow School to people grouped according to these subtypes.

The other feature of the system that adds to its potential danger — indeed, multiplies it — is the assumption, developed over the past decade, that each of the course forms represents, in essence, a separate illness, on one that has its own biological basis, which is, in turn, genetically determined. This implies that a person categorized as belonging in, say, the sluggish (mild) subtype of the continuous form has the same illness as anyone else in that form, including someone belonging in the malignant (severe) subtype; and, though he has a more mildly expressed version of that illness, he has it nevertheless — and for life. Such a person may therefore be subject to many of the same disadvantages, social and personal, as the person who is much more severely ill.

Now what is so troubling about this is clearly that the criteria given for the mild subtypes of schizophrenia apply to many people who would be seen by most psychiatrists as not schizophrenic. In fact, it could be predicted that, applied to a broad population, this system would draw into the schizophrenic fold precisely such people — people, that is, with neuroses, character (personality) disorders, affective illnesses, and no mental illnesses at all. And, in fact, there is evidence that this has indeed occurred.

Some of the evidence is impressionistic. Rollins, for example, reported in her book on child psychiatry in the Soviet Union that patients with primarily neurotic or psychopathic-like symptoms were typically given diagnoses by Soviet psychiatrists in the schizophrenic range.[24] More directly, Holland has reported, after a sojourn in Moscow's Institute of Psychiatry, that Soviet patients may be diagnosed as schizophrenic even if they exhibit no signs of the illness, and that, once the diagnosis is given, even if it is further subtyped as being of the mild variety, it continues to be used on the assumption that the patient has a life-long, genetically-based condition.[25-29]

But the most telling evidence has come from the International Pilot Study of Schizophrenia (IPSS). In that study, carried out during the late 1960s and early 1970s, nine centres around the world, including Washington, London, and Moscow, evaluated patients for schizophrenia and collected data about them. The centre in Moscow was Snezhnevsky's Institute of Psychiatry. As part of the study, a computer was programmed by John K. Wing to re-diagnose the patients originally diagnosed as schizophrenic at the various centres using data regarding the patients' symptoms that were gathered by the centre itself; the computer used strict criteria for its own rediagnoses, notably those formulated by Kurt Schneider.[30] While most centres did 'well' — that is, while the computer 'agreed' with most of the diagnoses of schizophrenia rendered at those centres — two centres did poorly.

One of these, Washington, did poorly, it turns out, primarily because its diagnosticians followed the rules of their own diagnostic system and, unlike the computer, tended not to differentiate between schizophrenia, schizophrenia-like psychoses, and paranoid psychoses; the computer gave them low marks only because it found their schizophrenics to be, by its criteria, otherwise psychotic. The agreement as to psychosis, however, was high.

The other centre that did poorly in the computer re-diagnosis exercise was Moscow's Institute of Psychiatry. But in that case, the reasons were different. A larger percentage of Moscow's diagnosed schizophrenics were re-assigned by the computer not to the psychotic but, rather, to the depressive and neurotic categories. Table 5.2 shows the computer classification (i.e., re-diagnosis) of patients who were originally diagnosed at the nine centres as belonging in those subtypes most likely to contain patients who would be considered by psychiatrists in many countries to be 'borderline schizophrenics' or, merely, 'borderline' — that is, patients who would be mildly ill, and possibly not psychotic. For eight of the centres, these subtypes were identified

Table 5.2 *IPSS computer classifications of schizophrenia subtype diagnoses*

IPSS Center	Schizophrenia subtype diagnoses	No of patients	Computer classifications (%)				
			Schizophrenic similar psychoses	Paranoid psychoses	Manic psychoses	Depressive psychoses	Depressive neuroses
Washington	Simple	4	50	33	17	0	0
	latent	2					
Moscow	Sluggish	12	0	0	33	8	58
Seven remaining centres	Simple	27	71	9	6	0	14
	latent	8					

as 'simple' and 'latent'. For Moscow, it was 'sluggish' (the mild subtype of the Moscow School's continuous form). Although the numbers are small, the difference seems striking. The patients classified as belonging in these subtypes in eight of the centres, including Washington but not Moscow, were classified by the computer as overwhelmingly schizophrenic or as having paranoid or schizophrenia-like psychoses, while the patients classified in the mild subtype by the Moscow diagnosticians, following the rules of the Moscow School, were classified by the computer as being primarily affectively ill or depressed, just as one might have predicted from an inspection of the system's broad diagnostic criteria.[31]

Finally, another confirmation of the tendency of the Moscow School's diagnostic system to overdiagnose schizophrenia has come from a Soviet psychiatrist, one working at Moscow's Serbsky Institute of Forensic Psychiatry. In an unprecedented article in a Western psychiatric journal, the psychiatrist, E. P. Kazanetz, used his own computer exercise to show that the Moscow School's system tended to overdiagnose as endogenous schizophrenics persons who were only exogenously ill — that is, it tended to diagnose as chronically ill people whose illnesses were primarily of an acute, externally caused type. Furthermore, Kazanetz added the observation that such over-diagnosis could be harmful to persons with acute illnesses assigned irrevocably to psychiatric registers of the chronically ill. Together with the evidence from the IPSS, Kazanetz's study reveals the degree to which an overly broad diagnostic scheme can result in overly broad diagnostic practice.[32]

What is so extraordinary about the Soviet experience, and ethically so significant, is that the patients who were misdiagnosed in the IPSS and in the population studied by Kazanetz were misdiagnosed — that is, diagnosed as schizophrenic despite the fact that almost all other psychiatrists would diagnose them as belonging in less severe categories of mental illness — only because of the dictates of the official diagnostic system. Those Soviet psychiatrists really *saw* the patients as schizophrenic; or, to put it another way, *the system created a category, first on paper and then, with training, in the minds of Soviet psychiatrists, which was eventually assumed to represent a real class of patients and which was inevitably filled by real persons.* Those diagnosticians came to see schizophrenic pathology as including very mild forms, and diagnosed accordingly. People who should not have received those diagnoses did, to their detriment; and psychiatrists who should not have given them did, in apparent full faith. Had those psychiatrists been sensitive to the capacity of diagnostic systems to shape the way psychiatrists understand, categorize, and perceive psychopathology, they might have been able, one hopes, to avert this result.

Nor should the Soviet experience be seen as an exotic or unique occurrence. The Soviet diagnostic scheme represents an extreme spectrum system — a system that posits a spectrum of schizophrenic illness ranging in severity from the most mild to the most severe, and caused by a genetic deficit of variable clinical expression. Such diagnostic schemes are, in fact, under active consideration in the West.[33-43] To be sure, they remain under examination, and have not been introduced yet into formal diagnostic systems. But, given the Soviet experience, it would be valuable to weigh the potential of such systems for similar overdiagnoses; not to do so at this point would, it seems, constitute a kind of ethical trespass.

The beauty of diagnosis as a solution to human problems

A third source of non-purposeful psychiatric misdiagnoses, and probably the most significant, is the attractiveness of the diagnostic process as a means of solving or avoiding complex human problems. With remarkable ease, diagnoses can turn the fright of chaos into the comfort of the known; the burden of doubt into the pleasure of certainty; the shame of hurting others into the pride of helping them; and the dilemma of moral judgement into the opaque clarity of medical truth. Because of their nature, functions and meanings, diagnoses can do such things in efficient and powerful ways; and the fact that they can make their use by psychiatrists for such ends remarkably irresistible, enormously unrecognizable, and, in the final analysis, utterly and failingly human.[44]

Diagnosis as explanation, mitigation, and exculpation
Perhaps the most fetching beauty of diagnosis is its capacity to instantly explain; behaviour that is odd, objectionable, troublesome,

or illegal can be, through the mediation of diagnosis, suddenly understood, explained, and explained away. To be sure, such behaviour may indeed be the product of diagnosable mental illness. But the capacity of a diagnosis to perform this function makes its use a temptation even in cases in which such illness does not exist, or is at best, only marginally present.

The arena in which this diagnostic temptation has been most evident has been the law (see Chapter 14). For years, psychiatrists have been asked to testify as witnesses in cases of people accused of various crimes. Often, both the prosecution and the defence have called upon such witnesses, who, in turn, have presented conflicting testimony about whether or not the actions carried out by the accused were a product of mental illness. While such conflicts have occasionally embarrassed the profession by suggesting that either side in a case can get psychiatric testimony in support of any diagnosis it wishes, at least they have been straightforward. Generally, the clinical questions have had to do with the presence or absence of some kind of psychosis, a group of mental conditions that can render a defendant legally not responsible for his actions; and the testimony has usually involved judgements about whether or not the defendant's behaviour and history met certain widely accepted criteria for these, the most agreed-upon areas of psychopathology. Naturally, defendants and defence counsels have often sought findings of 'not guilty by reason of insanity', even when they have suspected or known insanity not to have played a role, because of their belief that, at least in cases of such serious crimes as murder or rape, confinement in a hospital may be shorter than the sentence that would likely be imposed should the defendant be found guilty and not insane. Still, some people *do* commit crimes because they are insane: the law recognizes that insanity compromises free will and classifies someone without free will as legally not responsible for his actions; it is the right of defendants to use that defence; and psychiatrists have a role, as a result of their expertise in recognizing such mental illness, in testifying on the substance of that defence.

The trouble is that, in recent years, attempts have been made to expand that role into realms in which psychiatrists do not have expertise. The pressure for that expansion has been the wish diagnostically to explain — and legally explain away — criminal behaviour that does not involve classical psychotic states. Instead of insanity, the clinical questions have involved issues about which psychiatry has almost no validated knowledge: questions primarily of coercion, persuasion, and influence. In a series of cases, defence attorneys have turned to psychiatrists to testify about the effects of certain environmental pressures on individual development and judgement, and on the role these factors played in the genesis of the criminal behaviour. The defence argument has usually been that these factors created a diagnosable mental condition, one that explained the behaviour and, in a legal sense, either mitigated, or totally exculpated it.

The best-known case of this sort is the 1976 bank robbery trial of Patricia Hearst, in which the defendant was said to have been incapable of criminal intent because she had undergone a process of 'coercive persuasion', a process that had affected her capacity for free will. In a sense, not only the defence, but also many observers, favoured such a diagnostic exculpation: it made it possible to understand how such an ordinary, peaceful, apolitical, and utterly American young woman could have turned so suddenly into such an extraordinary, violent, ideological, and anti-American revolutionary. The court allowed that novel defence — novel because it stepped beyond the traditional realm of insanity into the broader arena of persuasion — and a battery of psychiatrists supported it with their testimony. The jury, however, rejected it, despite its attractive advantages: diagnostic explanation, they found, was not, at least in their eyes, a basis for legal exculpation.[45–46]

The attractiveness of the diagnostic process as a means of explanation and exculpation has revealed itself in the legal arena a number of times since the Hearst trial. In each instance, the defence contended that environmental factors had influenced or determined the criminal act; and, in each instance, psychiatrists took the stand to issue their supporting diagnostic opinions. In one celebrated Florida case, for example, a young boy who was accused of having killed an old woman was defended with the explanation that his mind had been affected by television violence. As in the Hearst trial, the jury found such use of diagnosis inadequate to the task of explaining away the defendant's behaviour.

Despite these setbacks, it seems likely that the beauty of diagnosis will continue to be appreciated in the legal arena, and that psychiatrists will continue to expand the ambit of their diagnostic expertise into realms about which almost nothing certain is known. In time, it seems possible that psychiatric testimony will offer itself in support of psychosocial defences of all kinds — defences, for example, that attribute criminal actions to the defendant's early childhood rearing or to the pressures of his adolescent peers. While such influences undoubtedly exist, almost nothing is known about how they affect the capacity for individual judgement and the existence of free will. That psychiatrists are willing to testify on these matters in the belief that they have such knowlege demonstrates not only the settled habit of psychiatrists to opine on issues beyond their scientific domain, but also, it seems, the satisfaction gained from finding in the storehouse of the profession some explanation that will transform a person's criminal act into a symptomatic one, and that will turn a painful moral question into a painless medical one.

Nor should the turn to diagnosis in such cases on the part of psychiatrists occasion any wonder. It is a natural turn when an explanation for unwanted behaviour is needed, and is accomplished every day, outside the arena of the law, by non-psychiatric laymen as well. For example, journalists and other observers turn to it for simplifying explanations when political figures engage in behaviour that is inexplicable in ordinary political terms.[47–52] Still others call upon diagnostic explanations to justify forgiveness or elicit sympathy in situations ranging from breaches of airline etiquette [53] to more serious transgressions of industry ethics [54] and literary propriety.[55] That psychiatrists similarly turn to diagnoses in the search for satisfying explanatory simplification, ones that substitute medicine for morals, is therefore not surprising; the satisfactions and advantages are the same except that, in the hands of psychiatrists, diagnoses achieve official status and recognition and result in lasting effects which are not always, even in these cases, salutary.

Diagnosis as reassurance

A second beauty of diagnosis is its power to reassure. When acts are committed whose implications are disturbing — acts that suggest vulnerabilities in ourselves, our institutions, or our communal beliefs — diagnoses often come to mind, both in the layman and in the psychiatrist, which serve to shift the frame of the behaviour from the threatening personal or social arena to a safer medical one.

In one widely publicized case, for example, this shift was effected toward its reassuring end through the co-operation of all concerned, psychiatrist and laymen alike. In 1974 Dr William T. Summerlin, a young researcher hired by the Memorial Sloan Kettering Cancer Centre on the basis of his promising work in transplantation immunology, reported that he had been successful at grafting skin from genetically unrelated animals. When other researchers were unable to confirm these astonishing results, Summerlin, in response, repeated his experiments, inking in the skins of his mice to make it appear as if the grafts had taken.

When this scientific fraud was revealed by Summerlin's research assistant, a special in-house committee was constituted to investigate the matter. The major threat posed by the Summerlin affair was the possibility that the American public might conclude that not only that researcher, but research itself, was suspect. To a community that depended on the magnificent largesse of its various constituents and supporters — a largesse which from US government sources alone approached, at that time, more than two billion dollars a year — such a prospect was indeed distressing. Moreover, there were other concerns. Summerlin's story, after all, did violence to the new American dream: he was a young man from the country's heartland who had been embraced by the eastern scientific establishment only to prove himself shamefully unreliable. What of that dream? And, besides, what was to become of young Summerlin himself?

The solution to all these distressing concerns was quick in coming. First, the investigating committee issued its findings: Summerlin's 'unusual behavior involved at least a measure of self-deception, or some other aberration, which hindered him from adequately gauging the impact and eventual results of his conduct'.[56] Then, at a press conference, the cancer centre's president, Dr Lewis Thomas, a researcher and physician himself, went on to elaborate. 'The fraud in this work', Dr Thomas informed the assembled reporters, was 'a result of mental illness.'[57]

At one stroke, all concerns were eased. Summerlin's actions were the result not of a vulnerability in research, or of the habits of researchers, but, rather, of a fault in the man. Moreover, that fault was not moral, but, rather, medical. And, besides that, it was short-lived. At his own news conference, four days later, Summerlin offered that he had been suffering from an acute depression, a condition that accounted for his 'irrational act' and for which he had already begun psychiatric treatment. The psychiatrist, Summerlin explained, had prescribed rest and physical exercise, and he was already feeling much better. And so, indeed, did those who had been so distressed by the implications of Summerlin's act: the diagnosis preserved not only the good name of science, and not only the integrity of the scientific community, but also Summerlin, who could be seen now, in more reassuring terms, not as a person who would be forever morally tainted, but, rather, as one whose treatment would leave him clean, whole and good, and ready to resume his professional life.

Whether Summerlin's behaviour was or was not, in fact, the result of an acute depression cannot, of course, be confirmed here; but the case is important because it illustrates the ease with which a turn to diagnosis can, at the same time, allay multiple concerns. When a psychiatrist is faced by such a case, when a means — the diagnostic process — is available that can accomplish so much, and when others are themselves inclined to think that mental illness can or should be used to explain the behaviour, then it is hard to imagine that the psychiatrist will not look seriously at that option, and even find himself considering it with greater favour than ordinarily he might in other cases involving similar behaviour which, however, in those cases, pose no threat or raise no concerns.

Diagnosis as the humane transformation of social deviance into medical illness

Another beauty of diagnosis is its power to reclassify whole categories of socially unacceptable behaviour as the product of psychiatrically diagnosable conditions. This kind of reclassification derives, in essence, from a liberal Utopian impulse: people are naturally good, and if someone acts to the detriment of society he must be ill. Hence, the social response should aim not at punishment, and not merely at control, but, rather, at treatment. If this approach is taken, everyone presumably benefits: the deviant, the 'root causes' of whose transgressions are thereby recognized and cured; society and its authorities, which are no longer in the position of exacting harsh punishments; and psychiatrists, whose re-definitions make all this possible and who can feel themselves in the noble position of healing where others would have only hurt.

Probably the most striking examples of such reclassification may be found in connection with sexual behaviours that traditionally have been classified as socially undesirable (see Chapter 9). As a result of developments in medical technology, as well as shifts in popular views, some of these behaviours have been reclassified in psychiatric — and therefore diagnostic — terms. One such development, the synthesis of drugs that reduce sexual drive, has resulted in calls for their use in cases involving sexual offenders. One drug company, for example, advertised in the *British Journal of Psychiatry* that its product 'has proven to be of value in treating men who have been guilty of sexual offences such as exhibitionism; paedophilia; indecent assault; rape; incest; voyeurism; bestiality and paederasty'. In addition, the company pointed out that other types of 'aberrant' sexual behaviours, even those not considered illegal, may also be 'controlled', including 'homosexual activities; fetishism; transvestism; compulsive masturbation; and sexual aggression in senile or mentally defective hospital patients'. In the United States, prisoners serving jail sentences for rape have gone to court demanding that they be treated with similar agents.[58] Other technological developments, those of a surgical type, have made still other 'treatment' options available, with individuals and their doctors rushing in to reclassify the aberration or malady in medical terms that have been tailored to fit the new treatments — and the increasing demands.

The danger here is that, despite their humanitarian goal, it is not at all clear that such reclassifications serve that end. Attributing to an exhibitionist, a rapist, or a voyeur an underlying diagnosable psychiatric condition — hypersexualism — and then treating that condition by pharmacological or surgical means is not necessarily humane, and, in fact, has not yet been proved to work. Indeed, the surgical approach to transsexuality, a darling of 1960s medical technology, has only recently been shown to be seriously questionable.[59] Certainly, it is not at all clear that such redefinitions have improved the lots of the persons redefined.

Analagous attempts at reclassification have also occurred in other areas of psychiatry, with equally questionable results for both the professionals and their newly classified patients. Young offenders, for example, have been told by courts and other authorities that they would not be punished for their drug-taking or other social trespasses if they submitted to psychiatric treatment; and psychiatrists and psychiatric hospitals sometimes have acquiesced to this process by making their practices, facilities, and diagnoses available to this population, usually in good faith and full belief. Instead of being recorded as criminals, such people have been hospitalized as sociopaths or, sometimes, as latent or mild schizophrenics, with the result that they have been labelled and treated as such, with inadvertently worse effects to the individuals than would have resulted from their original designations as deviants or criminals.

Diagnosis as exclusion and dehumanization

So far, we have examined the beauty of diagnosis as a means of accomplishing ends that in some sense reflect the universal wish to be or do good. From time to time, we all have an urge to exculpate, to reassure, and to turn deviance into illness; diagnosis does these things, does them magically and utterly, and, in turning to it, whether as lay men or as psychiatrists, we have what we think are the interests at heart of the person being diagnosed.

But the diagnostic process has a beauty that leads us well beyond the realm of generous human interest. We also use it because it helps us to do things we otherwise could not bring ourselves to do.

The roots are primitive, powerful, and universal. When we want to do unto others as we would not have them do unto ourselves, we find some way of turning them into others. We usually do that by labelling them, by excluding them from our own group, and by dehumanizing them — by defining their status as less than ours and, therefore, less human.

Stalin knew that, and did it on a national scale when he wanted to turn popular opinion against those who disagreed with him. Krushchev, in his 1956 Twentieth Party Congress speech,[60] described the process well. Stalin, he said,

originated the concept of 'enemy of the people'. This term automatically rendered it unnecessary that the ideological errors of a man or men engaged in a controversy be proven; this term made possible the usage of the most cruel repression, violating all

norms of revolutionary legality, against anyone who in any way disagreed with Stalin
. . . [p. 566].

Stalin understood that a person labelled 'an enemy of the people'
would be seen by a wary and besieged population as a dangerous
outsider who must be excluded from Soviet society. So seen, the
outsider would be suddenly transformed into someone who is different, not truly a member of society, not truly a man — and, therefore,
into someone who could and should be imprisoned, shot, or otherwise
silenced without the sympathy that ordinarily would be accorded a
non-labelled fellow comrade.†

Even more graphic examples of the dehumanizing power of labelling, and the universal tendency to use it, can be drawn from the
context of war. In the Second World War, both sides had ways of
turning each other into objects whose deaths would be less than
tragic, somehow almost deserved. In the Second World War, the
Nazis pushed this stratagem to its limits, using labelling to transform
Jews, gypsies, homosexuals, and sometimes Slavs into vermin whose
extermination would be a blessing and should certainly occasion no
discomfort in the heart of a good Aryan.

And even in Vietnam the martial advantages of labelling, exclusion, and dehumanization revealed themselves. American soldiers
sent there were given the task of fighting an enemy that was often
indistinguishable from the general population. In Vietnam, any man,
any woman, and any child was potentially lethal. And so they all
became the enemy; one had to be ready to kill them. And, in order to
be able to do that, one had to see them as not being in the same class
as oneself. One called them 'dinks' and 'gooks'; one saw them as
'nothing but whores or thieves' [p.194].[62] These terms reflected
perceptual changes that enabled American soldiers to transform the
Vietnamese population into objects that could be annihilated without
the danger of annihilating oneself through guilt. The power of this
process was illustrated by a soldier who had to move corpses found
after a battle. American corpses were bodies, while Vietnamese
corpses felt, to him, like 'potato sacks'. In carrying them, he told an

---

† In her remarkable memoir of her life with Osip Mandelstam, *Hope against hope*,[61] Nadezhda
Mandelstam, the poet's widow, locates the origin of the Soviet tendency to distinguish between
'one of us' and 'not one of us' (the second group commonly being known as 'alien elements') in
Lenin himself. Lenin, she points out, established that distinction during the Civil War with his
'Who whom', the phrase he used to summarize the difference between the Bolsheviks and their
enemies (p. 28). In the same memoir she also shows how widespread was the tendency under
Stalin, even among the intelligentsia, to exclude and dehumanize those officially cast out. Thus,
when an acquaintance would be arrested on unknown and usually arbitrary charges, people
would tell each other — probably to reassure themselves that they would not be next — that 'he
isn't one of us'. It was, for many, necessary 'to avoid those stricken by the plague' (p. 26).

interviewing psychiatrist, Robert Jay Lifton, he 'didn't feel a thing' [p. 192].[62]

Diagnosis is perfectly suited to label, exclude, and dehumanize in both its informal and formal usages. Informally, the terms 'crazy', 'mad', and even 'schizophrenic' often serve as exclusionary labels that are used in everyday language to identify others who are annoying, discomfiting, and different. Formally applied — that is, by psychiatrists — diagnoses can make a person into someone who seems wholly other and who *requires* exclusion. Depending on the severity of the diagnosis, he may be seen by others as disordered, polluted, and dangerous. In short, a diagnosis can turn him into another kind of human being, perhaps less than human, certainly not a fellow human being; and he not only has a need to be put away — he deserves to be put away. Such diagnostic transformation can serve the needs of psychiatric systems under certain conditions in exactly the same way that it can serve the needs of family and social systems when their peace and tranquility are disturbed by the symptoms of the mentally ill.

Psychiatric systems can benefit from the process of diagnostic exclusion and dehumanization because those systems subject individuals to experiences and conditions that would be difficult to impose without the advantages that such diagnostic transformation affords. Psychiatric hospitals may be unpleasant places; and some psychiatric techniques, such as the use of drugs, electric shock, restraints, and confinement to seclusion rooms, may be experienced by patients as highly noxious. The psychiatrist knows that in hospitalizing a patient he may be, in the service of treatment, also causing him a certain degree of harm. The awareness of possible harm is compounded if the patient is an involuntary one, if the most invasive or liberty-depriving techniques are used, and if the patient responds to those conditions and techniques with the insistence that he is not sick and with a plea that they should be altered or stopped and that he should be released. At such times, the psychiatrist must harden his heart. And what enables him to do this is, among other things, the diagnosis. With it, he can see the person as a patient, one whose pleas are not simple, soulful, human importunings but rather the routine and expected reactions of ill patients to the illnesses that have possessed them and to the treatments to which they have been subjected. With such a diagnosis, the psychiatrist can proceed and not have to see himself as a violator of human freedom and dignity. In fact, he can see himself as helping, through hospitalization and the use of such interventions, to transform a psychiatric case back into a human being, back into someone like himself: he can, in good conscience, allow himself to do unto the patient that which he would not have others do unto himself.

The advantage to the psychiatrist of diagnostic dehumanization is only a special instance of that advantage in everyday life. After all, psychiatric patients carry on the largest portions of their lives outside the psychiatric system and place non-psychiatrists in similar, even more vexing dilemmas. The behaviour of such patients may be extremely distressing to friends, neighbours, and relatives, who, in turn, seek help for themselves by persuading the individual to consult mental health authorities, by coercing him to do so in some way, or by enlisting others, such as the police, to carry out such coercion. Sometimes, having been successful, these friends, neighbours or relatives may recognize that their wish to be rid of the individual, and their actions to accomplish that end, are in part in the service of their own comfort; and, realizing the unpleasantness that may result to the patient because of their actions, they may feel some shame. That shame, however, can be dissipated if they can remind themselves that the person is, in fact, mentally ill, that his objectionable behaviour is caused not by him but by a disease, and that their purpose in bringing him to the attention of mental health authorities is related not to their own needs but to the needs of a person temporarily beset by a disease: a disease that has obscured his usual humanity and that makes it necessary and virtuous to do to him what, if done to others, would represent cruelty or a transgression of civil liberties, but what, in his case, represents only kindness, concern, and the desire to restore him to the normal community of man.

Of course, people do become psychotic, and do, in their psychoses, sometimes require intervention that we would not want done to ourselves. What is important here, though, is the capacity of diagnosis to enable people who respect and even love such individuals to suspend their ordinary tendency to honour their stated wishes — to reverse, that is, the usual meaning of compassion, so that what the person wants is precisely the opposite of what he is given. If diagnosis enables us to do that in such cases, then it has a great capacity to do it in other cases as well, ones that involve no respect or love. For example, in cases of marginal illness, when people annoy others by their socially unacceptable behaviour, it may become too easy to enlist the aid of diagnosis in response, so that, say, civil authorities can turn to the psychiatric system in the hope that it will aid them in removing the disturbance and in making them feel, through the issuance of a diagnosis, that they had been right in making that turn; and it may become too easy for those in the psychiatric system to acquiesce and issue a diagnosis — even when such a diagnosis may be somewhat doubtful, and even when the consequences may be unpleasant — on the basis of the self-deceptive rationale that a diagnosed person is not quite a person and probably needs to undergo this kind of treatment, at least until it has its effect, exorcises the disease, and brings him back to a fully human state.

Diagnosis as self-confirming hypothesis

Perhaps the most remarkable property of diagnosis, and sometimes, for the diagnosed patient, the most enraging, is its capacity for inevitable self-confirmation. That property is used in everyday life by persons who call others 'crazy' or 'weird': once they do so, everything that the receivers of such lay diagnoses do can be attributed to, and dismissed as a result of, those or similar epithets. In fact, everything they do subsequently can become a proof that the original assessment was correct.

This 'catch-22' quality of pathological naming functions with even greater efficiency and inevitability within psychiatry itself. An actual clinical case can illustrate this well. The chief psychiatrist at a medical school teaching hospital was asked to see a 65-year-old woman by the woman's son, a medical school faculty member, and by her husband, a physician in a nearby community. The woman, they explained, had become negative at home, disagreeable, more insistent than she previously had been about her views, and, in other ways as well, had undergone changes in personality. The chief psychiatrist, who tended to interpret behaviour and its aberrations as direct products of brain functioning or malfunctioning, concluded that, in the case of this woman, a malfunctioning had in fact taken place. He diagnosed an organic brain syndrome, one caused, probably, by the aging process, and admitted her to the hospital to confirm the diagnosis.

The trainee psychiatrist assigned to the case, however, could find no objective evidence of such malfunctioning. Meanwhile, the patient — finding herself in the strange circumstances of a therapeutic community, in which staff and patients were expected to aid each other in recognizing illness and in promoting health — became extremely distressed. She repeatedly insisted, to all who would hear, and in every community or group meeting, that she was not ill and should not be a patient. The response she received was consistent: she would certainly not have been admitted to the hospital had she not been ill, and the only way for her to achieve health was to acknowledge her illness. At first, she tried quietly to accept the ward routine in the hope that she would be discharged rapidly. When this failed, she complained loudly, angrily, and at length. The senior medical and nursing staff, observing her behaviour, cited it to the trainee psychiatrist as a 'catastrophic reaction' so typical of persons with her diagnosis who are challenged by tasks they can no longer master. Given fluphenazine, she quieted; and the drug-induced response was then cited as an improvement that further demonstrated the validity of the original diagnosis.

Of course, the diagnosis may indeed have been correct: the trainee psychiatrist may have been wrong and the chief right. But, given the authority structure of the ward, and the nature and effects of diagnoses, particularly those issued in such settings, it became almost inevitable that the chief's clinical pronouncement would confirm itself no matter what occurred. In the absence of objective, physically-based criteria, many psychiatric diagnoses are capable of such self-confirmation, whether they derive from a psychoanalytic orientation or, as in this case, an organic one. Indeed, even in this case, in which a diagnosis was issued that is more susceptible to physical confirmation than most, the lack of such confirmation failed to derail the inevitable train of events. In such a climate, it becomes simply too easy to diagnose: one is rarely proved wrong, and the penchant for rapid assessment, valued so highly in general medical settings (especially academic ones) as an emblem of knowledge and expertise, has few means of objective checks in the psychiatric arena, and can result in too cavalier an issuance of diagnoses — diagnoses that, because they may be wrong, and because they have so pronounced a tendency to persist, can be highly distressing and, ultimately, damaging. Of course, this dilemma is made worse still under circumstances in which the diagnoses are issued not in the spirit of academic showmanship, or as an expression of ideological bias, but, rather, as a result of hasty or uncaring judgements. But whatever the spirit, the results to the patient are the same.

Diagnosis as discreditation and punishment

And, finally, the ultimate function of diagnosis in everyday life, classical in every respect, is as universal as the species and as old as man: diagnosis as discreditation, the attribution of a person's views, politics, actions, or conclusions to a mind gone sick: diagnosis as a weapon.

We see it everywhere. In the Middle East, for example, the Shah, before losing power, identified Libya's Colonel Qadaffi as a 'crazy fellow'.[63] In turn, Ahmed Zaki Yamani, the Saudi oil minister, described the Shah as 'highly unstable mentally'.[64] Egypt's President Sadat diagnosed Ayatollah Ruhollah Khomeini 'a lunatic',[65] a compliment the ayatollah then passed on to President Carter.[66] In Israel, the Labour opposition had similar views about Prime Minister Begin,[67] while, on the West Bank, Ali Jabari, the Palestinian mayor of Hebron, campaigned to have the leaders ot the PLO locked up in insane asylums.[68]

And elsewhere, too, and at other times. Thus Lenin, in 1919, to

Gorky: 'all of your impressions are totally sick . . . your nerves have obviously broken down . . . Just as your conversation, your letter is the sum total of sick impressions carrying you to sick conclusions. This is all a pure sick psyche . . . It is clear that you have worked yourself up into sickness . . .'[69] The Soviet press on the dissident physicist Sakharov: 'pathological individualism'. A West German political leader on the Carter administration's reported plan to produce a neutron bomb: 'a symbol of mental perversion'.[71] And Eldridge Cleaver's former friends on Eldridge Cleaver, after learning of his shift from black radical militant to capitalist religious conservative: 'schizophrenic'.[72]

Within psychiatry, diagnosis has also surfaced as a weapon. In 1964, some American psychiatrists diagnosed a presidential candidate with whose views many of them disagreed, Barry Goldwater, as mentally ill. A decade earlier, members of the profession, supporting the Alger Hiss defence, diagnosed Hiss's accuser, Whittaker Chambers, a psychopath without ever having examined him. And the CIA, understanding the power of diagnosis to discredit, made plans in 1954 to use it in its covert operations.[73] Its hope was to administer LSD to those it wished to make mad — or, more to the point, to those it wished to be diagnosed by others as mad. Under the influence of the drug, these enemies of the United States would seem psychotic, with the result, presumably, that their own people, having come to that diagnostic conclusion, would reject or depose them.

But the most flagrant setting for the raw use of psychiatry to discredit — and, indeed, to intimidate and punish — is probably Russia (see Chapter 18). During the past decade, probably several hundred dissidents have been arrested for political trespasses, sent to psychiatrists, found mentally ill, and committed for involuntary stays at psychiatric hospitals for the criminally insane.[74-83] Of these, a number have been truly ill.[84] A number almost surely have not.[85] To the extent that they have not, and to the extent that the diagnoses in those cases were rendered at the direct or indirect request of governmental authorities, these actions represent the worst expression of psychiatric abuse. The motivations behind the misdiagnoses are probably mixed, and in many cases they were probably issued in full if misguided sincerity;[84,86] at least some may have resulted from, or may have been made possible by, the availability or influence of the Moscow School's overly broad and overly inclusive criteria for the diagnosis of schizophrenia. But the fact that those misdiagnoses *could* be issued, and the fact that psychiatrists were asked to examine these dissidents in the first place, also has something to do with the beauty of diagnosis in all its array — not only as a means to discredit, and not only as a means to punish, but also as a way of dehumanize, to transform social deviance into medical illness, to reassure, and to explain.

Comment

If we turn to diagnosis because of its non-medical beauty we are at risk, whether we are laymen or psychiatrists, for being injured by that beauty. For years people have been coming to psychiatrists to circumvent the law: they have sought diagnoses to help them get abortions or to help them evade the military draft. Psychiatrists often saw little danger from such humanitarian deeds, and responded to the requests willingly. But the danger was there, and we need only look to Russia to appreciate its extreme potential. Things went awry in that country because a powerful tool was just too attractive and too capable of misuse to be protected from it; the fear of governmental power was too great, the respect for the law too weak, the diagnostic scheme too broad and the opportunities for self-deception on the part of both ordinary bureaucrats and well-trained psychiatrists too available. But the same attraction to diagnosis, the same appreciation of its multiple beauties, exists in the West, too; and though our laws so far have protected us from succumbing to a similar fate, the law itself has a certain weakness for diagnosis, tends to be partial to its charms, and is exquisitely susceptible to its inroads. Eventually psychiatrists will have to understand that diagnosis plays a poweful, varied, and unrecognized role in the lives of all people; that that role is equally powerful and no less varied and unrecognized in the lives of psychiatrists; and that all abuses of diagnoses — and, ultimately, all abuses of psychiatry — are a psychiatric problem in considerable measure because they are a human problem, and probably stem less from the corruption of the profession than from the needs and vulnerabilities of us all.

Naturally, psychiatrists must be expected not to misdiagnose knowingly. But in order to avert non-purposeful misdiagnoses, psychiatrists must come to appreciate the limitations of the diagnostic process itself, the capacity of diagnostic theories and schools to influence and shape psychiatric perceptions of behaviour, and the inherent beauties of diagnosis that make it so enticing to use that only the most stringent efforts on the part of the psychiatrist, and the most serious attention on the part of those who teach and train him, will keep him from yielding unknowingly to those beauties — indeed, will keep him from failing to recognize that they even exist.

References

1. BALINT, M.: *The doctor, his patient, and the illness.* New York, International Universities Press, 1957.
2. SCHEFF, T.: *Being mentally ill: a sociological theory.* Chicago, Aldine, 1966.
3. LEVENE, H. I.: Acute schizophrenia: clinical effects of the labelling process. *Archives of General Psychiatry* 25:215–22, 1971.
4. MÜLLER-HEGEMANN, D.: Psychotherapy in the German Democratic Republic, in *Psychiatry in the communist world.* Ed. Kiev, A. New York, Science House, 1968, pp. 51–70.
5. MEHLMAN, P.: The reliability of psychiatric diagnoses. *Journal of Abnormal and Social Psychology* 47:577–8, 1952.
6. OVERALL, J. E. and HOLLISTER, L. E.: Comparative evaluation of research diagnostic criteria for schizophrenia. *Archives of General Psychiatry* 36:1198–1205, 1979.
7. CANTWELL, D. P., RUSSELL, A. T., MATTISON, R. *et al*: A comparison of DSM-II and DSM-III in the diagnosis of childhood psychiatric disorders. I. Agreement with expected diagnosis. *Archives of General Psychiatry* 36:1208–13, 1979.
8. BABIGIAN, H. M., GARDNER, E. A., MILES, H. C., *et al*: Diagnostic consistency and change in a follow-up study of 1,215 patients. *American Journal of Psychiatry* 121:895–901, 1965.
9. PASAMANICK, B., DINITZ, S., and LEFTON, L.: Psychiatric orientation in relation to diagnosis and treatment. *American Journal of Psychiatry* 116:127–32, 1959.
10. KATZ, M. M., COLE, J. O., and LOWERY, H. A.: Studies of the diagnostic process: the influence of symptom perception, past experience, and ethnic background on diagnostic decisions. *American Journal of Psychiatry* 125:937–47, 1969.
11. TEMERLIN, M. K.: Diagnostic bias in community mental health. *Community Mental Health Journal* 6:110–17, 1970.
12. PLUTCHIK, R., CONTE, H., and LANDAU, H.: A comparison of symptom evaluations by psychiatrists and social workers. *Hospital and Community Psychiatry* 23:13-14, 1972.
13. JASPERS, K.: Eifersuchtswahn: ein Beitrag zur Frage 'Entwicklung einer Persönlichkeit oder Prozess. *Zeitschrift für Gesamte Neurologie and Psychiatrie* 1:567,1910.
14. FISH, F.: *Schizophrenia.* Bristol, John Wright and Sons, 1962.
15. ASTRUP, C. and ODEGARD, O.: Continued experiments in psychiatric diagnosis. *Acta psychiatrica scandinavica* 46:180–212, 1970.
16. LANGFELDT, G.: Diagnosis and prognosis of schizophrenia. *Proceedings of the Royal Society of Medicine* 53:1047–52,1960.
17. ZIGLER, E. and PHILLIPS, L.: Psychiatric diagnosis and symptomatology. *Journal of Abnormal and Social Psychology* 63:69–75, 1961.
18. RÜMKE, H. C.: Signification de la phenomenologie dans l'étude clinique des délirants. *Psychopathologie Générale* 1:125, 1950
19. ASTRACHAN, B. M., HARROW, M., ADLER, D., *et al*: A checklist for the diagnosis of schizophrenia. *British Journal of Psychiatry* 121:529–39, 1972
20. SNEZHNEVSKY, A. V. and VARTANYAN, M.: The forms of schizophrenia and their biological correlates, in *Biochemistry, schizophrenia, and affective illness.* Ed. Himwich, H. E. Baltimore, William and Wilkins, 1970, pp. 1–28.
21. SNEZHNEVSKY, A. V.: Symptom, syndrome, disease: a clinical method in psychiatry, in *The world biennial of psychiatry and psychotherapy.* Ed. Arieti, S. Vol. 1, 1971, pp. 151–64.

22. SNEZHNEVSKY, A. V.: The symptomatology, clinical forms and nosology of schizophrenia, in *Modern perspectives in world psychiatry*. Ed. Howells, J. G. New York, Brunner/Mazel, 1971, pp. 423–47.
23. NADZHAROV, R. A.: Course forms, in *Schizophrenia*. Ed. Snezhnevsky A. V. Moscow, Meditsina, 1972, pp. 16–76.
24. ROLLINS, N.: *Child psychiatry in the Soviet Union*. Cambridge, Mass. Harvard University Press, 1972.
25. HITE, C.: Bridging the US–Soviet psychiatric gap. *Psychiatric News*, **9**(pt 1); 6–17, **19**(pt 2): 30–1, 40, 1974.
26. HOLLAND, J. and SHAKHMATOVA-PAVLOVA, I. V.: Concept and classification of schizophrenia in the Soviet Union. Unpublished, 1974.
27. HOLLAND, J.: Draft of pilot study of joint classification of schizophrenia, Psychiatric Research Institute USSR/Academy of Medical Sciences and NIMH/USA. Unpublished, 1975.
28. HOLLAND, J.: 'State' hospitals in the USSR: a model of governmental psychiatric care, in *Future roles of state hospitals*. Ed. Zusman, J., and Bertsen B. Toronto: Lexington Books (D. C. Heath), 1977, pp. 373–85.
29. HOLLAND, J.: Schizophrenia in the Soviet Union, in *Annual Review of Research in Schizophrenia*. Ed. Cancro R. New York, 1977.
30. World Health Organization. Report of the International Pilot Study of Schizophrenia. Geneva, WHO, 1973, Vol. 1.
31. REICH, W.: The spectrum concept of schizophrenia: problems for diagnostic practice. *Archives of General Psychiatry* **32**:489–98, 1975.
32. REICH, W.: Kazanetz, schizophrenia and Soviet psychiatry, *Archives of General Psychiatry* **36**:1029–30, 1979.
33. ROSENTHAL, D.: *The Genain quadruplets*. New York, Basic Books, 1963.
34. KETY, S. S., ROSENTHAL, D., WENDER, P. H., et al: The types and prevalence of mental illness in the biological adoptive families of adopted schizophrenics, in *The transmission of schizophrenia*. Ed. Rosenthal, D. and Kety, S. S. London, Pergamon Press, 1968, pp. 345–62.
35. ROSENTHAL, D., WENDER, P. H., KETY, S. S., et al: Schizophrenic's offspring reared in adoptive homes, in *The transmission of schizophrenia*. Ed. Kety, S. S., Rosenthal, D., and Wender, P. H. Oxford, Pergamon Press, 1968, pp. 377–91.
36. ROSENTHAL, D., WENDER, P. H., KETY, S. S., et al: The adopted away offspring of schizophrenics. *American Journal of Psychiatry* **128**:302–6, 1971.
37. WENDER, P. H., ROSENTHAL, D, KETY, S. S., et al: Crossfostering: research strategy for clarifying the role of genetic and experimental factors in the etiology of schizophrenia. *Archives of General Psychiatry* **30**:121–8, 1974.
38. KETY, S. S., ROSENTHAL, D., WENDER, P. H., et al: Mental illness in the biological and adoptive families of adopted individuals who have become schizophrenic: a preliminary report based upon psychiatric interviews, in *Genetic Research in Psychiatry*. Ed. Fieve, R., Rosenthal, D., and Brill, H. Baltimore, The Johns Hopkins University Press, 1975, pp. 147–65.
39. FOWLER, R. C., TSUANG, M. T., CADORET, R. J. et al: Non-psychotic disorders in the families of process schizophrenics. *Acta Psychiatrica Scandinavica* **51**:153–60, 1975.
40. REICH, W.: The schizophrenia spectrum: a genetic concept. *Journal of Nervous and Mental Diseases* **162**:3–12, 1976.
41. RIEDER, R. O.: The schizophrenia spectrum. Presented at the 131st Annual Meeting of the American Psychiatric Association, May 8–12, 1978.
42. KETY, S. S., ROSENTHAL, D., WENDER, P. H., et al: The biologic and adoptive families of adopted individuals who became schizophrenic: prevalence of mental

illness and other characteristics, in *The nature of schizophrenia*. Ed. Wynne, L. C., Cromwell, R. L., and Matthysse, S. Wiley, New York, 1978, pp. 25–37.

43. KETY, S. S., WENDER, P. H., and ROSENTHAL, D.: Genetic relationships within the schizophrenia spectrum: evidence from adoption studies, in *Critical issues in psychiatric diagnosis*. Ed. Spitzer R. L. and Klein D. F., Raven Press, New York, 1978, pp. 213–23.

44. REICH, W.: The diagnosis of everyday life. *Harper's Magazine*, February, 1980.

45. REICH, W.: Brianwashing, psychiatry and the law. *The New York Times*, 29 May, 1976.

46. REICH, W.: Brainwashing, psychiatry and the law. *Psychiatry*, **39**:400–3, 1976.

47. SINCLAIR, W.: After the upheaval: who's running what? *The Washington Post*, 21 July, 1979.

48. *The Washington Post*, Weicker suggests Carter not run. 22 July, 1979.

49. QUINN, S.: Rosalynn's journey. *The Washington Post*, 25 July, 1979.

50. SCHRAM, M.: The troubled times of a different Billy Carter. *The Washington Post*, 25 February, 1979.

51. GUP, T.: Brooding replaces clowning. *The Washington Post, 25 February, 1979*.

52. EVANS, R. and NOVAK, R.: Brother Billy: political blunders. *The Washington Post*, 2 March, 1979.

53. *Newsweek*, The stewardess and the 'witch', 30 April 1979.

54. BERRY J. D., and EGAN, J.: Alleged embezzling, maneuvering in moviedom. *The Washington Post*, 25 December, 1977.

55. MITGANG, H.: Greene calls profile of him in New Yorker inaccurate. *The New York Times*, 12 May, 1979.

56. BRODY, J. E.: Inquiry at cancer centre finds fraud in research. *The New York Times*, 25 May, 1974.

57. BRODY, J. E.: Scientist denies cancer research fraud. *The New York Times*, 29 May, 1974.

58. COLEN, D.: Drug for sex offenders called success. *The Washington Post*, 5 December, 1975.

59. MYER, J. K. and RETER, D. J.: Sex reassignment: follow-up. *Archives of General Psychiatry* **36**:1010–15, 1979.

60. KHRUSCHCHEV, N.: *Khrushchev remembers*. Translated and edited by Strobe Talbott. Boston, Little, Brown, 1970.

61. MANDELSTAM, N.: *Hope against hope*. New York, Atheneum, 1970.

62. LIFTON, R. J.: *Home from the war*. New York, Simon and Schuster, 1973.

63. *The New York Times*, Libya helping terrorists with arms and training, 16 July, 1976.

64. ANDERSON, J., and WHITTEN, L.: Saudis suspect an Iran–U.S. plot. *The Washington Post*, 17 September, 1976.

65. *The New York Times*, 10 November, 1979.

66. KHOMEINI, R.: The world is not on your side. *The Washington Post*, 22 November, 1979.

67. FARRELL, W.: The furor surrounding Begin: he fights harder and doesn't budge. *The New York Times*, 25 July, 1978.

68. RANDAL, J. C.: Role in U.N. session builds confidence among Palestinians. *The Washington Post*, 12 January, 1979.

69. LENIN, V. I.: *Sochineniya* [Works], 4th edn. Moscow State Political Literature Publishing House, 1951–67. Letter to Gorky of 31 July, 1919. Quoted in Lev Navrozov, *The education of Lev Navrozov*. New York, Harper's Magazine Press, 1975, p. 164.

70. *The Washington Post*, Mrs. Sakharov flies home, 24 November, 1977.

71. GETLER, M.: Bonn party aide calls U.S. bomb a "perversion." *The Washington Post*, 18 July, 1977.
72. ALLMAN, T. D.: The 'rebirth' of Eldridge Cleaver. *The New York Times Magazine*, 16 January, 1977.
73. HORROCK, N. M.: Drug tested by C.I.A. on Mental Patients. *New York Times*, 3 August, 1977.
74. Committee on the Judiciary. Abuse of Psychiatry for Political Repression in the Soviet Union. Hearing before the Subcommittee to Investigate the Administration of the Internal Security Act and Other Internal Security Laws of the Committee on the Judiciary, United States Senate, Ninety-Second Congress, Second Session. Washington, DC., US Government Printing Office, 26 December, 1972.
75. STONE, I. F.: Betrayal by psychiatry. *The New York Review of Books*, 10 February, 1972, pp. 7–14.
76. CHODOFF, P.: Involuntary hospitalization of political dissenters in the Soviet Union. *Psychiatric Opinion*, **11**:5–19, 1974.
77. Amnesty International: *Prisoners of conscience in the USSR: their treatment and conditions.* London, Amnesty International Publications, 1975.
78. GRIGORENKO, P.: *The Grigorenko papers: writings by General P. G. Grigorenko and documents on his case.* London, C. Hurst; Boulder, Colorado, Westview Press, 1976.
79. YEO, C.: The abuse of psychiatry in the U.S.S.R.: the evidence. *Index on censorship*, Vol. 4, No. 2 (Summer 1975).
80. BLOCH, S. and REDDAWAY, P.: *Psychiatric terror.* New York, Basic Books, 1977.
81. LADER, M.: *Psychiatry on trial.* Harmondsworth, Penguin Books, 1977.
82. PLYUSHCH, L.: *History's carnival.* With a contribution by Tatyana Plyushch. Ed. and trans. Marco Carynnyk. New York, Harcourt Brace Jovanovich, 1979.
83. BUKOVSKY, V.: *To build a castle: my life as a dissenter.* Trans. Michael Scammell. New York, Viking Press, 1979.
84. REICH, W.: Diagnosing Soviet dissidents. *Harper's Magazine*, August, 1978, pp. 31–7.
85. REICH, W.: Grigorenko gets a second opinion. *The New York Times Magazine*, 13 May, 1979.
86. REICH, W.: Soviet psychiatry on trial. *Commentary*, January, 1978, pp. 40–8.

6

Ethical aspects of psychotherapy

Toksoz Karasu

IT has recently been suggested that we have evolved from an 'Age of Anxiety' to an 'Age of Ethical Crises'.[1] Progressive loss of faith in traditional institutions and the erosion of authority are now being met with increasing challenge of existing standards set by the 'establishment', and widespread concern for the retrieval of human values and rights. The main cultural background events include (a) the advances and perils of rapid technological innovation which have enormously expanded the ability to modify the behaviour of man, and simultaneously created critical dilemmas with regard to behaviour control and influence; and (b) pervasive currents of sociocultural change or the so-called 'social egalitarian revolution',[2] marked by increasing democratization of power relations across all segments of society, — male to female, young to old, bureaucrat to citizen, provider to consumer, and more pertinent for our purposes here — doctor to patient.

This climate of anti-establishment, anti-professional, and anti-rational sentiment has had direct implications for the field of psychiatry including the roles and responsibilities of the psychotherapist. Growing scepticism about the sanctity of scientific, medical, and psychiatric domains now means that these highly endowed fields can no longer be considered above reproach or exempt from active moral review. The psychotherapist, once left relatively undisturbed in the private confines of his office, has now been besieged 'from within'[3] and 'from without'.[4] The 'siege from within' reflects psychiatry's own members who extol widely different models and criteria of mental illness and its treatment, which are confusing and divisive to the field and its future; the 'siege from without' reflects the public confusion regarding the functions, procedures, and powers of the psychotherapist. For both patient and profession, there has occurred an increasing expectation and demand for accountability: that the patient be granted health care as a right, with greater participation in determining and assessing his treatment; and that the therapist, responding to rising social and political pressure (e.g. in the US the prospect of a national health service), reviews the nature of his practices and their effects upon his patients. The profession's current failure to stave off challenge and criticism has been attributed to

several compounding factors, including a fundamental disappointment with the limitations of science and reason in answering the
problems of mankind; an anti-élitism which aims to mitigate the
power of professionals as symbolic representations of the inequitable
distribution of resources in society; and most potently in the moral
context *per se*, the fear of overgeneralization of professional authority
from scientific to ethical areas.[5]

The interface between science and ethics

Indeed, the relationship of science to ethics in psychotherapy may be
considered the conceptual heart-of-the-matter. Ethics has been
defined as 'the system or code of morality of a particular person,
religion, group or profession' (morals as 'relating to, dealing with, or
capable of making the distinction between right and wrong in
conduct'); science (which psychotherapy presumes to be) defined as
'a branch of knowledge or study concerned with establishing or
systemizing facts).[6] Theoretically, science and ethics have been
conceived as two distinct and separate entities, almost antithetical, —
science as 'descriptive' and ethics as 'prescriptive'; science relying on
'validation', ethics on 'judgement'; and science concerned solely with
'what is' whereas ethics addresses 'what ought to be'.[7] But the lines
become less sharply drawn when the complexities of social reality are
considered, as when the psychotherapist is obliged to act as a 'double-
agent' to accommodate conflicts of interest between not only patient
and therapist, but also involving third parties to whom the therapist
holds allegiance (e.g. family members, school, hospital, military);[8,9]
and as the therapist straddles the ambiguous line between the science
and art of psychotherapy, dual attitudes of his identity which differ
both in degree and quality.[10] There is still a question whether
psychotherapy is a science at all, in that it deals with hermeneutics
rather than explanation, is humanistic rather than mechanistic, seeks
private rather than public knowledge, — in all, is not a science but a
body of knowledge with a special status, which frees it from obligations that other sciences have.[11]

   In addition, as London[12] has pointed out, while the distinction
between the principles of science and those of ethics may more readily
hold for the researcher inside his laboratory, it is less applicable to the
clinician in his daily practice. Lifton[13] especially highlighted this
point in describing his work with Vietnam veterans, which required
him to combine sufficient detachment to enable him to make
psychological evaluations, with involvement that expressed his own
personal commitment and moral passion (i.e. he had previously taken
an active anti-war position). He aptly concluded, 'I believe that we

(therapists) always function within this *dialectic between ethical involvement and intellectual rigour*' (p. 386).[13] He further recommended that
'bringing our advocacy "out front" and articulating it makes us more,
rather than less, scientific. Indeed, our scientific accuracy is likely to
suffer when we hide our ethical beliefs behind the claims of neutrality
and that we are nothing but "neutral screens"' (p. 386).

With the above in mind, it is inevitable that in psychotherapy the
boundaries between science and ethics are blurred. Indeed, there has
been a greater recognition of the inevitable constraints upon the
presumed purity of objective treatment by the pulls of subjective
commitment (unconscious if not conscious). More specifically, the
idyllic notion of psychotherapy and the psychotherapist as 'value-free'
is now widely accepted as a fallacy.[14] This is supported by current
research which has demonstrated many contradictions in expressed
belief and reported practices in psychotherapy.[15] One could
hypothesize the existence of a 'two-tier' system, — one, the ideal or
correct (i.e. value-free, non-suggestive); the other, the practical or
applied view (i.e. includes direct suggestion, encouragement of
specific goals) which interferes with a value-free frame of reference. In
brief, the application of psychotherapy represents neither pure science
nor pure ethics, but a branch of the healing profession which resides
somewhere in between. Therefore, it is likely that psychotherapy will
only find its ethical place by locating a legitimate and unique area
between the two ideological extremes, — that of being an objectively
applied science, and that of representing an ideology of healthy
conduct.[16]

Concern with the interface between science and ethics is not new to
psychotherapy. Major controversies since Freud have long pivoted
upon the question of whether psychoanalysis inherently propounds
particular values, especially values which may be immoral or biased.
Some believe it does not do so.[17,18] Others point out its political and
repressive nature by virtue of its very existence, [19,20] or more
specifically, view it as an enemy of morality and religion (see
refutation,[18]) or take exception to particular biases, e.g. its favour of
certain social classes or patient types over others[21] or discrimination
against women[22] (see Therapist-patient sex and sexism, p. 107). Still
others, while accepting that psychotherapy cannot be value-free, and
even believing that in its overall goals it *should* not be,[23] see the basic
issue as whether imposition of such values is 'deliberate and avowed'
or 'unrecognized and unavowed'.[16]

In this regard, the ethical impact of psychoanalysis has occurred on
several fronts. One major front was Freud's discovery of unconscious
motivation and conflict, which posed fundamental ethical questions of
psychic determinism versus free will and responsibility. But for Freud

the doctrine of exceptionless psychic determinism did not preclude moral responsibility. As he put it: 'One must hold oneself responsible for the evil impulses of one's dreams'.[18] As for the therapist's ethical position, Freud foresaw the inevitable influence of therapist on his patient, and his unique power within the transference relationship both to cure and to be resisted. Classic here, of course, have been the devoted analytic attempts to maintain the purity of the therapeutic relationship through the technical neutrality of the therapist; and when inevitably violated, the full exploration and understanding of the therapist's countertransference. In addition, a legacy of analytic techniques are said to necessarily preclude the therapist's assumption of roles, or his conscious manipulation and control of the patient because this is antithetical to the development of insight.[24] Certainly Freud held an overriding ethical ideal about the conduct of psychotherapy when he wrote: 'One must not forget that the relationship between analyst and patient is based on a love of truth, that is, acknowledgment of reality, and that it precludes any kind of sham or deceit' (p. 248).[25]

General ethical issues in psychotherapy

The following section on 'general' ethical issues in psychotherapy refers to those which are global and pervasive to its goals and to the therapist–patient relationship. Unfortunately, they often involve implicit and ubiquitous values, which, because of their complex, covert, and often intangible nature, have been least amenable to recognition and discussion, no less legislation.

The goals of psychotherapy

The principles of medical ethics of the American Medical Association has set down standards of practice for physicians.[26] Although 'psychiatrists are assumed to have the same goals as all physicians,' these principles have recently been revised 'with annotations especially applicable to psychiatry'.[27] The rationale was that 'there are special ethical problems in psychiatric practice that differ in coloring and degree from ethical problems in other branches of medical practice'. The format of these annotations meant no alterations in the original AMA standards; only additional qualifying statements were made.

Firstly, it may be pointed out that Section 3 of the AMA principles was the only one not annotated for psychiatry. It states that the physician (and therefore the psychiatrist equally) 'should practise a method of healing founded on a scientific basis; and he should not voluntarily associate with anyone who violates this principle' (p. 1061).[27] Further, the psychiatrist in particular is advised that 'he should neither lend endorsement of the psychiatric speciality nor refer patients to persons, groups, or treatment programs with which he is not familiar, especially if their work is based only on dogma and authority and not on scientific validation and replication' (p. 1062).[27]

Fisher and Greenberg's recent book[28] on *The scientific credibility of Freud's theories and therapy* certainly suggests that this question, despite extensive exploration, has not been decisively settled in the minds of psychiatrists themselves (though their hearts may tell them otherwise). Moreover, the proliferation of well over one hundred supposed schools of psychotherapy,[29] each presumably with its own theory of mental illness and health, therapeutic agents, overall goals, and specific practices,[30] reflects the massive nature of investigating therapeutic efficacy and the complexity of establishing 'scientific' guidelines. Given the stunning diversity of therapeutic forms now being offered to potential patients, how does one ethically equate the goals, practices, and effectiveness of a 'screaming cure' (Janov's Primal Therapy), a 'reasoning cure' (Ellis's Rational Therapy), a 'realism cure' (Glasser's Reality Therapy), a 'decision cure' (Greenwald's Direct Decision Therapy), an 'orgasm cure' (Reich's Orgone Therapy), a 'meaning cure' (Frankl's Logotherapy), and a 'profound-rest cure' (Transcendental Meditation)? Slavson,[31] for example, in assessing 'feeling therapy, nude therapy, marathon therapy, and other new remedies of the ailing psyche,' concluded that 'these activities [are] untested, theoretically weak, and potentially very dangerous . . .'; more specifically that 'latent or borderline psychotics with tenuous ego controls and defenses may, under the stress of such groups and the complete giving up of defenses, jump the barrier between sanity and insanity'. But the data on the efficacy of these practices are not yet available. Does the psychotherapist have an ethical responsibility to force closure on these therapies, especially if his judgement may be premature?

Such tremendous confusion in the state-of-the-art has led to a virtual 'identity crisis' for psychiatry and the psychotherapist,[32–34] highlighted negatively in the rise of the recent anti-psychiatry movement,[35] which now makes it possible for a psychiatrist to be a psychiatrist by training, accreditation, affiliation, and status, but at the same time, an anti-psychiatrist in ideology and action. (All this under one ethical psychiatric roof.)

At this point the goals and responsibilities of the psychotherapist are so broadly and vaguely defined that it has been said that his profession is one 'without a role-specific function',[36] and that his practice runs the gamut 'from science to social revolution'.[37] Recent observers of the field are in a quandary as to whether the purpose of psychiatry (and the psychotherapist as one of its agents) is 'to diagnose, treat, and prevent a relatively defined number of (mental illnesses); . . . to make unhappy and incompetent persons happy and competent; or to tackle poverty and civil and international strife' (p. 134).[9] While these issues are not beyond the legitimate concern of psychotherapists in their aim to improve the psychological welfare of their patients, there is a question as to whether some of these goals are beyond their competence. But, at what point among these purposes is the psychiatrist no longer competent?

While broadly recognized goals include Freud's 'love and work', and variants of growth, self-realization, self-sufficiency, security, and freedom from anxiety, all of which may be noble aspirations, ethical issues are inherent in the practices which are conducted in their name. Across a spectrum of possibilities have been posed questions such as freedom to change (or not change) versus coercion, helping versus imposing the therapist's influence, and issues of 'cure' of illness versus positive growth. Thomas Szasz, probably the most prolific and vocal anti-psychiatrist, views conventional therapy by definition as 'social action, not healing,' and as 'a series of religious, rhetorical, and repressive acts'.[38] At bottom is the medical model's designation of 'patient' which presupposes a restricted concept of normality and health. More radical models, on the other hand, presume to free patients from such stigma by suggesting that they may be behaving in a reasonable way to an unreasonable environment.

A fundamental ethical dilemma directly related to these various models is whether to encourage the patient to rebel against a repressive environment or to adjust to his current condition.[39] The issue has been recently highlighted in American psychiatry's definition and traditional treatment of homosexuals, for example. On a purely diagnostic level, the nomenclature of 'homosexuality' as a 'sexual deviation'[40] has been ardently challenged by gay rights caucuses; sufficient pressure was brought to bear on the American Psychiatric Association that the official designation was subsequently changed to a presumably less stigmatizing 'sexual orientation disturbance'.[41] Yet, a recent review of the literature on psychotherapy and behaviour therapy indicates that therapists still regard homosexuality as undesirable, if not pathological.[42] On a less theoretical plane, the therapist may be obliged to take a position, implicitly if not explicitly: is heterosexuality the ultimate goal for his patient, or does he wish the patient to maximize the quality of his homosexual life. The latter stance, often unpopular, was recently subject to debate when a behaviour therapist treated a man sexually attracted to boys and provided him with methods to transfer that attraction to *men*, not women![43,44] Obviously, definition of goals varies not only between therapists, but also changes with the evolution of the concept of normality.

The knotty issue of setting therapeutic goals by the therapist, who must achieve a balance between the needs of the individual, his family, and society, was highlighted by Malev and his co-workers[45] and Lifton.[13] In the former case, a woman, married to a permanent invalid, was torn between her loyalty to her husband, and guilt lest she leave him to deteriorate; and her own personal development which necessitated that she find a life of her own. The therapist, as the patient's advocate, may have been tempted to veer towards the latter goal for the patient in serving her best interests. He chose, as an ethical psychiatrist, not to advise her directly one way or the other, but to assist her to explore the alternatives and implications of either decision. (This may have been more complicated had he also brought in the husband for treatment.)

The dual allegiance of the therapist, not only to the patient and his family, but to other of society's representatives, was placed in bold relief in the case of psychiatrists who treated soldiers in Vietnam.[13] Lifton felt that in this situation the therapist was forced to tread a thin line between advocacy and corruption. Referral to a therapist meant to Lifton that the troubled soldier was likely to be 'helped' to return to military duty and to resume the daily commission of war activities (i.e. adjustment as the goal). Thus, the psychotherapist's goals became inseparable from those of the military authority. Likened to a 'catch-22', the ethical dilemma of patients and psychotherapist in the context of military commitment therefore meant that one's very sanity in seeking to escape from the environment via a psychiatric judgement of craziness rendered one eligible for the continuing madness of killing and dying.[13]

Aside from conflicting goals in psychotherapy posed by the particular interests of the individual, family, or society, Hadley and Strupp[46] found in a survey of practitioners and researchers in the field that a major aspect of negative effects of psychotherapy was that of 'undertaking unrealistic tasks or goals'. In a compendium of such tendencies, all with profound ethical implications, were false assumptions concerning the scope and potency of therapy's goals. Misleading impressions may be given by the therapist when his need to instil hope in the patient, and the omniscience endowed him (by himself and/or the patient) become intertwined. While some degree of positive expectation is said to be a requisite element for producing therapeutic effects in all psychotherapies,[47] the patient may get the erroneous impression that therapy and the therapist can solve everything. This can perpetuate unrealistic expectations and goals which are ultimately deleterious to the patient. Such tendencies are often compounded by the therapist's failure to discuss, describe, or even acknowledge the reality of goals during treatment; or by goals which are specified but are too broad or obscure.

Special technical problems, with ethical implications, also arise when goals set explicitly or implicitly exceed the patient's capability, fostering a false estimate of speedy progress which cannot be realized (i.e. in reality the patient requires longer treatment). Conversely, the patient may have accomplished certain goals, but the therapist alters them and so prolongs treatment because he, the therapist, is unwilling to terminate (i.e. the patient in reality requires briefer treatment). Greenson[48] has aptly warned that any form or aspect of therapy that makes the patient an addict to treatment is undesirable.

The following case illustrations highlight some of these issues, especially the ethical conflict in providing short versus long-term goals (Case 1); and the confusion between ends and means in treatment (Case 2).

Case 1: How ethical is it to set limited goals when the needs of the patient may evolve as therapy progresses? Can ready-made interpretations, in the interests of time, short-change patients?

A 24-year-old woman was seen during a crisis over her one-and-a-half-year relationship with an older married man. A similar crisis had occurred two years before with another married man, and was resolved with brief treatment. Her recognition of the fact that he was not about to leave his wife and children prompted her to sever her ties with him. Two weeks following the breakup, the patient was depressed and tearful and couldn't sustain her decision; she went back to her boyfriend. In treatment, she described her suicidal ideas and her confusion regarding her love and need for him, despite her better judgement that this relationship had no future. In the ensuing 14 sessions the patient recovered from her depression, understood better her ambivalence, and learned to cope with the constraints of the relationship. Attempts were made for the patient to comprehend the unconscious nature of her conflict, unresolved attachment to her father, and her search for an inaccessible and unavailable man. Despite some intellectual recognition on the patient's part the therapist knew well at termination that she would repeat this pattern unless a fortunate turn of events occurred in her life.

Case 2: The psychotherapist tends not to prescribe medication for mild to moderate insomnia, anxiety, or depression, with the presumed justification that discomfort and suffering have a potentially motivating aspect for psychological work. The ethical question is where one draws the line? And has the patient been informed about the means and ends of treatment?

A 28-year-old professional woman with a long history of chronic depression was being treated with psychoanalytical psychotherapy twice a week. Her presenting difficulties were identified: not enjoying her work, her friends; having sexual difficulties with men; getting into highly dependent relationships. During four years of treatment in which she made good progress in working through some of her basic conflicts, she complained that her depression was not relieved. As a result of consultation, the therapist recommended a trial of medication concomitant with psychotherapy. The patient responded surprisingly well to the medication, her depression diminished, and she became socially and professionally more active. The therapist, with hindsight, realized that he might have prescribed drugs at some earlier point, which may have prevented needless suffering. But he also observed that medication, used as a crutch to provide quick or premature relief, sabotaged interest in exploring the psychological aspects of her depression.

In summary, the goals of psychotherapy are complex and subtle and include professional versus personal goals, long- versus short-term, non-specific versus specific, and overt versus covert. As we shall see, it is the last which is ethically most problematic, and potentially the one most under the therapist's (and patient's) control.

The therapeutic relationship

Section 1 of the psychiatric annotations to the Principles of Medical Ethics[27] states that 'the doctor-patient relationship is such a vital factor in effective treatment of the patient that the preservation of optimal conditions for development of a sound working relationship between a doctor and his patient should take precedence over all considerations.' Furthermore, 'The patient may place his trust in his psychiatrist knowing that the psychiatrist's ethics and professional responsibilities preclude him from gratifying his own needs and exploiting the patient. This becomes particularly important because of the essentially private, highly personal, and sometimes intensely emotional nature of the relationship established with the psychiatrist' (p. 1061). What are these 'optimal conditions', and what are their ethical implications in psychotherapy?

Regardless of goal, the therapeutic relationship between doctor and patient, constitutes both psychotherapy's strength as well as its weakness. This duality is related to the concept of authority which may be multiply defined.[49] In its most pure sense, it refers to an individual who is a specialist in his field, and who is therefore entitled to credit or acceptance; in another sense, it refers to power that requires submission. Different types of therapeutic relationship have been formed with various therapies,[30] or at different times in the process of the same therapy.[50] In each instance, the ethical issue of concern for the therapist is how to use his power justly:[51-53] the degree to which the therapeutic relationship is 'authoritarian' or 'egalitarian', or more specifically, to what extent the pervasive power of the 'transference' relationship, which offers the therapist a unique vehicle for exercising enormous influence over another person, is balanced by a true 'therapeutic alliance'[48] or 'therapeutic partnership'.[53] In general psychiatry, it has been pointed out that the fiduciary system, in which a patient puts his trust in the physician's ability and willingness to make crucial decisions, is being replaced by a contractual system (p. 126);[9] this trend also applies to the psychotherapies.

An egalitarian therapeutic relationship (i.e. adult-to-adult or peer-to-peer) is gaining in prominence and is considered more humanitarian and facilitative of free exchange between patient and therapist than the traditional medical model (i.e. doctor-to-patient) or the behavioural model (i.e. teacher-to-student),[30] but might some aspects of this model have negative implications for the therapeutic endeavour? Myerhoff and Larson[54] have examined the major change in the image of the physician in recent times, and suggest that 'The physician . . . has been traditionally depicted as a charismatic hero, a harbinger of progress, and a self-sacrificing, uniquely gifted, semi-divine figure . . . Presently, this portrayal appears to be changing and the doctor can be seen to be losing his charisma' (p. 189). Of what importance, if any, is this change? Parsons,[55] in his analysis of the social structure and the dynamic process of medical practice, identified certain requirements of the doctor–patient relationship as necessary for successful treatment; one of the most essential was the 'social distance' between practitioner and client. A study of human organization in hospitals concluded 'we are coming to understand that faith in the doctor is a necessary element in cure, that he will not be able to exercise therapeutic leverage if we, as patients, regard him in too prosaic a light' (p. 71).[56] The authors suggested that the therapist's power to claim the patient's confidence as well as the therapist's effectiveness would be impaired by the growing familiarity between the two. Where, then, does one draw the line between the good use of power in the traditional medical model and its abuse? Where do the new boundaries of partnership end and those of 'real' familiarity and friendship begin? More importantly for the times, will there be new ethical dilemmas for the egalitarian therapeutic relationship?

Goldberg's[53] exposition of the equitable 'therapeutic partnership' suggests that not only is the nature of the therapeutic alliance (i.e. its power distribution) critical, but the degree to which it is made explicit. Often within its non-explicit nature lies the ethical rub of psychotherapy. He recommends that a therapeutic contract be established with an explicitly agreed working plan (comparable to that in the medical model), the essence of which is how each agent will use his power. This should consist of agreed goals, established means to reach them, evaluation of therapy during its course, and methods of addressing dissatisfaction in the working alliance. But applying in practice what one intends in theory is not easily accomplished. In addition to ambiguity in aims noted earlier, theory has not always been applied in new treatment modalities such as encounter group therapy, where, despite the appearance of therapeutic virtues like openness, autonomy, and mutuality, there is often little attention given to the participant's specific needs;[57] and treatment is often begun without inquiring about the participant's expectations.[58]

Conflict between the two models of therapeutic relationship was also highlighted in Lifton's[13] work with Vietnam veterans. Early on, most therapists felt that the essential model for the sessions was traditional therapy; Lifton held a minority view which emphasized a sustained dialogue between professional and veteran based upon a common stance of opposition to the war. This latter model did not abolish the traditional roles, but placed more emphasis upon mutuality and shared commitment. It is usually assumed that the patient knows what he wants from such a therapeutic relationship, and knows what is good for him. Lifton aptly pointed out that those in therapy were most clear about what they opposed — hierarchical distance, medical mystification, and psychological reductionism; they were presumably less clear about what they wanted and expected. Indeed, the factors they objected to may have been reminiscent of other conflicts with authority that they were grappling with in the military context. Here, the therapists — as a model of non-authoritarianism — may have contributed in a crucial way to the development of a therapeutic relationship which enabled clients to change through the process of identification.[59]

A prominent negative effect of the traditional therapeutic relationship can result from its insufficient regard for the patient's intentionality or will.[46] This may manifest, for example, in the therapist's fervent search for unconscious determinants so that therapy soon becomes an end in itself; the therapist may thus assume priority over all other people in the patient's life. This may occur in an even more extreme form in some of the newer, large group therapies which can, in the context of group influence, encourage a godlike belief in the therapist. With or without peer pressure, the therapist's power is greatly exaggerated for reasons which have more to do with the therapist's needs than those of the patient.

The following case illustrates how close are ethical and technical aspects by examining the issue of excessive dependency and unresolved transference of patient toward therapist, and the role that the therapist may play in its maintenance.

Case 3: A 55-year-old woman had been in treatment for the last 17 years. She was first seen for difficulties with her husband who neglected and frustrated her, and could not meet her dependency needs. Concerns about the prospect of separation or divorce precipitated exploration of her need for him, though chronically frustrated by his shortcomings, and most recently by his sexual inadequacy. During the last two years of treatment, her emotional dependency shifted on to the therapist, thus diluting the pressure on her husband. Although the therapist privately complained about the patient's excessive phone calls, constant advice-seeking, and magical expectations of him, he did not actively put an end to them. The therapist's rationale for continuing to treat this woman without a more identified goal of treatment was that he provided a therapeutic 'benign dependency' where she could not be harmed, and that gradual maturation would occur.

Was the patient being exploited? Dependency may be one of the most common characteristics of all patients, and allows for the early establishment of the helper-recipient relationship. In treatment other relationships develop such as transference and a working alliance which help to lessen that dependence and ultimately enable the therapist to encourage independence in the patient. There are, of course, patients who need lifelong supervision even after much of the psychotherapy work is done; some of them may take the initiative and terminate treatment. But, it is also possible that a therapist, because of his lack of experience, or for less benign reasons (e.g. financial or psychopathological needs) perpetuates the dependency and unresolved transference of the patient. While most often seen as a technical problem in treatment, the question remains: when does a technical problem in therapy become an ethical issue as well?

Special ethical problems of behaviour modification

The basic ethical aspect of behaviour modification is no different from that of other therapies, that is, the 'judicious use of power'.[51,52] However, behaviour modification has been regarded as having some specific ethical problems, both conceptually and methodologically. These ethical issues revolve around behaviour therapy's underlying concept of man, and its alleged potential for contribution to a dehumanization or diminution of the individual; more specifically, its failure to view the patient as-a-whole by separating the person from his problem or symptom. For many, it fosters a 'machine model of man',[51] and portrays the therapist as a technician or 'social reinforcement machine'[60] and the patient as his mechanical tool. Experimental evidence of the potency of stimulus–response patterns, and the extent to which human beings can be conditioned, have supported a view of the behaviour therapist as a possessor of extensive powers of social influence, and as an overt perpetrator of 'despotic control, brainwashing, and crass manipulation', largely irrespective of, or even against, the patient's will.[61]

In addition, behaviour therapy is said to have more profound ethical implications than other forms of psychotherapy expressly because it 'does not expand awareness';[62] in these other forms, like individual, family and group therapy, the therapist explicitly helps the patient to understand the meaning of his symptom. In fact, the principal merit of behaviour modification techniques resides in their efficient and impersonal application 'without the necessity to deal with the troubling implications of what the patient's behaviour might mean' (p. 387),[62] and, because the methods work quickly, there is little time for the patient to contemplate their repercussions.

Despite these special features — often disadvantages from an ethical point of view — some observers argue that the degree to which behaviour can be altered without the intervening influence of the patient's own cognitive valuation has been greatly exaggerated.[61] As with other treatment, behaviour therapy usually cannot succeed in a person who does not wish to change. Certainly, a person's proneness to influence is ultimately an individual matter, and depends upon the type of patient. Moreover, the ethical vicissitudes of behaviour control probably differ in 'the non-consenting patient', 'the patient under duress', and 'the voluntary patient'.[62] They are perhaps more pronounced in settings where a person is under civil or criminal commitment, and in penal institutions and state mental hospitals, behaviour modification methods have often been extensively applied in the absence of consent. Here, the most critical ethical problem may neither be the implications of behaviour therapy's concepts nor its coercive quality, but the therapist's role as double agent, serving both the patient *and* the institution. Indeed, behavioural methods are regarded as 'peculiarly adaptable to meeting the needs of society' (over those of the individual).[62] More specifically, these methods may be used to increase conformity and to reinforce certain social norms, and to reduce assertiveness and deviant behaviour.

The use of specific techniques in behaviour modification, notably aversive conditioning or negative reinforcement, raises a major ethical difficulty.[63] This is well illustrated in the case [64] of an institutionalized, primary schoolchild who was treated for headbanging. Perpetually bruised, a padded football helmet was placed on her head, and her hands tied down to her crib; none the less, the headbanging persisted. As an alternative plan, after all kinds of positive reinforcers had proved ineffective, the therapist slapped her sharply on the cheek and shouted 'Don't', whenever she began to toss her head. Soon slapping was no longer necessary. Although this method had been effective, the child's parents withdrew her from the behavioural programme on learning that she had been slapped. The inevitable ethical dilemma arises: When do the ends justify the means?

The obvious question of parental informed consent is equally important in this case.

The token economy approach has been criticized, particularly because informed consent is rarely obtained. Here, the issue may not be the type of method, but its utilization without consultation or consent. Invariably the staff take the decision about which behaviours they wish to reinforce, and the token rewards serve an essentially disciplinary function. Moreover, since the practice of token economy has traditionally relied on material incentives and 'behavioural productivity', it reflects, for some critics, an over-emphasis on the achievement ethic at the expense of a more humanistic approach.[61] The questions must be addressed: Who shall set the standards of behaviour to be rewarded or punished? the doctors? the nurses? the patients? and, to what extent shall these decisions be made with the consent of their recipients?

In the treatment of out-patients with neurotic symptoms, where the decision to undergo behaviour therapy is presumably voluntary, another issue emerges. In that these methods aim to abolish the symptom *per se* (in the belief that there is no underlying neurosis), does treatment merely provide superficial relief for more deeply concealed disturbance? When is the behaviour therapist obliged to refer certain patients to another form of psychotherapy, and to advise them that they need a different form of help? If he does not do so, is he deceiving the patient (as well as himself)?

In summary, although the behaviour therapist: may have an advantage of technical precision over other psychotherapies; may be spared having to deal with long-term goals; can be more explicit in setting goals and applying his methods, and can thus more easily establish a mutual contract with the patient; he is no less caught up with ethical dilemmas than other psychotherapists. Moreover, he also has to grapple with additional ethical problems, arising out of his unique philosophy and techniques: namely, to his molecular (but perhaps dehumanizing) view of man and psychopathology; his specific (but perhaps reductionistic) goals in treatment; and his efficient and precise (but perhaps aversive, coercive, mechanical, and materialistic) methods.

Specific ethical issues in psychotherapy

Confidentiality and privileged communication

Confidentiality in the practice of psychiatry has been defined as 'the relationship between a physician (psychiatrist) and his patient, in which the patient may assume that his disclosures will not be passed on to others except under certain circumstances, and then only for the specific purpose of lending necessary help. This takes place within the framework of the social role of the doctor as one who treats and helps his patients, and who is ethically committed to this role' (p. 89)[64] At the same time, privileged communication is 'a right, existing only by statute, whereby a patient may bar his doctor from testifying about medical treatment and the disclosures which are an integral part of it', that is, it is 'a legal right which belongs to the patient, and not to the doctor' (p. 89).[64]

The issues of confidentiality and privilege in psychiatry have had major implications in the last decade. We need only note, for example, the disclosure, after Senator Thomas Eagleton had been nominated as Democratic candidate for Vice-President of the United States, of confidential information regarding his previous psychiatric history, including treatment for a major depressive disorder (which ultimately forced his withdrawal from public office); and the break-in of the office of the psychiatrist of Daniel Ellsberg (who had released the Pentagon Papers) to seek his medical record for possible use against him in trial for treason. The question arises: Under what circumstances are disclosures to someone other than the patient and therapist ethical? Although both of the above events received national attention, issues of confidentiality and privacy in everyday psychotherapeutic practice are more subtle, but no less crucial to the therapeutic endeavour. And, while we are concerned here with the moral, rather than the legal aspects of confidentiality, the subject is often complicated by the spectre of legal sanction.

That confidentiality has long had a venerable place in the practice of medicine is seen in its inclusion in the Hippocratic Oath: 'Whatever, in connection with my professional practice or not in connection with it, I see or hear, in the life of men, which ought not to be spoken abroad, I will not divulge, as reckoning that all should be kept secret' [p. 154].[65] Its sanctity in psychotherapy is perhaps even more crucial because of the inherently personal nature of the patient's communications, which cover his innermost thoughts, fantasies, and feelings. Statutes in many countries grant the relationship between psychiatrist and patient the same absolute protection as those accorded to husband and wife, and to lawyer and client.[66] Indeed, the most elaborate clause (Section 9) of the American Psychiatric Association Annotations Especially Applicable to Psychiatry relates to confidentiality. It declares that 'Confidentiality is essential to psychiatric treatment' [p. 1063],[27] with statements: that the psychiatrist may reveal confidential information only with the patient's authorization or under proper legal compulsion; that he must apprise the patient of the implications of waiving the privilege of privacy; that when the psychiatrist is ordered by the court to reveal confidences entrusted to him by a patient, he may comply or may ethically hold the right to dissent within the framework of the law; that he should disclose only that information that is immediately relevant to a given situation, and avoid offering speculation as facts. All in all, the Annotations call for extreme care with regard to confidential material, both written and verbal, especially in instances of consultation with other professionals; with clinical notes and records; and in case presentations and in the distribution of teaching material. Some psychiatrists have also warned against the more insidious practice of 'gossip' among colleagues which may inadvertently harm the patient and the therapeutic relationship.

In recent years confidentiality of the traditional therapist–patient relationship has been under increasing pressure as third-party insurance and peer review organizations have required certain information about treatment. Plaut[67] points out three forces in the escalating conflict between the right to secrecy and the right to information: increasing involvement of government in areas that were previously considered private e.g. health, welfare, business regulation, and product control; the technological revolution in both data collection (wire-tapping, tape-recording), and data storage and retrieval (computerized records); and the suspiciousness of the individual of authority, for whom knowledge has always meant power.

In the face of these new pressures, major questions concerning confidentiality in psychotherapy are: Whose agent is the psychotherapist — the patient's? the family's? society's? the law's?; What are the goals in divulging a confidence — better treatment? evaluation? consensual validation? support?; and what are the risks — will the therapeutic relationship be jeopardized? will the patient terminate treatment? Conversely, can rigid adherence to a rule of confidentiality between therapist and patient blind the therapist to certain risks and dangers to himself or to others?

In part, the issue of the therapist's allegiance is related to the type of psychotherapy he practises. Although individual therapy may be limited to traditional goals within the private framework of the patient's inner thoughts and feelings, there may be other goals whereby information communicated between therapist and patient is used to influence the patient's social milieu. A serious question that often arises is the responsibility of the therapist to the patient's family. In general, the less healthy the patient, the more important this issue becomes. With a relatively stable and independent patient, there is usually no need to contact family members, and the therapist would not encourage any communication from them. Should the latter occur, it is usually in the patient's interests that he is promptly informed of the contact, and that this is fully discussed in the therapeutic sessions. A more disturbed patient may not only need his family's support, but also involve family members with the therapist as an expression of his disturbance. In such circumstances, each communication with the family both complicates treatment and also raises ethical questions about breaches of confidentiality and whose interests the therapist serves.

In family therapy, whose purported goal is 'to treat the family as the patient',[68] the situation is usually reversed in that an individual's confidence may be subverted in the interests of treating the married couple or family. Whether a therapist uses an individual or family approach may determine not only the goals of treatment, but the nature of the treatment of the individual within each approach. How does the therapist evaluate if it is in the patient's best interests to be seen individually, or within the context of his family? How justifiable is it for the therapist to impose marital and family therapy if he regards the problem as stemming from the family or marriage? The following case demonstrates the difficulties involved.

Case 4: A 45-year-old man with a serious obsessive–compulsive ritual which inter-fered with his work and social life, especially his marriage, was treated by a therapist with a family approach who saw the man and his wife weekly in joint sessions. The man made little progress over the course of two years, although his marriage seemed less stormy. When the husband was seen alone by a consultant at the therapist's request, he confessed that he was not able to talk about his 'secret life' lest it be conveyed to his wife; nor was he able to seek the therapist for himself. It was apparent that he had unwittingly begun to identify with the therapist's viewpoint, regarding the interpersonal communication between himself and his wife as the source of his difficulites, rather than exploring intrapsychic conflicts and concerns of his own. That he should talk about personal problems to the consultant was regarded as a betrayal of his therapist, so that he was too confused and guilty to seek individual assistance.

Here, the therapist's theoretical stance of responsibility to the couple over the husband, precluded in some ways, the best interests of the individual patient. On the other side of the coin are instances where dynamic psychotherapists so strongly believe in confidentiality and individual privacy in the dyadic relationship that they fail to divulge confidences or share information with family members which may prove vital to the welfare of the patient (see Case 5).

Indeed, the sole exception to the rule of confidentiality between therapist and patient is the possibility of 'dangerousness' to others. This is now stipulated in the famous 'Tarasoff decision',[69] which enunciated the maxim that 'Protective privilege ends where public peril begins'; it refers to the requirement that the therapist must warn both certain specified authorities and potential victims, of possible dangerous actions by his patients. The case *Tarasoff v. Regents of the University of California*, involved the confidential disclosure by a young patient to his therapist that he intended to kill his girlfriend. After the therapist had consulted with two psychiatrists and notified the police, the patient was detained. His release followed his denial of any violent intent. He broke off treatment in response to the therapist's breach of confidence. Two months later, he murdered his girlfriend. The therapist and his psychiatrist-supervisor were then sued by the victim's parents for failure to warn them of her peril.

The case, although unusual, places in bold relief the dilemma of the therapist in balancing the patient's right to confidentiality and society's right to protection. Many psychotherapists opposed the decision, regarding it as conceptually and practically flawed and carrying negative implications for psychiatry.[70,71] Roth and Meisel,[70] for example, feel that the decision assumes a degree of expertise in predicting violence or danger that the psychiatrist simply does not possess; that a lowering of the threshold of dangerousness for a warning to an intended victim will result, which will compromise the patient's right to confidentiality and possibly his treatment; that the psychiatrist is not only liable if he fails to warn, but risks liability for invasion of privacy or defamation by the patient if the threat of harm does not materialize; and lastly as happened in the Tarasoff case the patient's dangerousness will probably increase, because of his sense of betrayal by the therapist and because of his premature termination of the very treatment he needs. On a more conceptual level, Gurevitz[71] argues that the Tarasoff decision erroneously 'defines and reinforces a social control function for psychiatry' by allying the psychotherapist 'more with the goal of protecting society than with that of healing patients' (p. 291). It is not, Gurevitz points out, that psychiatrists reject the need to balance these functions; in fact, most psychiatrists attempt to fulfil both responsibilities.

No doubt because of the Tarasoff decision, alternative action that can be taken by psychotherapists short of actual warning, have been recommended. For example, due to their very strong conviction about the importance of confidentiality in the doctor–patient relationship, in no instance have Roth and Meisel[70] directly warned the potential victim without first obtaining the patient's permission. Since violence is rare, they feel it is prudent to 'rely on odds and not warn' (p. 510). In addition, they advocate that the therapist inform the patient of the boundaries and limits of confidentiality. If danger seems imminent, the therapist should first consider social manipulations which might reduce its likelihood, before he makes the decision to compromise confidentiality. When confronted with a potentially violent patient, options include: continued treatment of the patient; involuntary hospitalization; notification of police; and notification of potential victim. Each action places a different weight on the competing values of confidentiality versus protection of society. The authors cite several cases of uncompromised confidentiality with 'happy endings'.

The following case in which the therapist also maintained a strong adherence to patient confidentiality and privacy, reflects an instance not of 'public peril' (i.e. danger to others), but of the more private peril of danger to oneself.

Case 5: A middle-aged executive was in psychotherapy for depression following a myocardial infarction, and presented suicidal thoughts, fears of dying, sexual avoidance, and other related symptoms. He was also considering leaving his twenty-year marriage and his children, and moving elsewhere to seek a less competitive job. The patient was seen for the first time in the hospital when recovering from his MI; the patient's wife remained at his bedside during most of this time. While the psychiatrist expressed appreciation of her availability to the patient, he did not encourage further communication between himself and the wife. When the patient did not respond to weekly psychotherapy, sessions were increased to three times per week, and the patient was given antidepressant medication after consultation with a physician colleague. During three months of combined pharmacotherapy and psychotherapy, the patient's improvement was modest. During that time, his wife had phoned the therapist on a few occasions, but the therapist chose not to return the calls. Rather, the calls were discussed with the husband in the context of their marital relationship, e.g. her over involvement, his dependency needs and desire to be controlled. Four months later, the therapist received a letter from the wife citing his non-response to her calls and mentioning that the patient had not taken his medication. The therapist shared this information with the patient, who confessed that he had only taken the medication for one week because he could not tolerate the feeling of being 'removed' that it gave him; and that he had kept the rest of the pills in case he decided to commit suicide. The patient reassured the therapist that he was not considering suicide despite the fantasy, and that he would, as the therapist requested, throw the pills away. Three weeks later, the patient suicided with an overdose of the medication.

The case throws up several questions: Can the therapist predict danger to the self any better than he can predict danger to others? If not, does he have a duty to inform family and friends? Could contact with the wife have better served the therapist, and ultimately, the patient? Where does one draw the confidentiality line when the patient is a threat to *himself*?

The above may also ethically relate to the therapist's position regarding suicide and its prevention. Recently, publicized cases of so-called 'rational suicide', especially in the context of terminal illness suggest that the psychotherapist may be faced increasingly with the need to respect decisions by patients to commit suicide. In these instances, therapist and patient alike are obliged to confront and resolve their ethical dilemmas together (see Chapter 10).

Therapist–patient sex (and sexism) (see Chapter 9)

The Hippocratic Oath includes a pledge that 'with purity and holiness I will practice my art . . . into whatever houses I enter I will go into them for the benefit of the sick and will abstain from every voluntary act of mischief and corruption, and further from the seduction of females or males, of freeman and slaves' (p. 236).[72] The Annotations Especially Applicable to Psychiatry (of the Principles of Medical Ethics), less eloquently but no less unequivocally, uphold this moral tradition by stating simply, 'Sexual activity with a patient is unethical' (p. 1061).[27] Indeed, it is the only activity deemed unethical between doctor and patient which is presented so unambiguously. As part of the requirement that the doctor 'conduct himself with propriety in his profession and in all the actions of his life' (p. 1061), the dictum regarding sex is stated to be especially important in the case of the psychiatrist because his patient tends to model his behaviour after that of his therapist. Further, the necessary intensity of the therapeutic relationship may activate sexual and other fantasies in both patient and therapist, while weakening the objectivity required for treatment. In so far as it has earned a position of such priority (Section 1 of Psychiatry's Annotations), therapist–patient sex may be considered the quintessence of the overt misuse and exploitation of the transference relationship.

Yet sexual activities, including sexual intercourse and various forms of erotic contact between therapist and patient, have been increasingly reported in the literature; and have involved clinicians at all levels of training, from psychiatric trainee to training analyst.[73–80] This is not a new problem for therapists who have reported erotic transferences and their vicissitudes since the dawn of psychotherapy. No less than Mesmer, Breuer, Janet, Charcot, and Freud have described the emergence of strong sexual feelings in treatment, and the inevitable problems wrought by their presence. While sexual affairs between therapist and patient were never sanctioned by Freud or his followers, they did occur. Often the therapist was saved from moral indictment, as he still is, by his marriage to his patient. But such a 'shotgun' resolution is an extreme and limited option to deal with sexual 'acting-out'. The question remains: What are the therapist's ethical options if he *does not* marry the patient?

In a recent review of legal and professional alternatives to deter discipline or punish sexually active therapists,[81] four possible avenues of approach are mentioned: criminal law (e.g. a charge of rape by fraud or coercion); civil law (e.g. a malpractice suit); medical board (e.g. revoked licensure); and professional association (e.g. pressure to limit referrals, threaten career opportunities). Each in its turn has been virtually ineffectual as a system of control. In the instance of criminal law, a rape charge, as strongly recommended by Masters and Johnson[82] is rarely brought and rarely sticks; most cases entail psychological and not physical coercion. Both force and fraud are required and the prevailing judicial view is that if the patient consents, and the therapist has never claimed that sexual activity was treatment, there has been neither force nor fraud. In the instance of civil law malpractice cases, again no legal course may be available if the therapist has not misidentified sexual activity as treatment. In a publicized incident recently, two factors were also held in the therapist's favour: the patient did not press charges until one and a half years after their relationship had begun, and she presumably did not have a normal transference. Medical licensing boards, at least in the United States, are not consistent from state to state, and may not have a close relationship with psychiatric members. Lastly, professional associations have no subpoena power and little expertise in evidentiary investigation, either to protect the due process rights of the therapist who is charged, or to cope with a therapist who sues them. Davidson[42] points out that entry into treatment may be another way for the seductive psychiatrist to escape censure, as well as serving to sabotage efforts to discipline him. Given the above failure of sanctions from without, Stone[81] concludes that ultimately 'patients must depend on the decent moral character of those entrusted to treat them' [p. 1141].

But what is deemed to constitute 'decent moral character' may change with the times, at least according to the findings of some current psychotherapists. In contrast to Masters and Johnson's position on the matter — that therapists who have sex with their patients should be charged criminally with rape, no matter who initiated the seduction — are attitudes of relative sexual permissiveness. Recent evidence suggests that the psychiatrist's value system has moved in the direction of sexual permissiveness both in terms of what is acceptable for the self and for others.[83] There is, for example, an overt endorsement of touching and so-called 'non-erotic' physical behaviour, by advocates of the human potential movement[84,85] which, far from being regarded as unethical or harmful, are felt to enhance the therapeutic relationship and to promote personal growth.

Attitudes to sex between professional and patient reflect not only individual predilection, but also theoretical orientation[86] and medical speciality.[87] Kardener's[76] survey of physicians' erotic and non-erotic physical contact with patients suggests that psychiatrists offended less commonly compared to some other medical specialities. Their reported rates of erotic contact by 10 per cent of psychiatrists and sexual intercourse by 5 per cent were lower than those of general practitioners, surgeons, and obstetrician–gynaecologists. Significant differences regarding psychotherapist–patient sex were found between 'psychodynamically oriented' and other theoretically oriented therapists. For example, whereas 86 per cent of the former group believed that erotic contact was *never* of benefit to the patient, this figure was significantly lower for humanistic and behavioural therapists (71 per cent and 61 per cent respectively). That there is widespread ambivalence on the subject even after the fact is seen in Taylor and Wagner's[87] review of cases of therapists who had actually had intercourse with their patients. About half reported that the experience had had negative effects on either patient or therapist, 32 per cent that it had mixed effects, and 21 per cent that it had positive effects (the authors did not question the patients). Butler[77] however found that 95 per cent of therapists who had had sex with their patients reported conflict, fear and guilt; only 40 per cent of them sought consultation for their problem.

We are left with some crucial ethical questions: Is sexual contact between therapist and patient unequivocally unethical regardless of outcome? If it is unethical, what about 'non-erotic' kissing, hugging, and touching, that more than 50 per cent of psychiatrists engage in with patients? When, if ever, are these appropriate?

A related issue concerns *sexism* in psychotherapy. Are sexual relations with the patient — virtually always female — the tip of an iceberg of a more pervasive practice, not of sex, but of sexism in psychotherapy?[88,89] The ethics of psychotherapy in relation to patient gender has implications not only for specific abuse, such as sex between male therapist and female patient, but for other forms of sexual exploitation and discrimination. Particularly pertinent are the underlying theory, training practices, and the nature of the doctor--patient relationship that typify many schools of therapy. Broverman and his colleagues[90] suggest that therapeutic theories have usually supported rather than questioned stereotypical assumptions about sex roles and different standards of mental health for men and women. Thus, therapists have commonly accepted that dependency and passivity are normal qualities in women whereas assertiveness and independence are typical of men; or designated a woman's dissatisfaction with her traditional role as evidence of psychopathology.[88] Aside from the unfortunate legacy of an 'antifeminine Freudian position',[88] women may also be harmed by a 'blame-the-mother' tradition, especially by a family therapist who regards them as potentially 'schizophrenogenic' to their children.[89] Such sex bias is often reinforced during training in which androcentrism is unlikely to be corrected by a male supervisor[89] (female therapists are much less likely to have had supervisors of their own sex as role models during training).[91]

The most insidious aspect of sexism in psychotherapy practice is the dominance of the profession by male therapists and the resultant tendency to replicate within the therapeutic relationship a 'one-down' position, a position in which women typically find themselves. This form of relationship may encourage the fantasy that an idealized relationship with a powerful man is a more desirable solution to problems than taking autonomous action;[75,89] it may also set the stage for the kind of sexual exploitation that we discussed earlier.

The new feminist psychotherapies can provide ethical guidelines to deal with sexism in psychotherapy. The egalitarianism between therapist and patient that typifies these treatments should be replicated in all forms of psychotherapy.

The promotion of proper ethical practice

While ethical concerns have long faced the psychiatrist (and hence the psychotherapist), codes of ethics are of recent origin, e.g. that devised by the American Psychiatric Association was published only in 1974 and the World Psychiatric Association's Declaration of Hawaii in 1977 (see Appendix). These sorts of codes have been criticized by some observers for setting arbitrary standards of professional behaviour; the weakness of presentation which is likened to a description of etiquette rather than a professionally honoured document; and the lack of moral substance to their tenets.[9,92] They are therefore felt to have serious limitations in assisting the psychotherapist to make ethical decisions in his daily practice; and they are understandably disappointing to those who confuse codes with covenants, or to those who expect to produce morally scrupulous psychotherapists.

Other observers insist that the pressing problem is not the establishment of a set of guidelines, but of enforcement.[93] The contention is that a code can always be revised to better meet the professional's needs, but that problems of peer review will still exist: the voluntary nature of complaint investigations; conflicting roles in which peer review committees are required to act, as investigator, prosecutor, judge and jury; inaccurate (and insufficient) case reporting; fear of liability by the professional reviewer; and over-concern with confidentiality which often takes precedence over other ethical considerations and can be used as a rationalisation to resist investigation.[2] In practice, it is exceedingly difficult to know what really occurs within the therapeutic relationship. Moreover psychotherapists like other professionals are naturally reluctant to judge their colleagues; nor may they feel morally or technically equipped to do so. The ethical conduct not only of the profession, but also of the peer review process is of concern;[94] an important criticism is that the patient has been excluded from the process and has been poorly informed about the procedures. Consequently, it is a commonly held view that psychiatry (and psychotherapy) is unable to police itself[93] and that peer review, as currently designed is 'bound to fail'.[95] None the less, positive headway has been made, and there is still hope that peer reviews can serve some purpose.[96]

Expectations of what a code of ethics and peer review can achieve may have been unrealistic. Perhaps their primary purpose should be education rather than control. Newman and Luft,[97] for example, have suggested that an educational peer review system which promotes cooperation among professionals is of greater utility and more acceptable to clinicians than a bureaucratic system of control. The difficult question still remains as to how much authority should be vested in peer review committees.

Conclusions and recommendations

As has been suggested throughout this chapter, ethical problems in the practice of psychotherapy are not easily soluble: dilemmas which face the psychotherapist are varied and complex. He is virtually never a single agent. He cannot rely on codified instruments as more than broad guides to behaviour. Ultimately he must seek specific remedies to ethical problems that inevitably arise in his practice. The following points may help the psychotherapist to exercise his ethical judgement:

(1) Greater exploration of the philosophical foundations of psychotherapeutic practice;
(2) self-awareness by the therapist through, for example, constant examination and analysis of his attitudes within and outside the therapeutic relationship;
(3) active development in treatment of a 'therapeutic alliance' or partnership, in which there is equal power and participation by both parties towards mutual goals and responsibilities;
(4) greater allegiance to a code of ethics and its development, in order to better sort out ethical choices and their implications for both patient and therapist;
(5) grater responsibility by the therapist for the maintenance of professional competence in himself and his peers;
(6) openness to consultation with others and a receptiveness to outside opinions in making proper ethical decisions in treatment; and
(7) greater understanding of human nature and morality from which timely and productive ethical alternatives can be derived.

As one author has aptly put it, 'by definition, ethical problems remain unresolved. By their unresolved quality, they provoke a continuous anxiety in the practicing psychiatrist and concomitantly a desire to search, to oppose, to think, and to research' (p. 2546).[98]

References

1. SPIEGEL, R.: Editorial: On psychoanalysis, values, and ethics. *Journal of the American Academy of Psychoanalysis* **6**:271–3, 1978.
2. MOORE, R. A.: Ethics in the practice of psychiatry — Origins, functions, models and enforcement. *American Journal of Psychiatry* **135**:157–63, 1978.
3. OSMOND, H.: Psychiatry under siege: The crisis within. *Psychiatric Annals* **3**:59–81, 1973

4. FREEDMAN, D. and GORDON, R.: Psychiatry under siege: Attacks from without. *Psychiatric Annals* **3**:10–34, 1973.

5. MICHELS, R.: Professional ethics and social values. *International Review of Psychoanalysis* **3**:377–84,1976.

6. GURALNIK, D. B. (ed.): *Webster's new world dictionary of the American language.* New York, World Publishing Co., 1970.

7. FLETCHER, J.: Ethical aspects of genetic control. *New England Journal of Medicine* **285**: 776–83, 1971.

8. POWLEDGE, F.: The therapist as double-agent. *Psychology Today* **11**:44–7, 1977.

9. REDLICH, F. and MOLLICA, R.: Overview: ethical issues in contemporary psychiatry. *American Journal of Psychiatry* **133**:125–6, 1976.

10. JASNOW, A.: The psychotherapist — Artist and/or scientist? *Psychotherapy: Theory, Research and Practice* **15**:318–22, 1978.

11. EDELSON, M.: Psychoanalysis as science: Its boundary problems, special status, relations to other sciences, and formalization. *Journal of Nervous and Mental Disease* **165**:1–28, 1977.

12. LONDON, P.: *The modes and morals of psychotherapy.* New York, Holt, Rinehart and Winston, 1964.

13. LIFTON, R. J.: Advocacy and corruption in the healing professions. *International Review of Psychoanalysis* **3**:385–98, 1976.

14. STRUPP, H.: Some observations on the fallacy of value-free psychotherapy and the empty organism: comments on a case study. *Journal of Abnormal Psychology* **83**: 199–201, 1974.

15. BUCKLEY, P., KARASU, T. B., CHARLES, E., and STEIN, S.: Theory and practice in psychotherapy: Some contradictions in expressed belief and reported practice. *Journal of Nervous and Mental Disease* **167**:218–23, 1979.

16. ERICKSON, E.,: Psychoanalysis and ethics — Avowed and unavowed. *International Review of Psychoanalysis* **3**:409–15, 1976.

17. MARCUSE, H.: *Eros and civilization.* Boston, Beacon Press, 1955.

18. HOLT, R: Freud's impact on modern morality. *Hastings Center Report*, April 1980, 38–45.

19. SZASZ, T.: *The myth of mental illness.* New York, Hoeber-Harper, 1961.

20. TORREY, F.: *The death of psychiatry.* Radnor, Pa., Chilton Book Co., 1974.

21. HOLLINGSHEAD, A. and REDLICH, F.: *Social class and mental illness: a community study.* New York, Wiley, 1958.

22. HORNEY, K.: *New ways in psychoanalysis.* New York, Norton, 1939.

23. FROMM-REICHMANN, F.: *Psychoanalysis and psychotherapy.* Chicago, University of Chicago Press, 1959.

24. GREENSON, R.: *The technique and practice of psychoanalysis.* Vol. 1. New York, International Universities Press, 1967.

25. FREUD, S.: Analysis terminable and interminable. *The complete psychological works of Sigmund Freud, Volume XXIII (1937–9).* London, Hogarth Press, 1964.

26. Judicial Council, American Medical Association: *Opinions and reports of the Judicial Council.* Chicago, American Medical Association, 1971.

27. The principles of medical ethics with annotations especially applicable to psychiatry. *American Journal of Psychiatry* **130**:1057–64, 1973.

28. FISHER, S. and GREENBERG, R. P.: *The scientific credibility of Freud's theories and therapy.* New York, Basic Books, 1977.

29. PARLOFF, M.: *Twenty-five years of research in psychotherapy.*, New York, Albert Einstein College of Medicine Department of Psychiatry, 17 October, 1975.

30. KARASU, T. B.: Psychotherapies: An overview. *American Journal of Psychiatry* **134**: 851–63, 1977.

31. SLAVSON, P.: *The New York Times,* 9 January, 1969.

32. BRILL, N.: Future of psychiatry in a changing world. *Psychosomatics* **14**: 19–26, 1973.
33. KETY, S.: From rationalization to reason. *American Journal of Psychiatry*, **131**: 957–63, 1974.
34. YAGER, J.: A survival guide for psychiatric residents. *Archives of General Psychiatry* **30**:494–9, 1974.
35. CERROLAZA, M.: The nebulous scope of current psychiatry. *Comprehensive Psychiatry* **14**:299–309, 1973.
36. RASKIN, D.: Psychiatric training in the '70's — Toward a shift in emphasis. *American Journal of Psychiatry* **128**:119–20, 1972.
37. VISPO, R.: Psychiatry — paradigm of our times. *Psychiatry Quarterly* **46**: 209–19, 1972.
38. SZASZ, T.: *The myth of psychotherapy*. New York, Anchor/Doubleday, 1978.
39. BLATTE, H.: *Evaluating psychotherapies*. Hastings Center Report, September 1973, pp. 4–6.
40. *Diagnostic and statistical manual of mental disorders*, 2nd edn. (DSM 11). American Psychiatric Association, 1968.
41. *Diagnostic and statistical manual of mental disorders*. 3rd edn. (DSM 111). American Psychiatric Association, 1978.
42. DAVIDSON, V.: Psychiatry's problem with no name: Therapist–patient sex. *American Journal of Psychoanalysis* **37**:43–50, 1977.
43. GARFIELD, S.: Values: An issue in psychotherapy: Comments on a case study. *Journal of Abnormal Psychology* **83**:202–3, 1974.
44. DAVISON, G. C. and WILSON, G. T.: Goals and strategies in behavioral treatment of homosexual pedophilia: Comments on a case study. *Journal of Abnormal Psychology* **83**:196–8, 1974.
45. MALEV, J. S., KAPLAN, E. A., HOLLENDER, M. H. *et al*: For better or for worse: a problem in ethics. *International Psychiatry Clinics* **2**: 603–24, 1966.
46. HADLEY, S. W. and STRUPP, H. H.: Contemporary views of negative effects in psychotherapy: An integrated account. *Archives of General Psychiatry* **33**: 1291–1302, 1976.
47. FRANK, J.: *Persuasion and healing: a comparative study of psychotherapy*. Baltimore, Johns Hopkins Press, 1961.
48. GREENSON, R.: *The technique and practice of psychoanalysis*, Vol. 1. New York, International Universities Press, 1967.
49. MILLER, D.: The ethics of practice in adolescent psychiatry. *American Journal of Psychiatry* **134**:420–22, 1977.
50. KARASU, T. B.: General principles of psychotherapy, in *Specialized techniques in individual psychotherapy*. Ed. Karasu, T. B and Bellak, L. New York, Brunner/Mazel, 1980.
51. LONDON, P.: *Behaviour control*. New York, Harper and Row, 1969.
52. STRUPP, H.: On the technology of psychotherapy, in *Psychotherapy and behaviour change, 1972*. Ed. Marks, I. M., Bergin, A. E., Lang, P. J. *et al*. Chicago, Aldine, 1973, 3–27.
53. GOLDBERG, C.: *Therapeutic partnership: ethical concerns in psychotherapy*. New York, Springer, 1977.
54. MYERHOFF, B. G. and LARSON, W. R.: The doctor as culture hero: The routinization of charisma. *Human Organization* **24**:188–91, 1965.
55. PARSONS, T.: Social structure and dynamic process: The case of modern medical practice, in *The social system*. Glencoe, Free Press, 1951, 428–79.
56. BURLING, T., LENTZ, E. M., and WILSON, R. N.: *Give and take in hospitals: a study of human organization*. New York, Putnam, 1956.
57. YALOM, I. D.: *Encounter groups and psychiatry*. Task Force Report, American Psychiatric Association, Washington, DC, 1970.

58. GOLDBERG, C.: *Encounter: group sensitivity training experience.* New York, Science House, 1970.

59. OFFENKRANTZ, W. and TOBIN, A: Psychoanalytic psychotherapy. *Archives of General Psychiatry* **30**:593–606, 1974.

60. KRASNER, L: The therapist as a social reinforcement machine, in *Research in psychotherapy,* Vol. 2. Ed. Strupp, H. and Luborsky, L. Washington, DC, American Psychological Association, 1962, 61–94.

61. BANDURA, A: The ethics and social purposes of behaviour modification, in *Annual review of behaviour therapy theory and practice,* Vol. 3. Ed. Franks, C. M. and Wilson, G. T. New York, Brunner/Mazel, 1975, 13–20.

62. HALLECK, S.: Legal and ethical aspects of behaviour control. *American Journal of Psychiatry.* **131**:381–7, 1974.

63. GOLDIAMOND, I.: Toward a constructional approach to social problems: Ethical and constitutional problems raised by applied behaviour analysis, in *Annual review of behaviour therapy theory and practice,* Vol. 3. Ed. Franks, C. M. and Wilson, G. T. New York, Brunner/Mazel, 1975, 21–63.

64. Commentary: Ethical and related issues in behaviour therapy, in *Annual review of behaviour therapy theory and practice,* Vol. 3 Ed. Franks, C. M. and Wilson, G. T. New York, Brunner/Mazel, 1975.

65. CASTIGLIONE, A: *A history of medicine.* New York, Alfred A. Knopf, 1947.

66. DUBEY, J.: Confidentiality as a requirement of the therapist: Technical necessities for absolute privilege in psychotherapy. *American Journal of Psychiatry* **131**: 1093–6, 1974.

67. PLAUT, E. A.: A perspective on confidentiality. *American Journal of Psychiatry* **131**: 1021–4, 1974.

68. BLOCH, D. A.: Family therapy, group therapy. *International Journal of Group Psychotherapy* **26**:289–99, 1976.

69. Tarasoff vs the Regents of the University of California, 118 California Reporter 129, 529, P 2d 553, 1974.

70. ROTH, L. H. and MEISEL, A.: Dangerousness, confidentiality, and the duty to warn. *American Journal of Psychiatry* **134**:508–11, 1977.

71. GUREVITZ, H.: Tarasoff: Protective privilege versus public peril. *American Journal of Psychiatry* **134**:289–92, 1977.

72. BRACELAND, F. J.: Historical perspectives of the ethical practice of psychiatry. *American Journal of Psychiatry* **126**:230–7, 1969.

73. DAHLBERG, C.: Sexual contact between patient and therapist. *Contemporary Psychoanalysis* **6**:107–24, 1970.

74. TRUAX, C. B. and MITCHELL, K. M.: Research on certain therapist interpersonal skills in relation to process and outcome, in *Handbook of psychotherapy and behaviour change: an empirical analysis.* Ed. Bergin, A. E. and Garfield, S. L. New York, Wiley, 1971, 299–344.

75. CHESLER, P: *Women and madness.* Garden City, Doubleday, 1972.

76. KARDENER, S., FULLER, M., and MENSH, I.: A survey of physicians' attitudes and practices regarding erotic and non-erotic contact with patients. *American Journal of Psychiatry* **130**:1077–81, 1973.

77. BUTLER, S.: Sexual contact between therapists and patients, doctoral dissertation, California School of Professional Psychology, Los Angeles, 1975.

78. ROBERTIELLO, R.: Iatrogenic psychiatric illness. *Journal of Contemporary Psychotherapy* **7**:3–8, 1975.

79. STONE, M.: Management of unethical behaviour in a psychiatric hospital staff. *American Journal of Psychotherapy* **29**:391–401, 1975.

80. MARMOR, J.: Some psychodynamic aspects of the seduction of patients in psychotherapy. Presented at the 129th Annual Meeting, American Psychiatric Association, Miami Beach, Fla., May 10–14, 1976.

81. STONE, A. A.: The legal implications of sexual activity between psychiatrist and patient. *American Journal of Psychiatry* **133**:1138–41, 1976.
82. MASTERS, W. H. and JOHNSON, V. E.: Principles of the new sex therapy. *American Journal of Psychiatry* **133**:548–54, 1976.
83. ROMAN, M., CHARLES, E., and KARASU, T. B.: The value system of psychotherapists and changing mores. *Psychotherapy: Theory, Research and Practice* **15**:409–15, 1978.
84. LEVY, R. B.: *I can only touch you now*. Englewood Cliffs, Prentice-Hall, 1973.B
85. PATTISON, J. E.: Effects of touch on self-exploration and the therapeutic relationship. *Journal of Consulting and Clinical Psychology* **40**: 170–5, 1973.
86. HOLROYD, J. C. and BRODSKY, A. M.: Psychologists' attitudes and practices regarding erotic and nonerotic physical contact with patients. *American Psychologist* **32**:843–9, 1977.
87. TAYLOR, B. J. and WAGNER, N. N.: Sex between therapists and clients: A review and analysis. *Professional Psychology* **7**:593–601, 1976.
88. RICE, J. K. and RICE, D. G.: Implications of the Women's Liberation Movement for psychotherapy. *American Journal of Psychiatry* **130**: 191–6, 1973.
89. SEIDEN, A. M.: Overview: Research on the psychology of women. 11. Women in families, work, and psychotherapy. *American Journal of Psychiatry* **133**: 1111–23, 1976.
90. BROVERMAN, I. K., BROVERMAN, D. M., CLARKSON, F. E. *et al*: Sex-role stereotypes and clinical judgements of mental health. *Journal of Consulting and Clinical Psychology* **34**:1–7, 1970.
91. SEIDEN, A., BENEDEK, E., WOLMAN, C. *et al*: Survey of women's status in psychiatric education. A report of the APA Task Force on Women. Presented at the 127th Annual Meeting of the American Psychiatric Association, Detroit, May 6–10, 1974.
92. JONSEN, A. R. and HELLEGERS, A. E.: Conceptual foundations for an ethics of medical care, in *Ethics of health care*. Ed. Tancredi, L. Washington, DC, National Academy of Sciences, 1974, 3–21.
93. ZITRIN, A. and KLEIN, H.: Can psychiatry police itself effectively? The experience of one district branch. *American Journal of Psychiatry* **133**:653–6, 1976.
94. SULLIVAN, F. W.: Peer review and professional ethics. *American Journal of Psychiatry* **134**:186–8, 1977.
95. KLEIN, H.: Current peer review system bound to fail. *Psychiatric News*, 16 July, 1975.
96. CHODOFF, P. and SANTORA, P.: Psychiatric peer review: The DC experience, 1972–75. *American Journal of Psychiatry* **134**:121–5, 1977.
97. NEWMAN, D. E. and LUFT, L. L.: The peer review process: Education versus control. *American Journal of Psychiatry* **131**:1363–6, 1974.
98. BERNAL, Y. and DEL RIO V: Psychiatric ethics, in *Comprehensive textbook of psychiatry*. Ed. Freedman, A. M. and Kaplan, H. I. Baltimore, Williams and Wilkins, 1967, pp. 2543–52.

7

Ethical Aspects of Drug Treatment

Gerald Klerman and Gail Schechter

CONCERN over the effects of drugs on the human mind and behaviour and the medical, social, and ethical implications of their use are among the oldest preoccupations of mankind. Almost every society has developed potions, brews, and remedies capable of changing behaviour, normal as well as disturbed; and they have been used from the times of the oldest civilizations in the ancient Middle East, in ancient Greece, and in the cultures of South America and the Orient. Scientific interest in drugs in Western society began in the middle of the nineteenth century, and psychopharmacology emerged as a distinct scientific discipline after the discovery of the mind-alerting effects of LSD by Hoffman in 1947 and the synthesis of chlor-promazine in the early 1950s by French pharmacologists.

Psychopharmacology is the scientific study of the effects of drugs on the mind, behaviour and mood. These drugs are variously called 'psychoactive' or 'psychotropic'. Clinically, the development of psychotropic drugs was a significant contributor to the revolution in mental health care in the 1950s. Scientifically, efforts to relate the psychological and behavioural effects of psychotropic drugs to brain mechanisms have generated valuable research in the fields of neurochemistry, neurophysiology, neurobiology, and experimental psychology. In both clinical and research arenas, enormous strides in understanding have occurred in a short period of history. In the past three decades, the pace of development of psychotropic drugs has accelerated, and dozens of new compounds have been developed. Depending on the purpose for which drugs are used, they can be separated into two groups: therapeutic or non-therapeutic.

Therapeutic agents include drugs for the treatment of psychosis, depression, mania, and anxiety. Non-therapeutic drugs are used for recreation and personal enjoyment. Included in this group are alcohol, cocaine, marijuana, hallucinogens like LSD, psilocybin and mescaline, and opiates such as morphine and heroin. These drugs have in common the capacity to alter normal mood in a way that subjects find pleasurable, although they may be therapeutically useful in certain clinical conditions such as terminal cancer; they are not directly relevant to the treatment of defined mental illness.

The widespread use of psychotropic drugs — both therapeutic and non-therapeutic — raises a number of ethical issues. In discussing these issues it is valuable to distinguish between questions involving scientific knowledge and those involving value judgements. The scientific aspects are especially important in medical and psychiatric treatment where the major questions are the effectiveness of these drugs and their side-effects and dangers. Corollary questions are: 'Which drug is best for which disorder?' and 'What is the appropriate way of using the drug?' All these questions lend themselves to empirical investigation, and are thus possible of resolution by scientific methods. The questions involving value judgements, however, are more difficult to resolve; they range from whether or not to prescribe drugs at all to how much and under what conditions they should be used. An important question with both clinical and ethical implications concerns the relationship between the benefits conferred by drugs and the damage they may do.

In this chapter our focus is on the ethical issues raised by the therapeutic and non-therapeutic use of psychotropic drugs; we give attention to both value and scientific aspects as appropriate.

Cost–benefit ratio and informed consent

Ethical questions in psychopharmacology currently receiving a great deal of attention are the rights of a patient to accept or refuse medication and the allied issue of informed consent. When considering the prescribing of psychotropic drugs, the question of the patient's right to make free choices becomes immediately relevant. It involves not only the right to treatment and right to correct treatment, but also the right to refuse treatment. Recently, efforts to affirm the right of a psychiatric patient to participate in the decision regarding his treatment have intensified, particularly in the United States. Patients as well as civil rights advocates have succeeded not only in focusing greater attention on this issue but also in testing it in the courts. The patient ideally should have: the right to accept or refuse medication; the right to give informed consent prior to use of any medication; the right to have a voice in choosing the drug; and the right to decide under what conditions to take the drug.

Controlled clinical trials provide overwhelming evidence that psychotropic drugs are extremely effective in the treatment of many mental disorders. However, they are not without risk of serious side-effects and they bear the potential for physical and psychological addiction. Because of the current state of knowledge about psychotropic drugs, the psychiatrist, in certain instances, may experience great difficulty in coming to a decision as to whether particular medication is indicated, and this will be even more true for the patient concerned. A brief consideration of tardive dyskinesia will serve to illustrate. When the phenothiazine drugs were first introduced, little was known about their potential side-effects. Soon clinical observation began to show a number of severe side-effects, of which the most notable are repetitive, involuntary, choreoathetoid movements involving the lips, tongue, mouth, trunk, and limbs, the condition labelled tardive dyskinesia. Information about it is at present limited, sometimes contradictory.[1] Of unknown incidence, its prevalence in chronic mental hospital patients has been reported to range from 0.5 per cent to 40 per cent. There is no clear evidence at present concerning the course of the condition: it is likely to be non-progressive, severe cases are probably infrequent, and it is probably irreversible in some patients, particularly among the elderly who have been on anti-psychotic medication for a prolonged period. The treatment of tardive dyskinesia is unsatisfactory: safe, effective, and specific remedies are lacking. The clinician must also face the uncomfortable possibility that its presence may be masked by the very drug which is responsible for its occurrence.

In the face of this confusion, how should the clinician decide about prescribing a psychotropic drug in the case, say, of a schizophrenic patient? On the one hand antipsychotic drugs have proven their worth in the management of schizophrenic conditions; on the other hand, a side-effect such as tardive dyskinesia is a real and serious possibility in any patient receiving these drugs. It is clear that in addition to clinical-scientific considerations, complex ethical questions are also involved. Two principles, at least, can be applied to the situation. First, the psychiatrist is duty-bound to be as informed as he possibly can about the advantages and disadvantages of the drugs he prescribes. Thus, for example, he should be entirely familiar with what is known about tardive dyskinesia and other serious side-effects; he should keep abreast of current research and be well equipped to appraise critically any new data. This principle of acting only on the basis of carefully evaluated information may be all too obvious, but is unfortunately not always adhered to. The second principle is based on the ancient medical dictum: *Primum non nocere* — the principle of least harm. Any decision to use a psychotropic drug must pass a critical test — that the benefits to the patient are likely to outweigh the hazards. As we have seen earlier, this test can prove extremely difficult and it demands clinical judgement of the highest medical standard.

Furthermore, it is not sufficient for the psychiatrist to be aware of the risks and benefits; the patient must also be informed. He should be given the necessary information even if complex, in order to reach a decision about whether to accept or refuse the recommended drug.

But this is true only to a certain point. For instance, can the patient, no matter how much information he is given, really appreciate the cost–benefit ratio for a side-effect like tardive dyskinesia? It could even be argued that we do the patient a disservice when we provide him with a large amount of information, not all of it scientifically proved. He may well become confused rather than enlightened, and burdened with an even more difficult decision about whether to accept or refuse treatment.

The issue of informed consent is complicated enough in the case of the patient who is capable of comprehending the information given to him. The problem is compounded in patients whose mental state precludes or at least interferes with such comprehension. The psychiatrist is then faced with an even more difficult dilemma. Under such circumstances he must determine, as accurately as he can, whether his patient can appreciate the nature and the consequences of the proposed treatment and so render an informed judgement about its use. Can a severely disturbed patient choose his treatment rationally when his defect in cognitive and emotional functioning limits his capacity to make truly free and informed decisions? The thorny problem presents itself: under what circumstances should patients lose this right and come under the paternalistic umbrella of the therapist? Should the committed patient, for example, have the power to decide about his treatment? Can we assume automatically that we have a duty to prescribe medication we consider necessary in any patient who has already lost his basic right, the right to liberty, because he is regarded as too disordered to arrive at an informed judgement? (see Chapter 11).

Many psychiatrists argue that the current strong emphasis on the patient's civil rights does not adequately take into account his urgent clinical needs. These psychiatrists assert that patients' rights are not necessarily the same as their needs and indeed that they may be in conflict. Although in practice patients usually agree with their psychiatrists' recommendations regarding treatment, the issue of the right to privacy versus clinical needs remains a cogent ethical matter. In particular the question revolves around the committed patient's right to refuse treatment, usually medication. Two recent important legal decisions — in the States of Massachusetts and New Jersey — argue for the right to refuse. In the first case,[2] seven patients sued their psychiatrists and called for a ban on forced medication (and seclusion) for themselves and fellow patients at Boston State Hospital. The court ruled, in the patients' favour, that involuntary commitment to a psychiatric institution is not automatically a judgement of incompetence: the committed patient retains a wide range of basic rights such as to marry, vote, or make a will. The court disagreed with the defendants' argument that the State must act as *parens patriae* for patients who are incompetent and make decisions about treatment on their behalf. Most patients, Judge Tauro concluded, were able 'to appreciate the benefits, risks and discomfort that may reasonably be expected from receiving psychotropic medication'. If a psychiatrist feels it necessary to treat a patient forcibly, it is the court's responsibility to judge on the patient's ability to provide informed consent and to appoint a guardian to decide about treatment should the patient be found incompetent to do so.

The New Jersey finding[3] is based on a similar right to privacy but differs in how the problem of the incompetent patient is dealt with. Again, the potency and 'harsh side-effects' of psychotropic drugs are emphasized, with the patient accorded the right to exert control over their administration. The patient's rights are in the New Jersey ruling to be protected by an independent psychiatrist at an informal hearing; the patient may also be represented by counsel.

These legal developments are concerned with the crux of the current debate about involuntary medication among psychiatrists, who argue that the patient's clinical state is the paramount consideration and civil rights advocates, who regard the patient's rights as more important. Thomas Gutheil[4] argues the 'clinical' case with considerable conviction. For him, the pendulum has swung too far in the 'legal' direction — 'The way is paved for patients to "rot with their rights on" ' — and he would like to see a redress of the imbalance so that equal weight is given to the therapeutic dimension. He has also attempted to demonstrate, through case examples, that the guardianship approach to involuntary medication, acceptable in theory, is unworkable in clinical practice.[5]

Roth[6] has also highlighted the critical problems generated by the recent United States court judgements, and offered his own remedy. 'The issue of the committed patient's right to refuse customary treatment should be adjudicated at the commitment hearing itself'. The commitment order could then validly authorize the psychiatrist to treat the patient without his consent if necessary.

Whatever solutions are offered for the knotty problem of involuntary medication, it is clear that the inherent ethical dilemma will face psychiatry for a long time to come.

Psychotropic drugs and the boundaries of mental illness

There has been a trend in recent years in some psychiatric quarters to widen the definition of mental illness. It is useful to consider the movement from mental illness to mental health along a continuum: three main areas can be distinguished (see Fig. 7.1). The first area

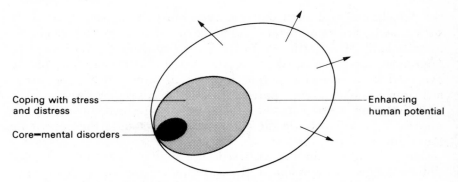

Fig. 7.1. Boundaries between mental illness and mental health.

includes the core mental disorders such as schizophrenia and affective illness. The most recent edition of the American Psychiatric Association's *Diagnostic and statistical manual of mental disorders* (DSM-III)[7] defines a mental disorder as a:

clinical significant behavioural or psychological syndrome or pattern that occurs in an individual and that is typically associated with either a painful symptom (distress) or impairment in one or more important areas of functioning (disability). In addition, there is an inference that there is a behavioural, psychological or biological dysfunction and that the disturbance is not only in the relationship between the individual and society. When the disturbance is limited to a conflict between an individual and society, this may represent social deviance, which may or may not be commendable, but is not by itself a mental disorder.

The second area encompasses mental health problems involving significant amounts of psychological and emotional distress associated with the stress of daily life but that do not meet the criteria for a diagnosable mental disorder. The third area includes people who do not see themselves as mentally ill but who seek to enhance their own potential, heighten their awareness, or improve their mental health.

The use of psychotropic drugs becomes increasingly problematic as we move from the core to the outermost area and thus raises certain ethical questions. Both scientific evidence as to the efficacy of treatment and the social mandate condoning medical intervention are clearest in cases of the definable mental disorder.

The blurring of boundaries between mental illness and mental health is most evident in the middle area of life stress which produces distress. Here, considerable debate exists about whether changes in emotional state such as depressed mood, anger, or increased anxiety should be defined as mental illness and be treated with drugs. Since this middle area encompasses a wide range of situations from life crises such as divorce or bereavement to the anxiety and tension associated with the routine stress of daily life, it is important to determine which of them will benefit from drug intervention. In the United States, in an effort to reduce the indiscriminate use of tranquillizers, the Food and Drug Administration has persuaded some drug manufacturers to warn physicians that psychotropic drugs are not indicated to relieve the stress and 'blues' of everyday life. This move comes in the wake of a growing reliance on tranquillizing and antidepressant drugs by a public which seems unwilling to 'suffer' distressing emotions and is prone to regard every unpleasant feeling state as a symptom and indicative of mental disorder. As Carstairs[8] puts it: 'Everyone nowadays expects to be happy. What is more, if anyone feels unhappy, he immediately thinks that something must be wrong either with him or with the state of the world, if not both.'

The diagnostic blur is particularly well illustrated with depression; there is no sharp boundary between normal mood and clinical depression warranting therapeutic intervention. Feelings of sadness, disappointment, and frustration are obviously a normal aspect of the human condition, and careful assessment and diagnosis is essential before prescribing medication. Recent research[9] indicates that only a proportion of patients with depressive symptoms meet the criteria for a depressive syndrome.

Elsewhere in this book, Philip Graham (see Chapter 13) has discussed the controversy over the drug treatment of children given the diagnosis of Hyperkinetic Syndrome. Here is another prime example of diagnostic blurring in relation to drug use. Methylphenidate and dexamphetamine sulphate have been found to diminish hyper-activity, distractability, impulsivity, and lack of persistence[10] — but it still remains uncertain whether these features together *actually* constitute a psychiatric syndrome, or whether a medical label has been conveniently applied to a social problem, thus facilitating the use of medical treatment.[11] Even if we were able to state definitively that the Hyperkinetic Syndrome is a distinct clinical entity, the potential for the abuse of methylphenidate and dexamphetamine sulphate would still be considerable; it is obviously tempting for some parents, teachers, and medical practitioners to 'medicalize' behavioural problems in children as evidence of illness. Thus, the 'difficult to manage' child in the classroom or at home becomes a psychiatric patient who needs medication.

Because of the imprecise nature of psychiatric diagnosis, as in the case of the Hyperkinetic Syndrome, the possibility always exists, particularly in psychiatric hospitals and in prisons, that 'awkward', 'unruly', 'troublesome', and 'difficult' people may be prescribed psychotropic drugs in the absence of diagnosable mental illness. The question then arises: in whose interest is the drug being given — the recipient's, the staff's, the institution's, other patients' or inmates'? Is the drug serving as a chemical restraint, as a form of social control? Many an inquiry on psychiatric hospital and prison practices, both formal and informal, suggests that psychotropic drugs have been given to deal with patients or inmates who threaten, act aggressively, fail to co-operate, or break institutional rules, and on occasion also as a punitive measure so as to prevent future disturbance.

It is helpful when considering the ethical implications of drug use in these circumstances to regard aggressive behaviour — verbal or physical — as merely a presenting feature and not as a clinical condition in its own right. Thus 'difficult' behaviour is not an indication for a drug unless it is a manifestation of some underlying psychiatric state: we should only prescribe drugs to treat the proved or probable (i.e. highly suspected) cause of aggression rather than treat the aggression *per se*. Obviously it is required of the clinician to attempt to make as accurate a diagnosis as possible when he encounters a patient who is 'difficult' or non-co-operative. Without this delineation of diagnosis and aetiology, we come perilously close to drug misuse and ethically questionable behaviour.

Does this approach mean that psychotropic drugs cannot be utilized at all for, say, a highly aggressive patient in a psychiatric ward who has committed some violent act or threatens to do so, and in whom the underlying cause of his behaviour is not established? An absolute position here is probably inappropriate — it depends greatly on the consequences of the aggression for that patient, his fellow patients, and the staff treating him. It could be argued that the interests of all parties are safeguarded if the aggressive patient is becalmed: others are protected from possible harm and injury and the patient himself is spared the likelihood of becoming alienated, even ostracized, from his social group on the ward. Prompt efforts to reduce the antisocial behaviour may thus help to facilitate the re-acceptance of the patient by both his peers and staff. But a caveat is in order: if at all possible drugs should still be avoided and psychological and social measures applied as appropriate; if a drug is regarded as essential, it should be given in close association with psychosocial therapeutic intervention. It is only too obvious that giving drugs in the above situation tends to be simpler and less demanding of time and effort than alternative methods, and therefore more attractive to a staff, which if under pressure and frustrated, seeks to restore institutional order as efficiently as possible.

The over-medicated society

The issue of what is a clinical symptom and therefore, possibly amenable to treatment with psychotropic drugs, overlaps with another issue which can conveniently be labelled as the over-medicated society.[12] This refers to the widespread tendency to rely on drugs in order to cope with life's vicissitudes. Ultimately we are dealing with philosophical and even religious criteria to determine what constitutes 'the good life': a far cry from the psychiatrist's office and his diagnostic manual.

Perhaps the minor tranquillizers when used as anti-anxiety agents best epitomize the over-medicated society. In the United States, they account for about one-half of all psychotropic drug prescriptions — over 75 million prescriptions each year, and the number is growing. Diazepam has achieved the dubious distinction of being America's most prescribed drug.

As the extent of the use of drugs like Diazepam has increased, so have expressions of concern by various groups — among them patients themselves, women, and physicians — about the possible abuse of chemical agent in order to cope with stress and distress. Some social critics have claimed that medical practices and forces in the pharmaceutical marketplace contribute to the abuse of psychotherapeutic drugs. Muller,[13] in a review of economic factors possibly associated with over-medication, points out how the increase in the number of prescriptions is the product of the converging interests of drug manufacturers, doctors, pharmacists, and others.

Lennard and his colleagues[14] go as far as to accuse the pharmaceutical industry and medical profession of the practice of mystification through their collusive redefinition of an increasing number of human and personal problems as medical, and thus appropriate for drug intervention. They note the variety of problems that previously were viewed as falling within the orbit of the normal trials and tribulations of human life and which are now labelled as medical or psychiatric.

Illich[15] has been a particularly strong critic of the medical profession, arguing that it undermines health and contributes to the 'medicalization of life'. More specifically in relation to drugs, he alleges that Western society has fallen prey to the 'pharmaceutical invasion': the current over-consumption of medical agents is part of the over-expansion of medicine. Although Illich's arguments tend to be exaggerated many of his points have merit. Certainly, the traditional therapeutic relationship is hierarchical and authoritative; the physician is dominant, the patient submissive and compliant. The expectation is that the doctor will act in his patient's best interests; but is this always so? Have doctors, including psychiatrists, been influenced by various forces such as those mentioned above, to regard more and more personal and social problems as falling within their sphere, and have they in turn reshaped their patients' perceptions about 'distress of living' into medical symptoms in need of medication? Thus, the isolated, overburdened housewife with three young kids in an urban high-rise flat, perhaps lacking her husband's support, becomes a case of 'depressive neurosis' in need of antidepressant medication. Or the young executive, determined and ambitious, and working under great pressure, most of it stemming from his own needs, becomes the 'anxiety neurotic', to be treated with tranquillizers.

Are physicians too ready to prescribe pills and patients too ready to consume them? Indeed, many patients expect to receive a psychotropic drug and are disappointed if their physician doubts their necessity and does not offer relief for their distress, in pill form. This expectation is heightened by persuasive advertising which proclaims that drugs ease a variety of problems of living such as stress at work or leaving home to attend college. So, the issue is not only what the medical practitioner does to his patients, but also what patients do to themselves. The important ethical question is whether the doctor, insufficiently aware of his tendency to 'medicalize' (perhaps through ignorance but more likely because prescribing a drug is easier than offering psychotherapy or solving major problems of society), fails via his prescription pad to act in his patient's best interests.

In part, we are brought back to the issue of informed consent, discussed earlier in this chapter. The medical practitioner's growing tendency to 'medicalize' and to turn too readily to the 'psychotropics' could be checked if he offered his patient accurate information about the use of these drugs including an account of their benefits and a cautionary word about their risks — of side-effects and dependence. This act in itself would soon remind the doctor that antidepressants and anti-anxiety agents have a relatively minor role to play in the management of problems which are more social in nature.

The doctor may indeed find himself pressed into providing this information by the rising tide of consumerism which appears to be lapping at his door. The contemporary consumer movement has helped to raise the public's consciousness about what constitutes fair, safe, and ethical practice in the professional relationship. The health field has, together with many other professional spheres, not escaped this intensified public scrutiny. Although it may come as a shock to some doctors when they are severely criticized by consumer advocates like Ralph Nader and Martin Gross,[16] the long-term effect on their practice is likely to be salutary. With regard to medication, patients may become less prepared to accept unquestionably prescriptions for psychotropic drugs, and may request full justification for their use in terms of appropriateness, effectiveness, and safety.

Ethical issues in the use of non-therapeutic drugs

Our discussion of the over-medicated society paves the way for consideration of the ethical issues relevant to the use by a significant proportion of society of non-therapeutic drugs. The psychiatrist is obliged to consider what attitude, both clinical and ethical, he should have to this form of drug use.

Many drugs — alcohol, tobacco, marijuana, and hallucinogens among them — are used solely for recreation and personal pleasure or to enhance intellectual, emotional, social, and sexual functioning. It is perhaps indicative of society's ambivalence to these compounds that no generally agreed-upon term exists for this use of psychotropic drugs. They are not considered therapeutic by psychiatrists, and are not prescribed by them in the treatment of defined mental disorders or psychological distress. Rather they have in common the capacity to alter a person's normal emotional state in a way that he finds pleasurable, and which usually leads him to seek repeated experience with them.

Veatch[17] believes that a fundamental aspect of the use of chemical agents to influence behaviour, mood, or experience is the challenge it poses to the world view of the person taking the drug and to the value system of the social group to which he belongs. Perhaps the most salient ethical issue in this context is that of personal freedom versus social regulation. Should a person have the right to do what he wishes to himself, in this instance the right to use any drug he pleases? Does the State have the right to regulate which drugs may be used and under what conditions?

These questions can be examined in a general way by considering two main value orientations, suitably labelled as 'pharmacological Calvinism' and 'psychotropic hedonism'.[18] Until recently, Western society has been dominated by a form of Calvinism that views drugs with distrust and believes that 'if a drug makes you feel good, it must be morally bad'; abstinence is the ideal. The current widespread use of psychotropics, according to the Calvinistic ethic, reflects society's increasing reliance on them to deal with the tensions and frustrations of everyday life. It is argued that this trend has undesirable consequences — principally, the erroneous belief that 'popping pills' offers a ready solution to complex personal and social problems (which should be faced through reliance on insight, will-power, and purposeful action) and that there is a potential danger of physical harm and of addiction, which outweigh any possible benefits.

Moreover, the harmful effects, it is feared, are not only on the adult drug-takers themselves but also on their children who, noting their parents' practices, accept such behaviour as a model for their own use of drugs. The ultimate concern, however, is not so much about the hazards to health or about the indirect stimulus to drug abuse among youth, but rather about basic moral degeneration: that the moral fibre of society is undermined by the inappropriate taking of drugs.

While pharmacological Calvinism still represents a dominant value in our society, it has undergone considerable erosion in recent years. One important factor in this erosion is the inconsistency that results from the exemption from prohibition of several widely used psychotropic substances. Alcohol and tobacco are clearly not taboo drugs despite the well-established facts that they are extremely hazardous and highly addictive.

Another factor derives from advertising: the commercialization of drug terminology and its incorporation into the mass media. As we noted earlier, the pharmaceutical industry has endeavoured to expand its market by extending the rationale for drug-taking to include relief of minor emotional symptoms related to stress. The industry has also sought to reduce the stigma attached to the use of psychotropic drugs in its advertisements by depicting those who take them as attractive and 'normal', rather than as deviant and abnormal. Furthermore, there has been an implicit promise that drugs will not only relieve symptoms but also enhance happiness, intelligence, sexual pleasure — in other words — the quality of life.

The most serious challenge to pharmacological Calvinism, however, stems from a notable contemporary youth culture and its adherence to a system of values embraced in the term 'psychotropic hedonism'. This sub-group culture (obviously we are not referring to all young people; the extent of the youth culture under consideration is difficult to estimate) distrusts the authority of adults with regard to drugs; increasingly incorporates drugs into its ethos; and sees drug taking as consistent with its hedonistic views.[19] In some ways, the current conflict harks back to the tensions between Dionysian and Apollonian values in ancient Greece. The cult of Dionysius emphasized pleasure and the use of drugs, including alcohol, to attain states of ecstasy and mysticism. There is a similar emphasis on pleasure in today's youth culture together with a tendency to devalue achievement and to be intolerant of delay in gratification. Professional and other achievement is less important than pleasurable experience in the immediacy of the moment. This world view contains a role for drugs such as marijuana, tobacco, and tranquillizers to enhance personal satisfaction and in no sense is their use seen as immoral. After all, if science and technology can produce a hydrogen bomb or propel man to the moon, why cannot chemistry make us all happy, serene, sexually potent, brilliant, and ageless?

These two opposing systems of values *vis-à-vis* drug taking are reflected in the ambivalence of society to adopt a consistent attitude to the taking of non-therapeutic drugs. Tobacco and alcohol are freely available and the State recoups enormous tax revenues from their use, whereas hallucinogens, coccaine, and marijuana — arguably less dangerous substances — are outlawed. The continuing intense debate in several Western countries over whether marijuana should be legalized illustrates sharply the complexity of the issues involved, in relation to health hazards and ethics. The psychiatric profession not surprisingly finds it difficult to speak with one voice on the questions of social regulation and individual freedom regarding non-therapeutic drug taking. Perhaps the questions are more appropriately directed to society as a whole (with the psychiatrist offering his opinion if he wishes, as one of its members); psychiatry has often been seduced in the past to proclaim its views on an issue which is realistically beyond its expertise and, as a result, has displayed muddled thinking and an obvious lack of authoritativeness. More appropriate a task for the profession is the diligent pursuit of scientific research in the subject of non-therapeutic drugs and the responsible dissemination of the results.

Conclusion

The last three decades have seen a rapid development in psychopharmacology. The discovery of psychotropic drugs with a wide range of therapeutic applications as well as with the capacity to enhance personal pleasure has had and will continue to have profound ethical implications. The psychiatrist, caught up in the midst of this development, has a central role to play in ensuring that while the therapeutic potential of psychotropic drugs is fulfilled, the ethical factors are kept under close and careful scrutiny.

References

1. GARDOS, G. and COLE J. O.: Overview: public health issues in tardive dyskinesia. *American Journal of Psychiatry* **137**:776-81, 1980.
2. ROGERS V., OKIN, Civil Action 75–1601 — T (1979).
3. RENNIE V., KLEIN, 462 F. Supp. 1131 (1978).
4. GUTHEIL, T.: In search of true freedom: Drug refusal, involuntary medication, and "rotting with your rights on". *American Journal of Psychiatry* **137**:327–8, 1980.
5. GUTHEIL, T., SHAPIRO, R., and ST. CLAIR, L.: Legal guardianship in drug refusal: An illusory solution. *American Journal of Psychiatry* **137**:347–51, 1980.
6. ROTH, L.: Mental health commitment: The state of the debate, 1980. *Hospital and Community Psychiatry* **31**:385–96, 1980.

7. *Diagnostic and statistical manual of mental disorders*. 3rd ed. Washington DC, American Psychiatric Association, 1980.
8. CARSTAIRS, G. M.: A land of lotus-eaters? *American Journal of Psychiatry* **125**:1576–80, 1969.
9. WEISSMAN, M. M. and MYERS J. K.: Rates and risks of depressive symptoms in a United States urban community *Acta psychiatrica scandinavica* **57**:219–31, 1978.
10. WENDER, P.: *Minimal brain dysfunction in children*. New York, Wiley Interscience, 1971.
11. BOSCO, J. J. and ROBINS, S. S. (ed.): *The hyperactive child and stimulant drugs*. Chicago, Chicago University Press, 1976.
12. KLERMAN, G. L.: Are we an overmedicated society? Annual Meeting of the American Psychiatric Association, Detroit, May 1974.
13. MULLER, C.: The overmedicated society: Forces in the market-place for medical care. *Science, New York* **176**:488–92, 1972.
14. LENNARD, H. L., EPSTEIN, L. J., BERNSTEIN, A., et al: Hazards implicit in prescribing psychoactive drugs. *Science, New York* **169**:438–41, 1970.
15. ILLICH, I.: *Medical nemesis: the expropriation of health*. New York, Pantheon, 1976.
16. GROSS, M. L.: *The psychological society*. New York, Random House, 1980.
17. VEATCH, R. M.: Drugs and competing drug ethics. *Hastings Centre Report* **4**:68–80, 1974.
18. KLERMAN, G. L.: Psychotropic hedonism versus pharmacological Calvinism. *Hastings Centre Report* **2**:1–3, 1972.
19. LASCH, C.: *The culture of narcissism*. New York, Norton, 1979.

8

Ethical aspects of the physical manipulation of the brain

Harold Merskey

In this chapter, I base my discussion of ethical issues in the physical manipulation of the brain upon some current attitudes which can be summarized in a banal way as follows:

(1) Physicians advise and do not impose their advice except in special circumstances. Thus the treatment of individuals to save their lives or relieve their own distress is normally highly ethical but it may be unethical to impose any such treatment (even though legally allowed).

(2) Children and others in a condition which precludes them from deciding rationally may have decisions taken for them by people (usually their next of kin) who have appropriate concern for their interests and welfare.

(3) Physicians may ethically give some treatments to those people who come under Rule (2) but the types of treatment which may be given require careful scrutiny and the status and motives of the other person who makes the decision require careful assessment.

(4) Ethical actions may or may not be sanctioned by law. Physicians normally do not consider themselves bound to pursue ethical treatments for the patient's benefit if they are forbidden to do so by law. (But a difficult situation arises, for example, with physicians who wish to treat injured persons in secret when police forces or other security agencies are pursuing.)

(5) Coercive treatments for the benefit of a third party are unethical. (To say 'You must have this behaviour modification or drug or lobotomy which you do not want because otherwise we expect you to murder your mother' is not a medically ethical approach.)

(6) The treatment of individuals against their wishes to change them for the sake of the needs of society or a political system is even more repugnant to ethical physicians than the previous conditions.

(7) Patients may consent to treatment which benefits either them-

selves or others but there are peculiar difficulties in confirming the presence of 'free consent' in some circumstances.

These rules partly reflect ethical considerations and partly reflect practical problems. The latter as will shortly be seen are capable of solution.

Clinical cost–benefit ratios

There are three major types of physical manipulation of the brain, namely, electroconvulsive therapy; surgical ablation by scalpel or other technique which deliberately damages tissue; and the insertion of recording or stimulating electrodes, which is an advanced form of surgery. Each of these types of procedure has been attacked on many grounds and often ignorantly. The purpose of this discussion is to sketch the reasonable basis for their use, if any, in terms of medical ethics. In all cases much of the controversy turns upon the usefulness or otherwise of the procedure and the morbidity due to it. Those are necessary aspects for any physician to consider in regard to any treatment. They do not determine the ethical justification for the use of a treatment. The decision about whether a treatment is justified must always pass the test of a clinical judgement that the chance of benefit outweighs the hazards. If the chance of benefit is held to outweigh the risk of suffering or loss from the morbidity and mortality of the treatment the recommendation is ordinarily that the treatment be given. As every clinician knows these matters are often difficult to put in quantitative terms. If radical mastectomy for carcinoma of the breast gives, say, an 80 per cent chance of five-year survival (with a 10 per cent chance otherwise), and less than a 1 per cent chance of immediate operative death the calculation is fairly simple even though the operation also gives a near 100 per cent guarantee of some days of pain and discomfort to say the least. It is harder to decide how a thalamotomy for chronic pain with perhaps a 70 per cent chance of significant relief for 12 months can be evaluated in relation to a 20–30 per cent chance of some exacerbation of the pain and a 5 per cent chance of stroke or aphasia (which may also improve or partly remit). Nevertheless, carcinoma of the breast continued to be treated by radical mastectomy so long as odds of the order quoted existed and no other treatment offered better prospects, whilst thalamotomy has largely or wholly been discarded for pain (and not at all because it was an operation on the brain).

Thus procedures are assessed or remain in vogue on the basis of informed knowledge of what they can do for patients. If ECT is attacked on grounds of seeming barbaric because it incidentally causes convulsions that is an irrational view by comparison with the acceptance of surgery in which a breast may be mutilated or a larynx removed. Each procedure can be done for the benefit of the patient and, in the light of the information provided to him, he may ordinarily choose if the disadvantages are more or less than the advantages.

Refusal of general surgery

If the non-psychotic adult does not choose to have some general surgical operation, despite his knowledge of the risks, an operation is not pursued. One important practical reason is that patients who undergo operation without some degree of acceptance often do badly. The patient who fears his operation excessively is dreaded by the surgeon. Clinical lore holds that such patients suffer serious complications and often die. The attitude of the patient thus becomes a factor in the cost–benefit equation. If it were not so, surgeons might be tempted to press necessary operations upon patients more vigorously. Practical wisdom reinforces the ethical position of not doing things to patients who refuse consent.

The wisdom of not operating on the strongly unwilling individual applies to psychotic patients also. If they refuse some general surgical operation there is usually no more chance of their doing well with it than if they are sane. Children however, are treated differently. Johnnie, aged 7, may protest he does not want an urgent appendectomy. He may be forcibly anaesthetized against his strongest expressed wishes and physical resistance, the operation is done and he recovers nicely. It would take an unusual person, medical or lay, to maintain he should have been allowed to refuse although death was otherwise likely.

We can conclude that practical wisdom limits the frequency with which extra-cerebral operations are undertaken against the patient's wishes. Nevertheless, in some patients, who cannot decide for themselves, namely children, practice and feeling both hold that it is right to disregard the patient's wishes and wrong to accede to them where life or perhaps disability is at risk. Even John Stuart Mill so often quoted by those who argue against compulsory treatment, has the following to say about the right of the individual to take actions which might be harmful to his physical or moral health:

It is, perhaps, hardly necessary to say that this doctrine is meant to apply only to human beings in the full maturity of their faculties. We are not speaking of children, or of young persons below the age which the law may fix as that of manhood or womanhood. Those who are still in a state to require being taken care of by others must be protected against their own actions as well as against external injury.[1]

The unique status of the brain

When procedures are considered which affect the brain an important fresh consideration arises. Even if the patient can consent we have to ask if it is right to alter, probably irreversibly, the structure of the organ on which the patient's volition and power to decide about treatment is based. If he cannot consent or refuses to agree to treatment is it justified at all to override his wishes in such a way that one may physically abolish the structural elements of his brain which have enabled him to sustain his objection? In either case, with or without consent, would we be in the position of chopping off the hands not of a thief but of a man who has created a work of art which we do not like, or perhaps an idol of which we disapprove?

Many psychiatrists past the age of 50 have no difficulty with one aspect of the question which is easily answered for them on the basis of a particular experience. Although the operation of frontal leucotomy was probably over-used, and sometimes crudely practised, there was a time when ECT was sometimes not sufficient to cure all cases of severe endogenous depression and antidepressant drugs were not available. During those years from approximately 1945 to 1959 a number of patients in chronic misery from prolonged depressive illness of the endogenous (or unipolar type) accepted leucotomy. In well-selected cases the cost–benefit ratio was such that in the view of patients, family, and physician the operation was usually held to have been a substantial success. Formal reports testify that the procedure, and especially some of its later modifications had a worthwhile cost–benefit ratio.[2–8]

Men and women who were ill had accepted that their structurally normal brains could be cut into, and had recovered, resuming happy and effective lives. Before operation the mood of many of them was appalling and their judgement of life and events was often made irrational by that mood. They had still perhaps enough command of their thoughts to be able to make a valid decision about whether they would have an operation, and the consequences were beneficial for many of them. Yet the brain was the organ of decision as well as the site of operation. In principle and in practice there should be no difficulty with the proposition that it is acceptable to operate on the brain to relieve emotional discomfort provided that the patient is able to make a valid decision about the risks and advantages and provided of course that those risks are small enough and advantages large enough.

A more specific argument could also be offered. The part of the brain subjected to treatment may not be involved in decision-making. Hence that portion is open to operation on the same terms as a limb or abdominal viscus. I find this argument unattractive however because profound disturbances of mood usually affect judgement and it may be specious to say that the site of operation does not have a function in the process of making decisions. It is better to rely on the presence of feelings and of reasoning which validate consent.

Similar considerations apply to the use of ECT for depressive illness which has not responded to medication and which is of the type known to be likely to respond to treatment. If the patient is willing, there is no ethical problem about giving it. Hazards to life are minimal, any impairment of brain function is minimal or temporary, it is doubtful if any recognizable structural disturbance results from well-conducted courses of treatment (up to 12 ECT in a course), and therapeutic results are frequently dramatic.

This situation, however, represents the optimal circumstances from physical manipulation of the brain. The anticipated cost–benefit ratio is highly favourable, the risk to life is low, significant personality change is not an issue, the patients are suffering intensely, and they can reasonably expect good results and minimal disadvantages. More difficult problems arise with patients who refuse treatment, with patients whose illness may pervert their judgement, with patients whose treatment may be recommended for the sake of others because of their aggressive or other unacceptable behaviour, and with patients who are constrained by circumstances such as imprisonment so that their consent or agreement to treatment may be felt to be forced upon them in some way by conditions which others impose. Some of these major problems require consideration with respect to each type of physical manipulation of the brain.

Electroconvulsive therapy (ECT)

The status of ECT has been assessed in the valuable report of the American Psychiatric Association Task Force on the subject.[9] ECT is now mainly used for severe depression in which suicide is a major risk.[10,11] Occasional other firm indications include some forms of schizophrenia[9] and mania.[9] The risk to life is very small,[12] as little as 1 in 28000 treatments in one survey.[13] In five other reports the death-rate ranged from nil to 0.8 per cent of patients treated.[9] The treatment is both scientifically proved for depression and highly regarded clinically. Compared with drugs ECT is the more effective treatment for depression particularly psychotic depression.[14,15,9] ECT compared with mock ECT is highly effective according to one report.[16] A double-blind controlled trial which did not show a good result from ECT in depression[17] has been criticized as inadequate[18] and also as allowing a possible favourable interpretation.[19] Another blind trial[20]

favoured ECT against placebo although the treatment was complicated by the use of active medication in some of the subgroups.
Costello[21] who notes the failure of trials to be methodologically
perfect, recognizes that ECT produces unique effects on memory
which might not be mimicked by placebo so that a truly blind
controlled trial may be impossible to achieve.

Controlled trials are perhaps not necessary if the long known work
of Cronholm and Ottoson[22] is accepted. They showed a quantitative
relationship between the amount of epileptic discharge produced and
the remission of depression. This is probably the strongest evidence
available for the significance and effectiveness of the actual convul-
sion. More recently a consistent relationship has been shown between
the dose response ratio with ECT and the overall results.[23] This has
long been observed by practising psychiatrists gauging the response
to treatments and looking for the typical stepwise improvement in the
successful case.

The main complication of ECT is a temporary impairment of
memory. Objective tests of memory indicate that after a conventional course of treatment (six to twelve applications, either bilateral
or unilateral) ECT produces no detectable permanent loss of memory
for the one or two years preceding treatment and for a still earlier
period in the patient's life.[9] Memory is lost for some events around the
time of treatment. New learning is not detectably affected six to nine
months after ECT.[24] However, two-thirds of patients who have had
ECT, especially bilateral ECT, do tend to complain of greater
memory difficulties prospectively. There is thus a suspicion that
bilateral ECT may produce some, not currently demonstrable, memory impairment. Extended courses of 250 bilateral ECT have been
shown to be associated with long-term memory impairment.[9] Three
retrospective reports[9] found impairment on tests of memory and
cognitive function but as the American Psychiatric Association Task
Force report indicates, there are alternative possible explanations in
terms of the patient's diagnosis or treatment which might have been
factors in causing the memory damage. It seems reasonable to assume
that after six months ECT will rarely cause more than mild memory
difficulty, but that the risk will increase with successive treatments,
particularly bilateral ones. Brain damage is known to result from
anoxia which may cause gliosis. There are no convincing reports of
these phenomena after ECT which can be dissociated from the
occurrence of anoxia due to more primitive methods of treatment than
are currently available.

Attempts have been made to forbid or curtail the use of ECT most
notably in Alabama where in state hospitals no less than three
specialists and five others have been required to approve the treat-

ment for a patient.[25] In California the law specifies that before ECT can be given to a voluntary patient, even in a private office, informed consent must be obtained from the patient according to a standard written consent form which shall be supplemented by the physician with appropriate information pertaining to the particular patient being treated. The information to be given includes 'significant risks . . . especially noting the degree and duration of memory loss (including its irreversibility) ' and that 'there exists a division of opinion as to the efficacy of the proposed treatment . . .'[26] Thus 'informed consent', as specified by the law, has to include a scientifically unproved criticism of the treatment and a misleading allegation about its efficacy which disparages the available scientific information. ECT may not be given in California to minors (under the age of 12) and only in emergency, as a life-saving procedure and after three child psychiatrists have approved it, to those between 12 and 16 years. It requires a court hearing as well as the consent of the appropriate relative or guardian to give ECT to a patient of any sort who is not competent to give consent.

Such political activity over a highly successful treatment owes little to knowledge of clinical practice and is also an interference with a patient's free choice of treatment. To some extent such measures are stimulated by claims that ECT is over-used for inappropriate conditions and to punish recalcitrant patients. But these are matters for technical decision and competent professional practice and not for arbitrary legislative interference. The currency which such wild law-making gains is to some extent due to irresponsible journalism. Psychiatry is a common subject for the news media and physical manipulation of the brain of any sort is a dramatic and appealing topic. In contrast with these political activities and legislative interference it can be noted again that ECT has a very favourable cost- -benefit ratio as demonstrated by the studies reported. When given unilaterally it involves only a very small risk of long-term memory impairment which for the great majority of people is of minimum importance compared with the suffering and hazards of depression.

Whether ECT should be given to patients against their will is a more troublesome issue. The problem was common but is now infrequent; yet occasionally it still arises with patients who have a severe (usually acute) depressive illness which is not adequately relieved by medication or other measures. A few such patients object strongly to having ECT. Some may have had it and developed fear of it even though it is beneficial. Some of these may yield to sympathetic persuasion. Others remain adamant. There may be a very serious risk of suicide or other self-damage, the distress of the patient is often severe or his or her judgement disordered. This situation can be compared with forcible appendectomy in children. The patient stands to gain far more than he will lose and cannot decide rationally for himself. The physician has an ethical commitment to attempt to relieve suffering and to prevent suicide. On the few occasions on which I have known it to be done the patient has continued to accept both ECT and a relationship with the physician long after the compulsory status has lapsed, the patient's family are grateful and there is no recrimination. It seems right to do so, and a legal system which fails to provide the patient with the opportunity to have his suffering relieved by such an effective available measure could be regarded as lacking in humane concern.

The American Psychiatric Association Task Force Report[9] allows the possibility of treatment in circumstances where the patient is incompetent but objects to treatment, and indicates that in some jurisdictions a court procedure may be required. It emphasizes rightly that the guiding principle should be good overall medical management with a minimum of delay and no unnecessary restrictions on the exercise of good clinical judgement. Edwards and Flaherty[27] in New South Wales, Australia, clearly imply that ECT may be given despite a patient's refusal but subject to review procedures.

The practical qualifications in this context are important. The diagnosis and alternative avenues of treatment should be double checked by independent physicians. Perhaps the patient does not respond because there is a dementia or physical illness underlying the depression and the treatment is less appropriate than might be thought. The agreement of the nearest relative is essential, not only on legal grounds as in some jurisdictions but also on ethical grounds. If those who are likely to be most concerned for the patient cannot also approve the treatment there should be doubts as to its justification. The physician should also be satisfied that even if he has the support of the patient's family that support is given out of love and not, as may happen, out of antagonism. We should be sure also that he is not himself responding out of irritation or frustration or other illegitimate motives. But granted that these conditions have been met and that the physician is supported by the law of the jurisdiction in which he practises it is humane and appropriate to insist on effective treatment being provided. Not to give it could be regarded as negligence.

In my view the decision to give treatment against a patient's wishes should always be validated or confirmed at least by a fully independent professional opinion.

The position adopted in this discussion is paternalistic. However, the paternalism is shared with colleagues, and just as to have good parents is valuable for children so to have good fatherly (or motherly) physicians can be valuable to psychotic patients. It is not necessary to reject paternalism totally because it is sometimes confused with authoritarianism. Some readers, particularly in the United States, may feel that a contractual relationship which relies on an ethic of mutual equality offers a better position than the above. My personal view is that the patient has more to gain from a 'scrupulous' and responsible fiduciary approach in which the professional does not take personal advantage of his inevitably greater knowledge of the illness and its treatment. Since physicians are expected anyhow to observe fiduciary self-restraint it seems mistaken to suppose that they are not influential in the outcome of the patient's decision.

Apart from depressive illness ECT is rarely needed today in psychiatry. A few excited manic or catatonic schizophrenic patients may require it briefly and the considerations which apply are essentially the same as those which relate to acute severe depression in which the patient directly refuses treatment and protests at being given an anaesthetic for the purpose. More often the question of consent is a paper issue. The patient will not sign a form, or is not competent to do so, but accepts preparation for treatment, fasts as required before the anaesthetic, knows that he or she will receive electricity to the brain, and receives the anaesthetic injection before treatment without complaint. As with depression, the doctor who will not proceed to give ECT after all the above qualifications are satisfied could be regarded as negligent morally, even if not legally.

Definition of psychosurgery

The main neurosurgical procedures which have been advocated for psychiatric illness are leucotomy and amygdalotomy, the former for the control of depression as already discussed, the latter for control of aggressive behaviour whether against the self or others. Occasionally, in Germany, operations on the hypothalamus have also been proposed for certain sexual offenders.

Neurosurgical operations undertaken on putatively healthy tissue to relieve psychiatric symptoms are generally called psychosurgery. The definition requires some care. A recent World Health Organization booklet[28] defines psychosurgery as 'the selective surgical removal or destruction . . . of nerve pathways with a view to influencing behaviour'. Bridges and Bartlett[7] point out that this definition is incorrect because most modern psychosurgery is concerned with the treatment of severe intractable affective illnesses without any intended effect on behaviour at all, although of course behaviour may alter where it is directly influenced by the illness. Unfortunately, the United States Department of Health Education and Welfare has taken the same view as the WHO booklet and has defined psychosurgery as: (1) surgery on the normal brain tissue of an individual not suffering from physical disease for the purpose of changing or controlling behaviour or (2) surgery on diseased brain tissue of an individual if the sole object of the surgery is to control change or affect behavioural disturbances.[29] As Bridges and Bartlett state[7] 'a better definition of contemporary psychosurgery is: the surgical treatment of certain psychiatric illnesses by means of localized lesions placed in specific cerebral sites'. This matter is important as will be seen since the incorrect definition has served as a basis for unreasonable conclusions which are likely to affect the availability within the United States of certain valuable operations.

Operations for disturbed affect

Psychosurgery as we know it began with an operation on the frontal lobes proposed by Egas Moniz, a neurologist, and undertaken by a surgeon, Almeida Lima on 12 November 1935.[30] However Burckhardt,[31] the medical superintendent of a small Swiss mental hospital, actually undertook operations on the intact brain in 1890, removing areas of cerebral cortex from six patients.[4] Freeman and Watts[32] pioneered the work in the English-speaking world, operating on their first case in 1936 and thousands of patients were leucotomized in the 1940s and 1950s. At the start of that time, according to Dax:[4]

Two aspects have to be mentioned to put the popularity of the operation in perspective. First, patients were much more disturbed than we know them now and the nursing staff was fewer in numbers. Barbiturates were fairly new and sodium amylobarbitone was greeted as the new wonder drug . . . Padded rooms were in frequent use, incontinence of urine and faeces was rife and many patients wore strong canvas clothing. Some were extremely violent and tube feeding was frequent. Depressives on suicide caution cards were stripped of their possessions, spoon fed and marched from one room to another. There was sentinel walking, echolalia, flexibitas cerea aı.d frequent stupor, with constant danger from the catatonics.

Personality changes from the operation were of course recognized.

The results of leucotomy and its modifications are today somewhat thoughtlessly despised. We should note however that it was introduced against a background of relevant neurophysiological and psychological information and that representative results obtained in England between 1942 and 1954 in 10 365 patients[3] showed that even with chronic schizophrenia and the old standard operation, 41 per cent approximately, were 'at least greatly improved' and only 3 per cent had marked deleterious changes of personality; 2 per cent were worse, mortality related to the procedure was 4 per cent and the incidence of chronic epilepsy was 1 per cent. The availability of antidepressants and phenothiazines together with ECT and improvements also in the environmental and psychological management of patients made leucotomy redundant for most patients. Nevertheless it was established as an effective treatment, particularly for affective illness. However, more sophisticated techniques have produced good results for anxiety (94 per cent) obsessional symptoms (49 per cent) and depression (79 per cent) in the few patients who still require operation, without submitting them to high rates of morbidity. For example, with stereotactic procedures, operative mortality has been reduced to 0.2 per cent, chronic epilepsy to 0.6 per cent, post-operative intellectual impairment to 0.6 per cent, and marked personality change to 0.5 per cent[33] These good results are confirmed in reports from independent and reliable studies.[5,6]

An even more advantageous technique has been developed and practised by Crow and his colleagues where the implantation of indwelling electrodes is accompanied by stimulation and subsequent ablation of successive small amounts of cortex so that any bad effects on personality can be almost totally prevented.[8]

The number of operations done in Britain is not large. Between 1974 to 1976 the rate was 3.4 per million population aged over 15 or 431 operations.[34] In the 240 patients operated on in the three most active units 21 (8 per cent) were for repeated violence whilst 85 per cent were for mood disorders. Thus the bulk of psychosurgery was undertaken for illnesses in which the patients' symptoms were primarily subjective and consent was quite likely to be informed and valid.

An enquiry in the United States[35] found that about 400 procedures, meeting the definition of psychosurgery which the Department of Health Education and Welfare has adopted, were being performed annually in the United States. No significant psychological deficits were attributable to the psychosurgery in the patients evaluated and the treatment was efficacious in more than half of the cases studied. The data presented did not indicate that the procedure had been used for social control (as had been alleged) or that the procedure had been applied disproportionately to minority or disadvantaged populations (as had been noisily claimed). Indeed from correspondence with the most active psychosurgeons in the United States, it was found that out of a combined total of 600 patients, one was Black, two were Oriental Americans, and six were Hispanic Americans. Seven operations were reported to have been performed on children since 1970 and three prisoners underwent psychosurgery in 1972. Most psychosurgery patients were middle class individuals referred to neurosurgeons by psychiatrists and were about equally divided between males and females. The National Commission for the Protection of Human Subjects of Biomedical and Behavioural Research in the United

States found that psychosurgical treatment constituted a minuscule proportion (estimated to be less than 0.001 per cent) of psychiatric treatment in general.

From the evidence reviewed it appears that at least some forms of psychosurgery are accepted procedures in the sense that many different physicians refer patients for these treatments at the hands of particular surgeons, recognize appropriate indications for the referral, and are able to anticipate the probable outcome with considerable accuracy. Thus in their opinion the treatment is 'accepted' on normal clinical grounds. It is therefore surprising that the United States National Commission cited came to the conclusion that 'the procedure' did not constitute 'accepted practice', seeming to confound indiscriminately a variety of different operations. The conclusion seems to have more to do with the political and social atmosphere in which the Commission worked than with the merits of the case, even though the Commission was regarded as having produced a surprisingly favourable report in respect of psychosurgery.

This is not to say that some psychosurgical procedures are not experimental — but rather that certain operations are indeed as well proved as many other valid medical or surgical procedures. Stereotactic subcaudate tractotomy[2] and varieties of limbic tractotomy[4] and Crow's procedure[8] surely constitute accepted forms of treatment as probably do a number of other modified leucotomy operations.

Operations for pain

Although cerebral operations have been carried out to alleviate pain and have been briefly mentioned they do not currently present an issue because they are almost never indicated and because, so far as I know, they were always done with consent. Pain may be due either to physical lesions or to an emotional state.[36-38] It is accordingly defined as 'an unpleasant sensory and emotional experience which we primarily associate with tissue damage and describe in terms of tissue damage'.[39] Whatever the cause the experience is subjectively the same, an unpleasant one in the body. Leucotomy for pain when done in the presence of an appropriate psychiatric illness such as depression was successful. However in the last 17 years in regular work with patients with pain, I have only seen one who seemed to require an operation for pain and depression and he had a stereotactic subcaudate operation. This modified version of leucotomy was used primarily because he was depressed. When depression was not the main cause, leucotomy for pain only worked if the lesion was so large as to damage the personality.[40,37]

Thalamic and mesencephalic operations have also been undertaken for pain but were largely unsatisfactory.[41] These were for patients presumed to have, usually, peripheral lesions causing pain. Hypophysectomy is currently undertaken with benefit for pain from carcinoma,[42] but no one talks of this organ as sacrosanct. Thus operations for pain can either be assimilated to the argument concerning those for affective disorder or are not in significant use. However should a new operation be discovered for pain due to peripheral lesions, or central lesions, it is hard to imagine anyone saying that they should not be done. This suggests that the wrong sort of distinction is made between psychiatric illness and physical illness, viz. that it is all right to operate on the brain for a physical illness arising elsewhere in the body, but not for a psychological disturbance. This seems unfair not only to the patient who has pain for psychological reasons but also to all those patients who might benefit psychiatrically from brain surgery.

Operations for aggression

The human brain, as much as the animal, has highly developed anatomical and physiological systems which subserve self-protective defensive and aggressive responses and are accompanied by emotional changes. It may also, like some animal brains, provide for cool predatory aggression.[43] Most human aggression is affect-laden. When it is not it is probably unpredictable by anybody other than the aggressor. Much human aggression also can be clearly linked to environmental triggers, to cultural patterns, to childhood experiences, and to a variety of social and psychological factors. Even so, the prediction of aggressive behaviour is extremely difficult and for clinical purposes often very unreliable, despite the fact that better prediction would be of enormous value for judges in passing sentence and in connection with offenders seeking parole. Nevertheless there are a few individuals who engage in violent repeated aggressive behaviour against themselves or others. As a result of animal work and from operations on patients who had temporal lobe lesions (often with epilepsy) it became evident that aggressive behaviour might be modified by means of surgical lesions, particularly in the region of the amygdala. Such stereotactic operations have been undertaken in retarded patients[44], on children who are overactive and self-damaging,[45] and on violent offenders.[46–48] As the earlier discussion indicated the number of operations in this group is small in Britain and the United States and the operations are comparably few in the rest of the English-speaking world. Several hundred operations on children in India apparently required consent not only from the children's parents but from grandparents as well.

The results of such operations have been reviewed by Kiloh.[44,48] Some apparently striking successes have been obtained[44-49] although the results are not nearly as good overall as those for the latest development of leucotomy. Nevertheless, Kiloh points out that these stereotactic procedures appear to be relatively safe and free from undesirable sequelae. The success rate is 50–75 per cent at 2 years or more and the successful cases become more effective and indeed happier human beings. Perhaps, given time, the results might become as good as those for the modern developments of leucotomy, but the opportunities for steady development of the technique in suitable patients are increasingly circumscribed because of public concern expressed by a variety of groups. The United States Department of Health Education and Welfare[29] points out that the National Commission for the Protection of Human Subjects of Biomedical and Behavioural Research was called into being after 'widespread expression of public and congressional concern . . . including allegations that these procedures were . . . being used for "social control" of dissidents and violence prone individuals and . . . were performed disproportionately on members of minority populations'. In the event the results already quoted indicate a truly enormous disproportion between the outcry and the facts. It is doubtful that any operation was done for 'social control' and minorities were under-represented, as already described. The main issues which remain are whether the social considerations form an invalid part of some decisions to operate, and whether operations may be done without consent.

The first of these questions relates mainly to psychosurgery for violence. The other two relate both to surgery for mood states and to that for violence.

Social definition of disease

For those who like it, as well as for those who do not approve, it is still a fact that the attribution of the word 'disease' to a set of circumstances is determined in many cases by social factors. Fabrega[50] has described how social behaviour is used as a criterion of disease in different societies. Conventionally doctors give disease labels to 'conditions' about which they are consulted. Those 'conditions' may be organic changes or disabilities (e.g. pneumonia), psychotic disorders with or without organic causes (delirium, mania), and neurotic and behavioural disorders (phobic anxiety, enuresis, sociopathic personality). Some conditions such as mania or depression may be 'spontaneous' or induced by organic change (steroid treatment, influenza, depression with dementia). The same phenomenology in mania or depression may have an overt organic cause or none.

Sociopathic behaviour may perhaps be 'constitutional'-XYY linked, induced by social conditions or childhood ill-treatment or a consequence of epidemic encephalitis or head injury. Without arguing the details of these particular instances it seems to me and perhaps to most psychiatrists that disease patterns are determined at least in part by social expectations combined with biological knowledge, and that biological knowledge is not the sole criterion. More precise definitions of disease (or health) have long eluded agreement. Physicians see themselves as trained to recognize 'diseases' or 'conditions'. If a physician has something to offer in the treatment or care of a 'condition' he is normally willing to provide his professional services. These may be along the lines of drug or other physical treatment, psychological treatment, and even manipulation of the environment. For example, patients with peptic ulcer or conversion hysteria alike might receive a recommendation for discharge from the armed services, and so on.

All this need not stop the physician from limiting his functions to those which are 'medical' and refusing to be involved primarily as an agent to deal with social issues. The physician who adheres to the traditional role will help a patient to get better social conditions but will not *qua* physician seek automatically to change the conditions. In some cases (cholera due to contaminated water) his view of a social arrangement will be deservedly accepted. In others (the advisability of conscription or imprisonment in general) he is wise if he is content only to exercise the role of an ordinary citizen.

This being said, let us consider the situation of the physician and of the patients who are recommended for treatment of disorders of thought, mood, or behaviour. The disorder may be recognizable to the physician as a syndrome with or without biological cause. There is no reason why he may not offer to treat it if that is what the patient asks. If it is not what the patient asks, the doctor may then determine if the failure to ask arises from a failure of reason. If so he might treat the patient who does not ask, but does not oppose, provided that the proper representatives of the patient (family, guardian, etc.) request him to do so and do not have a disproportionately selfish interest in the treatment. (The wife of a depressed man once asked me if leucotomy would help the impotence from which he had suffered even before depression supervened.)

If the patient is clearly opposed to treatment then the physician will only rarely if ever undertake it. Those special circumstances where this might happen in relation to the brain will be discussed shortly. At this point it is sufficient to have indicated that I take the following position: our notion of illness is partly biological and partly social; treatment by physicians is on the 'medical model'; we may recognize and sometimes act in relationship to social causes but only within the limits of our agreed function as physicians which is to diagnose and promote cure where we can, and to advise on how individuals and society may take the responsibility for prevention and control. It is from this standpoint that I consider the ethics of psychosurgery.

Brain surgery with consent

Relevant considerations for physicians include as always the cost--benefit ratio. Another consideration is more 'ethical' in nature: whether it is right to destroy putatively normal brain tissue in order to relieve emotional distress. Edgar[51] points out that there is no objection to operating on the brain as such e.g. to remove a tumour. He argues that in the face of evidence that a person's aberrant behaviour resulted from a tumour we would not reject operation because it might be at a brain site related to personality or the 'will'. Thus we are prepared to operate on the brain in circumstances where there is also evidence of structural change and we accept possible effects from this upon personality. If individuals who are able to give free and valid consent, wish to accept a surgical procedure which offers worthwhile benefit in the absence of overt pathology there is no reason why they should not do so, and it curtails their freedom if we refuse permission. General surgery also is not confined to abnormal tissue. Legs may be shortened, ears or noses reshaped (although healthy). Normal organs are removed — as in adrenalectomy for carcinoma or hypophysectomy for severe pain.[42] Also, operations have been performed on putatively normal brain tissue in order to relieve pain attributed to organic disturbances elsewhere in the body.[41] Although it is sometimes technically difficult to do useful surgery on the substance of the brain there should be no objection to brain surgery for psychological disorder solely because the brain controls thought, feeling, judgement, and personality. Logically it is the most appropriate site of intervention in a consenting individual. But it will be very necessary to consider in due course what constitutes consent or valid agreement.

The relevance of brain pathology is a practical issue. Mark and Ervin[49] and Mark and Neville[52] rejected psychosurgery for aggression except in patients with brain lesions. They seem to accept in principle that psychosurgery for aggression might be allowed without physical pathology but they rule it out in the short-run. Physical pathology may be one source of evidence that intervention at a particular site is 'good medicine', particularly if '(a) the patient's brain is damaged in a particular way, (b) most people who have such damage behave aberrantly as does the patient, and (c) this operation has worked to change that behaviour in other patients.[49] However, to limit brain operations for psychological illness to cases which only have brain pathology would make for a number of difficulties.

If a patient is distressed and regretful over his aggressive behaviour why should he not have the opportunity to receive surgical help, assuming it to be effective, just as much as a man with phobias or a lady with chronic pain due to an emotional disorder or to a lesion outside the brain? There are also problems in defining pathology broadly and yet perhaps it should be so defined. While EEG abnormality is less easily related to disease than histological change it could have valid associations with pathophysiological disturbances in the temporal lobes. Except in the dementias, relevant chemical abnormality cannot be shown by present techniques in any specific brain area in life but may well be significant. Micro-anatomical differences will not be found before surgery.

Brain pathology alone is too restrictive and uncertain as a criterion in consenting patients.

Brain surgery without consent

If it is humane and proper to undertake appropriate surgery to change the mood or behaviour in individuals who can make an appropriate judgement and therefore give valid consent would it not also be humane and morally unobjectionable to operate for the same purposes on individuals who cannot give consent because they are too disordered to be able to approve the situation? In principle the answer appears to be yes. Special precautions are of course required in such circumstances. It should first be abundantly clear that the patient really is not decided or able to decide about the matter. Any hint of reluctance perhaps expressed in behaviour like eating a meal before an anaesthetic is due, or failing to co-operate with preliminary procedures should be taken as an indication that consent is refused even though the patient does not explicitly put the matter into words. The decision should also obviously be made by more than one person, and should be subject to review and special supervision. As usual, it would require the approval of the next of kin. Perhaps too it should be agreed upon by some independent non-medical professionals. I do not think such people would be in a better position to judge than experienced physicians. But the need to present a case before intelligent disinterested parties should provide a helpful safeguard. In particular, those parties should establish that dependence upon the doctor's good-will is not the patient's reason for consent. Some of these conditions are essential, some of them optional. Given that enough of them were satisfied it should be acceptable to treat with brain surgery those patients who do not consent but who do not explicitly or implicitly refuse. If neither the patient's indifference nor his consent can be established then the case has to be seen as one in which consent is refused.

In my view it is unacceptable to perform leucotomy or other brain surgery on patients who are specifically or implicitly unwilling. This differs from the view offered on ECT. The first reason is the minimal or absent risk of permanent detrimental physical brain changes with ECT compared with the potential risk of such changes with surgery. It is unacceptable to enforce even such infrequent hazards as those of some brain surgery upon unwilling patients in the present context. The second reason is more fundamental. Even if there were no deleterious changes possible with surgery or if the manipulation was not a physical one, it seems wrong to impose potentially permanent changes in a man's mental state against his wishes. In case this should seem to be at variance with my willingness to recommend occasional ECT to patients who refuse it, I would point out that the effects of ECT are essentially temporary and may be required as emergency, even life-saving treatment. Although psychosurgery may also be life-saving it is inconceivable that its effects could usually be classed only as temporary (even though they are sometimes not sufficiently sustained to be therapeutically worthwhile). Thirdly, while the giving of ECT compulsorily also violates a man's mental state against his wishes it is done in conditions which give him later opportunities to protest at what was done. It does not carry any risk of permanently changing his original personality and basis of judgement or take away his opportunity later to seek redress for unfair treatment.

It may be the case that legal and social systems do sanction interventions on men's minds which change them permanently. All reformatories, correctional institutions, and penal establishments usually have some such aims for unwilling participants but they are not founded upon medical considerations. If we are considering procedures which depend on medical expertise the refusal of consent is a fundamental objection to all procedures which aim at irreversible personality change. If this position is accepted it should safeguard against the appalling possibility that procedures of psychosurgery would be used on unwilling political prisoners.

There remains an important issue to do with consent, namely that of men or women under legal constraints in prison or comparable institutions. Mark and Neville[52] argue strongly that no one in prison or prison-like conditions should receive psychosurgery. Against this view a hypothetical case may be postulated of a criminal who develops a depressive illness for which in freedom he would have a neurosurgical procedure. Provided that the conditions of his imprisonment and the length of his sentence have no bearing on the treatment recommended, which could, say, be a modified leucotomy, the question of whether he should have an operation should be decided on the same basis as for a free individual. However, psychosurgical operations suggested for prisoners sometimes do not satisfy these requirements. They are in any case few in number. It is likely that there is a ratio of a score of articles on the topic to every operated prison case. But what these operations tend to do is offer a treatment for aggressive behaviour; treatment which may change the personality as well as simply reduce the frequency of aggressive antisocial actions. Let us assume for the moment that such treatments are effective. The question then arises whether it is right to offer them to men in detention, and on what conditions. Some patients engage in self-mutilation and other harmful activities against their own persons; some of them may be glad to accept an operation which relieves them of this behaviour. If in frustration one day we are engaged in banging our head against a wall we may welcome some assistance which relieves us of the inclination to do so. Operation in those cases may be as valid and as justified as for depressive illness.

Still other patients might feel a deep regret at behaviour which they do not manage to control but which is harmful to others — say repeated assaults or fighting. One such man sought treatment for his aggressive outbursts by attending a hospital out-patient department. An oral phenothiazine was included in his treatment and was partly helpful, but supposing that surgery gave the best chance of success and that the risks were acceptable, would it have been justified to operate on his brain? A conditional yes seems the correct answer. If so, perhaps the treatment should be available also for prisoners with the same motives and wishes. Again the right answer appears to be in the affirmative. However, prisoners present great difficulties.

At this point let us consider only established procedures with known benefits and hazards. The problem is whether the prisoner is giving his consent not because he wants to change his behaviour and avoid harming others in future but because he wishes to alter the terms of his sentence. It can be presumed that a man who is at the end of a long sentence or only has a short sentence of less than 12 months will not be unduly influenced by the hope of early release. A prisoner with a longer sentence might well assent to operation for just that reason, that he wishes to shorten the sentence. While his consent might not be called free it might be valid in his own interests. But we are reluctant to accept that an external constraint should be influential in such a decision. In the one case the decision may be correct. But since constraints from the civil authority can be varied then a variety of new constraints might appear (perhaps with a new revolutionary government?) and psychiatrists would be asking surgeons to take on new cases because of new political changes. The thought is anathema. It is even not too far-fetched to imagine a society where imprisoned psychiatrists might be invited to accept some intracerebral lesion which would change their responses so that they would become more accepting of the tenets of the government of the day. Some of our colleagues have been tortured in Argentina, or vanished without a trace. Dr Gluzman languishes in the Soviet prison system because of his adherence to medical ethics (see Chapter 18). Less resolute physicians (and who can say he would be a hero like Gluzman?) might prefer the option of surgical treatment. It seems hard to assent to any brain operations under conditions of constraint.

In the United States a famous court action was brought to prevent psychosurgery on a prisoner.[53] The man in prison for 18 years for murder (followed by necrophilia), had satisfied an 'Informed Consent' Review Committee consisting of a law professor, a priest, and an accountant that he wanted the operation. Ironically the attorney who brought the case 'Kaimowitz representing himself and certain individual members of the Medical Committee for Human Rights on behalf of John Doe', had never consulted the prisoner. The lawyer appointed by the court to represent the man thought that he desperately wanted the operation[54] but proved to the court's satisfaction that the man was held unconstitutionally as a prisoner. Despite the fact that the prisoner was therefore freed, the hearing continued on the question as to whether a prisoner could give free informed consent to psychosurgery and it was held that he could not. It has been argued[55] that this conclusion violates the right to treatment so that it seems unlikely that the Kaimowitz case represents a definite conclusion in United States law.

The issue may be hard for American lawyers or judges. It also presents a problem in practical ethics for doctors. It seems that physicians, lawyer, priest, and accountant all believed, probably correctly, that the prisoner wanted the operation. But after he was released, he changed his mind. Burt's account[54] gives clear reason to think that the circumstances of imprisonment and medical surveillance at least contributed to the prisoner's consent without any attempt being made by physicians to press the prisoner to agree.

In the light of this finding it can be argued that no prisoner's consent should be accepted for psychosurgery related to the type of behaviour which has caused his imprisonment. That however might be called double jeopardy. It seems desirable to insist that the attempt should be made to avoid prisoners accepting operation with a view to facilitating release. In the case in question that condition was not apparently fulfilled.

Some arrangements might however be proposed which would allow long-term non-political prisoners (very strictly defined) to obtain treatment for repetitive violence or chronic maladjustment. One necessary condition could be that the prisoner is clearly aware that no immediate change in his sentence is to be expected. Only long-term evidence of change over, say, a minimum of three years, would be acceptable evidence leading to a reduction of the sentence. Such change should be equally helpful to him if it occurred in the absence of operation. It would be up to him to decide whether he wanted the procedure to facilitate his own efforts. Secondly, a substantial independent review of the proposal would be required for each case involving at least three expert psychiatrists and including preferably one from outside the country, and a substantial lay review body as well drawn similarly from beyond the institution. A hearing in open court could also be required. The consent of the prisoner and his relations would be obligatory and the review personnel would be specially required to assess if the individual's consent was reasonable and consistently held and was not dependent on the hope of release. With such safeguards very few operations might be done, but it is conceivable that they would be worthwhile for the patients. Prisoners too should have 'the right to treatment'. It is of course unthinkable that anyone who did not give consent should have psychosurgery.

On the basis that minors, prisoners, and civilly committed mental patients should not be denied the benefits of treatment the United States National Commission accepted that psychosurgery should be allowed for them provided their rights were rigorously guarded.[29] The American Psychiatric Assocation largely supported the Commission's report but opposed psychosurgery on children because of insufficient data and approved it only for prisoners if its indications were unrelated to criminal behaviour. The United States Department of Health Education and Welfare[35] decided not to fund psychosurgery research or treatment by any of the institutions which it supports, for any of these three groups. This action going against the recommendations of both the National Commission and the American Psychiatric Association seems to be like the Commission's conclusion that psychosurgery was not 'an accepted procedure' in that it is perhaps related more to considerations of public noise than to the facts or merits of the matter.

In regard to children and the mentally incompetent I suggest that stringent procedures, similar to some of those outlined for prisoners, might be used to establish that: (1) the procedure offered worthwhile benefit and appeared to be in the patient's interest, and (2) consent was not refused implicitly.

To sum up this discussion I have argued that psychosurgery should never be forced but it might be done with non-competent individuals or prisoners subject to stringent safeguards, some of which have been considered.

Depth electrical stimulation

Electrical stimulation offers similar problems to the longer established forms of surgery, and one additional problem. The similar problems arise because electrical stimulation is not without risk of permanent harm. Any electrode or sheaf of inserted electrodes might rupture a vessel. Indwelling electrodes, further, can give rise to a fibrotic reaction — particularly when used for repeated electrical stimulation. These risks require assessment in relation to any electrical stimulation procedures, those of a haemorrhage are perhaps minimal but those of fibrotic reactions may be greater than is currently anticipated. It is known that implanted electrodes used for dorsal column stimulation for the treatment of chronic pain have given rise to fibrotic reactions. Intra-cerebral electrodes, no matter how sophisticated, might do something like this, or promote some other form of continuing damage to cells. Nevertheless both Heath[56] and Crow[8] appear satisfied that this technology is minimally damaging, and it is not intended for permanent implantation. At present only occasional operations with indwelling electrodes in the brain have been done for pain[57] and they do not appear to be very successful.[58] They have been used for chronic pain from peripheral lesions. As with the unsuccessful thalamic operations it is hard to imagine moral objections being raised to these treatments in the event of their being successful.

The additional problem is that indwelling electrodes may provide the possibility of pleasurable self-stimulation. This is not often the case but if it were, someone would be sure to want to stop it. At the present time there are patients who have been given batteries which they can turn on and off and which deliver stimulation by the implanted electrodes. When this is done with animals which are taught to do certain acts, for example lever-pressing, to initiate self-stimulation the animals may work tremendously hard to stimulate themselves, and do little else.[59] Some neglect food, water, and natural functions. For a further account see Valenstein[60] who indicates that such phenomena are rare and difficult to reproduce in both animals and man consistently.

Apart from these practical considerations there is a theoretical issue. Medicine has so far aimed mostly at correcting abnormalities, not at obtaining a subjective Elysium. Self-stimulation which achieves the latter would be socially objectionable. Should we take heed of such a consideration? Perhaps not in principle if we accept the individual's right to self-determination. Again, in practice the operation would probably not get far since it would be biologically disadvantageous, leading to failure of reproduction as well as death. There appear sufficient reasons for physicians not to wish to support the achievement of super-normality by self-stimulation.

There are hypothetical situations in which surgery and especially self-stimulation could make people function more actively and with greater success. Perhaps intelligence could be improved. Mark and Neville[52] point out that this makes medical men authorities on what constitutes the good life. A case could be argued for that conclusion without suggesting that we are the sole authorities. But the profession is certainly neither ready nor prepared to assume such a role.

The dangerous attraction of electrical stimulation of the brain is that in the short-term it offers possibilities of scientific investigation of the brain in patients with psychoses and perhaps some others by means of recordings taken from the electrodes which are used for stimulation. We would clearly like to know more about the patterns of activity in different parts of the human brain in all sorts of psychiatric conditions — and even non-medical circumstances. This motive is not a legitimate guide to the ethical management of patients. The justifiable attraction of electrical stimulation of the brain is that firstly, it offers much improved chances of precision in placing lesions, and secondly, it allows graded ablation of tissue. After stimulation in a given part, tissue between the electrodes may be destroyed by increasing the current used. Only small amounts of tissue need be destroyed at one time. Careful, painstaking steps can be taken to secure relief without personality change. Such advantages are enormously attractive. Despite the problems outlined, this is presumably the optimum way to conduct psychosurgical ablations.

Surgical innovation

In the discussion so far reference has been made to operations where established knowledge is fairly extensive and to hypothetical situations where such extensive knowledge was postulated. Most controversy attaches to innovations in treatment. This is a difficult subject in any branch of medicine. Is the first patient to have a particular operation being treated ethically? If not, how can any operation be developed? Medicine is not alone with this problem. Everyone with a legal difficulty deserves an experienced barrister. If so, how can a new barrister be morally justified in getting experience?

It is clear that new procedures should not ordinarily be introduced on those who cannot give valid consent. This might be qualified to the extent that the new procedure is reasonably supposed to be less risky than other established treatment. A coronary patient may be able to give valid consent for a new type of graft if it is explained to him. But can any psychiatric patient needing treatment for his mood, thoughts, or behaviour give valid consent to an unproved treatment? The answer is uncertain but it is equally uncertain whether a patient with advanced carcinoma can make a free valid judgement on some last-chance new procedure. Some, for example Mark and Neville[52], recommend the criterion of physical pathology. In the development of techniques this is plainly sound. If we start from a base where verification of the facts is relatively easy, we have more chance of finding beneficial new procedures with least risk to patients.

However neither psychiatric nor carcinoma patients should be excluded from the possibility of being helped by an unproved treatment which has reasonable scientific justification. Innovations which carry hazards should therefore be allowed with due precaution for both of these groups. Innovations in treatment are now subject to increasing control with special review mechanisms. It seems best to argue that they may occur in consenting, free patients without physical disease, that the control procedures will be maintained and that they will not be done in prisons or on patients who are not competent in the usual sense: but if an innovation were suggested which could only help prisoners or the incompetent this conclusion might need to be revised.

Some practical issues

The theoretical issues have been considered so far, with reference to practical problems as required. We need next to discuss briefly some practical points. In all the procedures examined the outstanding pre-condition is that they should be capable of yielding the patient worthwhile benefit at minimal risk and that the benefit should be significantly greater than that from alternative less traumatic proce-dures. By this criterion ECT is outstandingly attractive. Its morbidity rate is much less than that of anti-depressant drugs (with perhaps one exception, flupenthixol, which is not yet approved in North America). It causes some transient memory disturbance, very few fatalities, and little else in the way of trouble. In contrast, anti-depressant drugs almost invariably cause discomfort (dry mouth, constipation, blurred vision), quite often cause hypotensive faint feelings, and can provoke a variety of significant illnesses such as prolapsed hemorrhoids from constipation, epileptic fits, retention of urine, and, theoretically, glaucoma. The cardiotoxic effects of the anti-depressants probably also cause fatalities several times more frequently than does ECT.

Although leucotomy-like procedures are rarely performed in North

America and in Britain, the modified versions have high standing, as has been described, because of their lack of morbidity and for their therapeutic success.[2,5,8] They still have a proper place in psychiatric treatment.

Among the major psychosurgical procedures amygdalotomy or amygdalectomy and hypothalamic operations[61,62] are less well-established. This is not only because of opposition to treating behaviour rather than distress, it is also because knowledge of their benefits and risks has been available for a much shorter time and the technology of investigation (criteria for selection of patients and for assessment of results, etc.) is still embryonic. There is further an inherent difficulty in assessing aggression compared with depression or obsessional neurosis or schizophrenia because the manifestations of aggression are frequently intermittent. Some patients are continuously assaultive of themselves or others. But major assaults are liable to be committed by individuals who have 'over-controlled hostility'.[63,64] Discussions in the literature[65] indicate that the prediction of dangerousness is handicapped by the infrequency with which dangerous behaviour occurs. Cocozza and Steadman [65] with a particular population developed a score which correctly predicted dangerous behaviour by eleven patients and no dangerous behaviour by three who did behave dangerously. Twenty-five were predicted by the score as dangerous and did not prove to be so. Thus the score produced statistically significant results (P <0.001) which were however clinically insufficient. The best conclusion we can draw is that operations for aggression should be developed first for those who are frequently assaultive so that a time span of one or two years will help to indicate significant improvement.

The difficulty in prediction also provides a further reason why operative intervention on prisoners should be avoided if possible in circumstances which would make the results of operation a condition for release. Psychiatrists normally operate on the principle that the patient who is interested in cure will be as frank with them as he is able. This does not hold for some aggressive prisoners. Psychiatric skill is reasonably good for the management of psychotic patients and neurotics. It is poor with deceivers and we need not be ashamed of this since we do not or should not purport to be detectives. We are another type of investigator. Assessing patients who might say they are cured by operation so as to promote their own release is fraught with difficulty. Nevertheless in principle it seems to be wrong to deny to prisoners the benefits of worthwhile operations, especially since not all of them present the above problems. Sufficient safeguards ought therefore to be sought to allow the performance of some psychosurgery on prisoners who consent. A novel safeguard would be one which follows from the Detroit case[53],[54] and that would be to call for a legal review of a prisoner's sentence, before psychosurgery, such that any neglected opportunity for him to challenge his incarceration could first be pursued.

Conclusions

The conclusions in this chapter can be stated briefly. ECT is a valuable treatment which on occasion may be given even to incompetent patients who object. Stereotactic types of leucotomy are of proved value but only rarely indicated; neurosurgical operations for aggression have some potential but need more evaluation; it is reasonable to operate on brain tissue which is not the site of known gross disease; it is not reasonable or ethical to undertake neurosurgery against the patient's wishes; prisoners may have appropriate treatment of any type for illnesses unrelated to their crime; operations on violent prisoners may only be considered with stringent precautions. Brain stimulation by implanted electrodes is a form of brain surgery and subject to the same considerations as psychosurgery; it has some advantages and no great practical disadvantages compared with other brain surgery.

References

1. MILL, J. S.: *On liberty* (1859), London, Watts and Company, 1929.
2. KNIGHT, G. C.: Further observations from an experience of 660 cases of stereotactic tractotomy. *Postgraduate Medical Journal* **49**:845–54, 1973.
3. TOOTH, G. C. and NEWTON, M. P.: Leucotomy in England and Wales 1942–1954. *Reports on Medical Subjects*. No. 104. London, Her Majesty's Stationery Office, 1961.
4. DAX, E. C.: The history of prefrontal leucotomy, in *Psychosurgery and society*. Ed. Smith, J. S. and Kiloh, L. G. Oxford, Pergamon, 1977, pp. 19–24.
5. MITCHELL-HEGGS, N., KELLY, D., and RICHARDSON, A.: Stereotactic limbic leucotomy — a follow-up at sixteen months. *British Journal of Psychiatry* **128**:226–40, 1976.
6. GOKTEPE, E. O., YOUNG, L. B., and BRIDGES, P. K: A further review of the results of stereotactic subcaudate tractotomy. *British Journal of Psychiatry* **126**: 270–80, 1975.
7. BRIDGES, P. K. and BARTLETT, J. R.: Psychosurgery: yesterday and today. *British Journal of Psychiatry* **131**: 249–60, 1977.
8. CROW H.: The treatment of anxiety and obsessionality with chronically implanted electrodes, in *Psychosurgery and society*. Ed. Smith, J. S. and Kiloh, L. G. Oxford, Pergamon, 1977, pp. 71–3.
9. AMERICAN PSYCHIATRIC ASSOCIATION: Electroconvulsive Therapy. Task Force Report No. 14, Washington, 1978.
10. GUZE, S. and ROBINS E.: Suicide and primary affective disorders. *British Journal of Psychiatry* **117**:437–8, 1970.
11. HUSTON, P. E. and LOCHER, L. M.: Involutional psychosis: course when

untreated and when treated with ECT. *Archives of Neurology and Psychiatry* **59**:385–94, 1948.

12. BERESFORD, H. R.: Legal issues relating to electroconvulsive therapy. *Archives of General Psychiatry* **25**:100–2, 1971.

13. BARKER, J. C. and BAKER, A. A: Deaths associated with electroplexy. *Journal of Mental Science* **105**:339–48, 1959.

14. BRUCE, E. M., CRONE, N., FITZPATRICK, G., FREWIN, S. J., GILLIS, A., LASCELLES, C. F., LEVENE, L. J., and MERSKEY, H.: A comparative trial of ECT and Tofranil. *American Journal of Psychiatry* **117**, 76, 1960.

15. MEDICAL RESEARCH COUNCIL: Clinical trial of the treatment of depressive illness. *British Medical Journal* **5439**:881–6, 1965.

16. SAINZ, A.: Clarification of the action of successful treatments in the depressions. *Diseases of the Nervous System* **20**:53–7, 1959.

17. LAMBOURN, J. and GILL, D.: A controlled comparison of simulated and real ECT. *British Journal of Psychiatry* **133**:514–19, 1978.

18. OTTOSSON, J. O.: Simulated and real ECT. *British Journal of Psychiatry* **134**:314, 1979.

19. WATT, J. A. G.: Simulated and real ECT. *British Journal of Psychiatry* **134**:314, 1979.

20. WILSON, I. C., VERNON, J. T., GUIN, T., *et al.*: A controlled study of treatments of depression. *Journal of Neuropsychiatry* **4**:331–7, 1963.

21. COSTELLO, C. G.: Electroconvulsive therapy: is further inevestigation necessary? *Canadian Psychiatric Association Journal* **21**:761–7, 1976.

22. CRONHOLM, B. and OTTOSSON, J. O.: Experimental studies of the therapeutic action of electroconvulsive therapy in endogenous depression. *Acta psychiatrica et neurologica Scandinavica* **35**: (Suppl. 145) 69–97, 1960.

23. PRICE, T. R. P., MACKENZIE, T. B., TUCKER, G. J., and CULVER, C.: The dose response ratio in electroconvulsive therapy. *Archives of General Psychiatry* **35**:1131–6, 1978.

24. SQUIRE, L. R. and CHACE, P. M.: Memory functions six to nine months after electroconvulsive therapy. *Archives of General Psychiatry* **32**:1557–64, 1975.

25. WYATT V. HARDIN, No. 3195–N (M. D. Ala. 28 Feb., 1975, modified 1 July, 1975): 1 Mental Disability Law Reporter 55, 1976.

26. CALIFORNIA WELFARE AND INSTITUTIONS CODE. 1979. SS. 5325.1, 5434.2, 5326.7, 5326.8.

27. EDWARDS, G. A. and FLAHERTY, B.: Electroconvulsive therapy: a new era of controversy. *Australia and New Zealand Journal of Psychiatry* **12**:161–4, 1978.

28. WORLD HEALTH ORGANIZATION: Health Aspects of Human Rights. Geneva: WHO, 1976.

29. Determination of Secretary Regarding Recommendation on Psychosurgery of the National Commission for the Protection of Human Subjects of Biomedical and Behavioural Research. Federal Register, 15 Nov., 1978. Part VI, pp. 53241–4.

30. MONIZ, E.: Les premières tentatives opératoires dans le traitement de certains psychose. *Encéphale*, **31**:1, 1936.

31. BURCKHARDT, G.: Ueber Rindenexcisionen, als Beittag zur operativen Therapie der Psychosen. *Allgemeine Zeitschrift fur Psychiatrie*, **47**:463–548, 1891.

32. FREEMAN, W. and WATTS, J. W.: *Psychosurgery*. Thomas Springfield Ill., 1942.

33. SMITH, J. S.: The treatment of anxiety, depression and obsessionality, in *Psychosurgery and society*. Ed. Smith, J. S. and Kiloh, L. G. Oxford, Pergamon, 1977.

34. BARRACLOUGH, B. M. and MITCHELL-HEGGS, N. A.: Use of neurosurgery for

psychological disorders in the British Isles during 1974–1976. *British Medical Journal* **iv**:1591–3, 1978.

35. US NATIONAL COMMISSION FOR THE PROTECTION OF SUBJECTS OF BIOMEDICAL AND BEHAVIOURAL RESEARCH INVOLVING PSYCHOSURGERY: Report and Recommendations with Appendix. Bethesda, Md: US Department of Health, Education, and Welfare Publication No. (OS)77–0001 and (OS)77–0002, 14 March, 1977.

36. BEECHER, H. K.: *Measurement of subjective responses*. New York, Oxford University Press, 1959.

37. MERSKEY, H. and SPEAR, F. G.: Pain: psychological and psychiatric aspects. London, Baillière, Tindall and Cassell, 1967.

38. STERNBACH, R. A.: *Pain: a psychophysiological analysis*. New York, Academic Press, 1968.

39. *Definitions of pain terms*. A report of the Subcommittee on Taxonomy of the International Association for the Study of Pain. Pain, (in press), 1979.

40. ELITHORN, A., GLITHERO, E., and SLATER, E.: Leucotomy for pain. *Journal of Neurology, Neurosurgery, and Psychiatry* **21**:249–61, 1958.

41. CASSINARI, V. and PAGNI, C. A.: *Central pain: a neurosurgical survey*. Cambridge, Mass, Harvard University Press, 1979.

42. MORICCA, G.: Pituitary neuroadenolysis in the treatment of intractable pain, in *Persistent pain: modern methods of treatment*. Ed. Lipton, S. London, Academic Press, 1977.

43. SHEARD, M. H.: Neurobiology of aggressive behaviour, in *Aggression, mental illness and mental retardation: psychobiological approaches*. Ed. Zarfas, D. and Goldberg, B. University of Western Ontario, London, Canada, pp. 76–93.

44. KILOH, L. G., GYE, R. S., RUSHWORTH, RG, BELL, D. S.,and WHITE, R. T.: Stereotactic amygdalotomy for aggressive behaviour. *Journal of Neurology, Neurosurgery, and Psychiatry* **37**:437, 1974.

45. BALASUBRAMANIAM, V. and KANAKA, T. S.: Amygdalotomy and hypothalamotomy in a comparative study. *Confinia neurologica* **37**:195, 1975.

46. NARABAYASHI, H., NAGAO, T., SAITO, Y., YOSHIDA, M; and NAGAHATA, M.: Stereotaxic amygdalotomy for behaviour disorders. *Archives of Neurology* **9**:1, 1963.

47. HEIMBURGER, R. F., WHITLOCK, C. C., and KALSBECK, J. E.: Stereotaxic amygdalotomy for epilepsy with aggressive behaviour. *Journal of the American Medical Association* **198**:741–5, 1966.

48. KILOH, L. G.: The treatment of anger and aggression, in *Symposium on psychosurgery and society*. Ed. Smith, J. S. and Kiloh, L. G. Oxford, Pergamon, 1977.

49. MARK, V. H. and ERVIN, F. R.: *Violence and the brain*. New York, Harper and Row, 1970.

50. FABREGA, H., JR: *Disease and social behaviour: an inter-disciplinary perspective*. Cambridge, Mass. MIT Press, 1974.

51. EDGAR, H.: Regulating psychosurgery: issues of public policy and law; In *Operating on the mind: The psychosurgery conflict*. Ed. Gaylin, W.M., Meister, J. S., and Neville, R. C. New York, Basic Books, 1975.

52. MARK, V. H. and NEVILLE, R.: Brain surgery in aggressive epileptics: social and ethical implications. *Journal of the American Medical Association* **227**:765–72, 1973.

53. KAIMOWITZ, V.: Department of mental health: Cir Ct Wayne City, Mich. Civil No. 73–19434 AW, July 10, 1973.

54. BURT, R. A.: Why we should keep prisoners from the doctors. *Hastings Center Report* **5**:25–34, 1975.

55. GREENBLATT, S. J.: New York Law School *Law Review* **22**, 961–80, 1976–77.

56. HEATH, R. G., JOHN, S. B., AND Fontana, C. J.: Stereotaxic implantation of

electrodes in the human brain: A method for long-term study and treatment. *IEE Transactions on Biomedical Engineering* Vol. BME–23, pp. 296–304, 1976.

57. HOSOBUCHI, Y., ADAMS, J. E., and LINCHITZ, R.: Pain relief by electrical stimulation of the central gray matter in humans and its reversal by Naloxone. *Science, New York* **197**:183–6, 1977.

58. GYBELS, J.: Electrical stimulation of the central gray for pain relief in humans. *Pain Abstract* 1:170, 2nd World Congress on Pain, Montreal. International Association for the Study of Pain, 1978.

59. DELGADO, J. M. R.: *Physical control of the mind: toward a psychocivilized society.* New York, Harper and Row, 1969.

60. VALENSTEIN, E. S.: *Brain control.* New York, Wiley, 1973.

61. SANO, K.: Sedative neurosurgery, with special reference to postermedial hypothalamotomy. *Neurologia medico-chirurgica* **4**:112, 1962.

62. SANO, K.: Sedative stereoencephalotomy: fornicotomy, upper mesencephalic reticulotomy. *Progress in Brain Research* **21**:350, 1966.

63. MEGARGEE, E. I.: A critical review of theories of violence, in *Crimes of violence.* Ed. Mulvihill, D. J., Tumin, M. M., and Curtis, L. A., Washington DC, US Government Printing Office, 1969.

64. QUINSEY, V. L., PRUESSE, M., and FERNLEY, R.: A follow-up of patients found "unfit to stand trial" or "not guilty" because of insanity. *Canadian Psychiatric Association Journal* **20**:461–7, 1975.

65. COCOZZA, J. J. and STEADMAN, H. J.: Some refinements in the prediction of dangerous behavior. *American Journal of Psychiatry* **131**:1012–14, 1974.

9

Ethical aspects of sexuality and sex therapy

John Bancroft

In general, the purpose of ethical guidelines for the psychiatrist are threefold: (1) to protect the patient from exploitation, incompetence, and pressures to conform; (2) to uphold the rights of that patient, his entitlement to make decisions about his own life and to have access to information that is important to his welfare; and (3) to foster, by the psychiatrist's own behaviour, desirable social attitudes and action.

The first two objectives, protection of the patient and the promotion of his rights, often coincide, but they may also conflict with one another, and present some of the most difficult ethical dilemmas that we have to face. These are circumstances when, in respecting the patient's rights, we may be acting against his interests or well-being. As members of a caring profession, we have to take that dilemma seriously. Fortunately such a dilemma is seldom involved in sex therapy though there are a few examples that I will consider. Problems do arise for the sex therapist when dealing with the sex offender, when there may be conflict between the interests of the offender and those of society.

In considering the third objective, the fostering of desirable social attitudes, we are acknowledging that the responsibilities of the psychiatrist extend beyond his patient to the society in which he lives. Public attitudes and social policy concerning many forms of behaviour have been extensively influenced by medical opinion, often, it seems, disadvantageously. For example, the medical condemnation of various kinds of non-procreative sex in the eighteenth and nineteenth centuries has been well documented.[1] Much more recently, the evidence of the British Medical Association to the Wolfenden Committee on prostitution and homosexuality involved the strong assertion of values that were quite unjustified by any rational medical appraisal.[1] Such influences not only stem from our explicit public statements as professionals, but also from our day-to-day work. The sex therapist has a special need to consider this aspect.

The ethical issues will be considered in this chapter under a number of headings. These include the sexuality of the patient-

–therapist relationship; the influence of the therapist on the patient; informed consent and the appropriateness of treatment; problems of confidentiality; and the professional qualifications of the sex therapist.

Three types of clinical situation will recur and require separate consideration. The first is treatment of sexual dysfunction and general problems in sexual relationships. Numerically, this is the most important, the large majority of patients seeking sex therapy coming into this category. Typically these are individuals or couples who complain of loss of interest or enjoyment in their sexual relationship or impairment of more specific sexual responses, such as erection, ejaculation, or orgasm. The second is the treatment of deviant or stigmatized sexual behaviour, and the third, a particular form of the second, the treatment of the sexual offender.

The sexuality of the patient–therapist relationship

This is not an issue confined to sex therapy. Any medically qualified clinician or nurse has to recognize that the involvement of nudity and physical contact in their dealing with patients has sexual implications that are not present in other types of professional relationship. Sexual feelings may arise in either the patient or the doctor. But in sex therapy there is not only the explicit focus on sex but also the need to increase comfort with sexual matters and to give permission to overcome sexual inhibitions. Hence sexual feelings that arise in the relationship may have therapeutic potential. Prolonged discussion of the patient's sexual history and current feelings inevitably introduces a degree of vicarious sexuality, even without a physical examination. Thus this issue has special significance for all sex therapists whether medically qualified or not.

As a result of the taboo against a sexual relationship between doctors and patients, any such relationship, even when occurring outside the professional context and when quite unrelated to sexual problems, may be regarded as grounds for withdrawal of professional status. Most doctors accept this without question; and yet it is not rare for doctors to engage in sexual activity with their patients on the grounds that it is therapeutic to do so.[2] In a survey of American physicians it was reported that approximately 13 per cent of respondents admitted to engaging in erotic behaviour with patients and approximately 7 per cent in sexual intercourse.[3] It is difficult to believe that this is a representative sample, but it at least indicates that such things do happen. The professional taboo has been likened to the taboo against incest.[4] Elsewhere, I have argued that the incest taboo may serve a useful function by permitting a degree of sexuality in the parent-child relationship which facilitates sexual development, while at the same time protecting from the destructive effects that a fuller sexual relationship might bring.[5] In a similar way, the security derived from the taboo in the doctor–patient relationship may allow sexual feelings to be used constructively in therapy either implicitly or explicitly. Certainly the argument that is most commonly put forward to support the professional taboo is that the special relationship that is required for effective, professional help, which perhaps combines caring and detachment, is incompatible with an overtly sexual relationship with its potential for emotional involvement and self-interest on the part of the professional. In particular, the requirement for the patient to lower his or her defences for the purpose of treatment produces a vulnerability that makes exploitation especially reprehensible.[6] It has been pointed out that such ostensibly therapeutic sexual interaction almost always involves a male therapist and a young female patient, and that there is little evidence of the therapist providing such help for the fat or ugly who might receive from it more benefit to their self-esteem.

If I declare my support for this taboo, I must admit to some uncertainty as to where to draw the line. Should you ever touch your patient except for obviously clinical purposes? An arm around the shoulder or a hug to comfort distress might be construed as sexual and professionals are often advised to avoid even these basically caring gestures if only to safeguard themselves from the occasional histrionic manipulative patient. I would find such limitations to my therapeutic relationships unacceptable and am prepared to take the risk, providing that I am quite clear of my own motives. Other professionals may hold different views.

Some doctors, anxious to avoid inducing any sexual feelings during their genital examination use a purposely brusque and mildly unpleasant examination technique. Whether intended or not, this conveys a negative message about sex. Others, by contrast, feel that the occurrence during physical examination of sexual responses which do not lead to overt sexual interaction not only reinforces the sexual security of the professional relationship but may provide information of therapeutic value. In Britain sex therapists trained in the Balint approach rely a great deal on the *emotional* reactions of the female patient to vaginal examination. Tunnadine[7] calls it 'the moment of truth'. This method involves female therapists treating female patients but that does not exclude sexuality of either a homosexual or a parent–child kind. Within the safety of the professional relationship such experience can lead to crucial permission — as Tunnadine puts it — with a shift from the fantasy: 'this part is bad, prohibited, still belonging to mother who has not handed over permission for a sexual life' — to the fact of a motherly woman saying: 'go ahead — it is yours to explore, use, love with, just like your lips or hands: a decent, beautiful organ of pleasure.'[7]

Concentration by this group of workers on the treatment of female problems has in part stemmed from their difficulty in finding an equivalent of the vaginal examination for the male patient. In the male, examination may not have the same potential for 'permission giving'. But it can nevertheless facilitate a special openness between the male doctor and the male patient if used appropriately. But are such factors relevant when the doctor and patient are of the opposite sex? The relevance is clear when the sexual problems stem from the patient's relationship with the opposite sex parent, although the therapeutic use of such factors may require considerable skill. Also, a therapist of the opposite sex may effectively desensitize the patient to sexual fears of the opposite sex within such a 'safe' relationship. A case can therefore be made for allowing and exploiting the sexuality of the physical examination when it occurs within the security of a professional relationship and when the purpose of the physical examination is not *explicitly sexual*.

What of direct sexual stimulation during such an examination? Hartman and Fithian[8] use what they call a 'sexological examination'. During examination of the female patient, both the male and female therapists take turns in stimulating the vagina. The woman is encouraged to regard any positive or erotic feelings that are elicited as acceptable. At a later stage, the male partner is called in to the room and encouraged to examine his wife and stimulate her vagina in a similar fashion. Their sexological examination of the male partner by contrast does not involve any attempt to stimulate and is much briefer. The reason for this discrepancy is not given. Hoch[9] reports a comparable approach in which the female patient is sexually stimulated by a male therapist during the course of a vaginal examination and in front of her husband. In both these cases, this form of examination is seen as therapeutically valuable. A modification which comes midway between the sexological examination and a 'simple' sexual relationship between therapist and patient has been euphemistically called 'body work therapy'.[10] Here sexual touching of the patient by the therapist or vice versa is encouraged and the patient's emotional reactions to the experience discussed at the time. Although one can recognize the obvious educational potential of this approach, the question that its proponents have not succeeded in answering is the effect that such predecures have on the therapist–patient relationship. Is the rationale of the therapy accepted at face value by the patient or does the relationship in the patient's eyes transform into a sexual game. It is far from clear that possible negative effects on the therapeutic relationship are outweighed by the assumed advantages.

The sexuality of the therapeutic relationship is perhaps most explicit as a result of physical contact, but as mentioned earlier, there are other manifestations. Both verbal and non-verbal behaviour of either therapist or patient may be seductive or sexual in meaning. The therapist may be influenced in his choice of questioning or advice by the vicarious sexuality that ensues. The patient's responses may be influenced in a similar way. Acceptance or rejection of a patient for therapy, or the allotment of time in therapy may be similarly affected. While there would be agreement that such tendencies on the part of the therapist should be both recognized and controlled, there are aspects of the structure of sex therapy which have a relevance not always acknowledged.

First, whether the sex of the therapist is the same or different from that of the patient is a therapeutic variable which ideally should be chosen to meet the needs of the case. The potential sexuality of the relationship may be desirable in one case, to be avoided in another. In practice, there is often limited choice in this respect. Secondly, the therapist may work either with an individual patient or with a couple. In the latter case, the sexual potential for the therapeutic relationship is reduced but not eliminated. Any sexuality that arises between the therapist and one of the patient couple may have an adverse effect on that couple's relationship. This provides one of the justifications for co-therapy — using two therapists, one male and one female. The above problem can then be minimized, particularly if the principal responsibility for relating to each member of the couple is taken by the same sex therapist.

Most of the points that have been raised so far have concerned heterosexuality in the patient–therapist relationship, but the homosexual parallel in each case should also be considered.

One of the most controversial issues in sex therapy is the use of surrogate partners. Here the therapist provides someone *other than himself* to become sexually involved with the patient. The advantages that are claimed are due to the surrogate being concerned and sympathetic as well as knowledgeable about sexual problems; in other words, all the advantages of having sex with your therapist without the disadvantages. One objection often raised is that such a procedure is indistinguishable from prostitution. This does not solve the problem as the ethical status of prostitution itself is far from clear. The similarity is beyond dispute and in fact therapists do sometimes use sensitive, caring prostitutes for this purpose. Such practice is by no means of recent origin.[11] But usually the women involved as surrogates in no way regard themselves as prostitutes. Their motives are of interest and not readily apparent. Masters and Johnson[12] reported that nine of the 13 female surrogates in their research studies justified their participation on the grounds of having had personal experience in helping a family member with sexual problems and wanting to extend that help to others. Only three openly declared that their motives were sexual. Masters and Johnson used only female surrogates but other therapists such as Cole have used males in this role.

The ethical acceptability of surrogate therapy is a complex matter. If the sexual distress of an individual can be overcome by a person who is motivated to help, what is the objection? The efficacy of such help remains obscure though both Masters and Johnson [12] and Cole[13] have claimed good results. Perhaps the ethical issue is related to the criteria of effectiveness. Is the success of such treatment based on the quality of the sexual performance with the surrogate or on the nature of the sexual relationship established with the surrogate? Do changes in that particular relationship generalize to other relationships? These questions highlight one of the most basic controversies among sex therapists — is treatment aimed at sexual function or the sexual relationship? Those who stress the primary importance of the former may be more inclined to accept surrogate therapy as a useful option. Those who favour the latter may reject this approach on the grounds that it either divorces sex from the relationship or leads to complications resulting from the relationship that does develop between the patient and surrogate. Problems of confidentiality with surrogates have also been stressed.[14]

A development in this area that is also causing concern is the emergence of surrogates as a form of helping professional, with their own organizations and codes of practice.[15] The distinction between surrogate partner and therapist is therefore becoming blurred and takes us into the problem area discussed above. This is well illustrated by Cole who refers to his surrogates as therapists. It is the main reason put forward by Masters and Johnson for ceasing to use surrogates.[16]

The influence of the therapist on the patient

For a number of reasons, the therapist is usually in a position to influence his patient. The patient, because of his presenting problem and his need to lower his psychological defences, is often in a psychologically vulnerable state. The therapist, as a member of a helping profession, will often be seen by him as having status and kudos. The esteem accorded to the therapist by the patient is likely to be enhanced by his understandable need to have faith or to put trust in the therapist. From this position of relative power, the therapist has to consider to what extent he is imposing his own values on the patient.

But there is a wider influence that also has to be considered. The therapist, because of his status, may influence a much broader range of opinion not only by what he says in the form of public statements, but also as a consequence of the types of treatment he is known to use. There may be considerable misunderstanding of his motives or opinions for which he cannot be held directly responsible, but it is his responsibility to recognize these wider influences so that he can modify them or amplify them according to this ethical principles. I will consider some specific examples below.

The doctor, working in a medical setting, is used to taking an advisory role with his patients. He is the expert on illness, and the 'sick' patient, if sensible, will put himself into the doctor's hands and do what he says. This is one aspect of the 'medical model' and there is no doubt that in many instances of severe illness, it is appropriate.[17] But such circumstances rarely prevail in the treatment of sexual problems. It is true that there are many medical factors which impinge on sexual funtion, and medical advice on their management will be needed. But the bulk of treatment should be seen as crucially different, as more of an educational process where the therapist helps the patient or couple to learn new ways of relating sexually. Although considerable psychotherapeutic skill may be required to help a patient to overcome the resistance to specific change, the primary purpose is still the change to new ways of behaving. Not only is the onus of change on the patients but they have to be clear that such change is what they seek. The treatment thus involves 'the negotiation of a contract', whereby patient and therapist reach agreement about goals of treatment and methods of reaching them. To use the concept of transactional analysis, the relationship between therapist and patient is of an 'adult–adult' type, rather than 'parent–child' or 'doctor–sick-patient'. I have argued elsewhere[18] that this type of relationship is necessary for effective treatment of sexual problems whereas the more dependent relationship which characterizes the medical setting is less conducive to the type of learning that is required. If that is so, the ethical implications of therapist influence are twofold. First, by wielding such influence, the therapist may unwittingly undermine the appropriate therapist–patient relationship and hence the efficacy of treatment. Secondly, and most obviously, the therapist is in a postiion to impose his own values or beliefs on the patient because of his influential postion.

Given this potential for influence, is it *necessarily* wrong for therapists to impose their own values? In the past, the medical profession has acted as the guardian of sexual morality to an extent second only to the Church. The usual justification stems from the confusion of health and morality, recently exemplified in the Mental Hygiene movement of the 1920s. There is no doubt that sexual values have been powerfully influenced by medical opinion. In the eighteenth and nineteenth centuries, warnings from doctors of the dire medical consequences of non-procreative sex — coitus interruptus or masturbation or homosexuality — added a particularly heavy load to sexual guilt that is still very much in evidence.[19] Members of the medical profession may be less naive about compounding medical advice with morality nowadays, but more subtle versions undoubtedly continue. There is a dilemma here. Are physicians to avoid using their position of influence to encourage attitudes that they believe are for the public good? Given this position, it is difficult for the medical profession to avoid criticism. They will be attacked for bolstering values which are regarded as unacceptable by the critic or they will be attacked for failing to encourage values that the critic upholds.

Whether a doctor is capable of remaining neutral is a matter of some doubt. The ethical requirement is perhaps that he should be clear when he is not doing so, that he should avoid the deceit of justifying his own morality on quasi-medical grounds, and that by the same token he should be active in countering similar deceit stemming from his medical colleagues. Before encouraging a patient to adopt values or attitudes that the therapist holds as important, he should consider carefully whether this would create distressing conflict with the patient's cultural or religious mores. Let us consider some specific examples.

One of the most debated issues of this kind is the treatment of homosexuality. In virtually all Western societies, homosexuality carries social stigma. This may range from outright hostility and ostracism to tolerance, rather than acceptance, of abnormality or more commonly of 'sickness'. Although there are many homosexuals who lead perfectly satisfactory and happy lives in spite of this, there are many others who at some stage experience unhappiness and depression that seems to be directly related to their homosexual lifestyle.[20] The extent to which their distress is a consequence of social stigma is not measurable but is likely to be substantial. When a person seeks professional help for distress of this kind, there are, in simple terms, two obvious goals: one, to learn to adapt more happily within a homosexual role, the other, to explore an alternative such as heterosexuality, asexuality, or bisexuality. What are the ethical issues facing the therapist in this situation? If he has a genuinely open mind about homosexuality, the problem is relatively straightforward. If, for instance, he feels quite comfortable helping people to adjust either to a homosexual or a heterosexual role, he can proclaim his neutrality and set about helping his patient to find the goal and life style that suits him best. If the therapist has more definite views — for example he believes that life as a homosexual is never satisfactory or acceptable and that an asexual or heterosexual alternative should be sought, or by contrast, he believes that someone with homosexual preference should *always* accept those preferences and not try to change them, he is faced with an ethical dilemma. In either case, he is in danger of pressing the patient to conform to his, the therapist's, own values. And yet he may feel strongly that pressure is justified.

In recent years, the view has been expressed increasingly that any therapeutic help aimed at establishing heterosexual feelings or relationships in someone with homosexual preferences is ethically and socially unacceptable. Davison[21] is the most eloquent proponent of this point of view. I have debated the matter more fully elsewhere[22,23] and will here briefly outline the three principal issues that are involved.

The first concerns the effect of such treatment on social attitudes to homosexuality. Any treatment aimed at helping homosexuals to be non-homosexual is regarded as reinforcing negative social attitudes to homosexuality and giving medical support to the notion that homosexuality is bad. Undoubtedly there is some truth in this idea. Greater tolerance of homosexuality in a social group is often attained only by an increase in the number who regard it as a 'sickness' rather than a 'sin'. The knowledge that there is a 'cure' for the 'sickness' encourages that tendency. Hence, it is argued, all such treatment should be avoided. And yet, what about the needs of the individual who seeks help? Can one justifiably deny him help because of the effects that help may have on society in general? Placing the needs of society before those of the patient seems to threaten a most basic principle of the caring professions. But does it have to be an either-or situation? Much depends on the aims of any specific treatment. If the aim is unequivocally to suppress or eliminate homosexual interest, the above argument carries weight. Over the past few years, clinical evidence has shown that such treatment is unlikely to succeed in this aim, providing a second powerful reason for its unacceptability. If, on the other hand, the goals of treatment are to extend the individual's scope for sexual relationships to include the heterosexual, the argument fails. It may be said, to sustain the argument, that therapists never help heterosexuals to establish homosexual relationships. This may be true, principally because such an objective is seldom, if ever, sought; no doubt because heterosexuality *per se* is not stigmatized. It is not unusual, on the other hand, for a therapist to encourage an individual to acknowledge and accept homosexual feelings which he, the therapist, believes to be present when that individual is striving unsuccessfully to maintain a heterosexual identity.

Opinion may remain divided on this issue, but I have no doubt that it is possible to help an individual to explore alternative sexual roles without reinforcing anti-homosexual feelings. A good example of a balanced approach is shown in the book on homosexuality[24], by Masters and Johnson, in which they describe two types of treatment, one aimed at improving homosexual relationships, the other at establishing heterosexual relationships in people with previous homosexual feelings. While their patients may not have been representative of homosexuals in general, they nevertheless sought help. Unfortunately, even a balanced and basically positive report on homosexuality such as that by Masters and Johnson can be taken out of context and used to support a totally opposite point of view. In a recent public debate, following prosecution of a British politician with previous homosexual experience, one commentator cited their report of therapeutic success as evidence that homosexuality is always 'learnt'; hence, it was justified to take steps to prevent it by fostering anti-homosexual values. Such gross misuse of clinical research data can hardly be taken as justification for condemning Masters and Johnson's efforts at treatment, though it certainly helps one to understand how opposition to their approach arises. Attitudes to the treatment of homosexuality have been confounded by this type of statement for some time. Since the late nineteenth century when the 'sinfulness' of homosexuality was being challenged by people with more humanitarian beliefs, evidence of treatability has been used by the opposing camp to demonstrate that homosexuality is acquired rather than innate and hence, for some curious reason, sinful.[1]

The second issue concerning the treatment of homosexuality is that the patient who seeks help does so because of social pressure. His apparent 'free will' is an illusion. The implication of this point of view is that one cannot freely choose to conform. If taken seriously, this argument would throw doubt on the 'free choice' of most forms of psychiatric treatment. Obviously in the capacity of professional advisers we have a responsibility to give as much relevant information as we can to someone who is confronted by such a choice. But to assume that a person is unable to make the most appropriate decision for himself is to take on a responsibility which raises other much more difficult ethical issues.

The third issue derives from the idea that homosexuality is the natural state for the homosexual. An attempt to conform or encouraging someone to conform to an unnatural state, such as heterosexuality, would therefore be regarded as unacceptable. 'Unnaturalness' (i.e. recourse to 'natural law') is often used to justify the moral unacceptability of homosexuality itself[26] and not surprisingly a similar argument is sometimes used to oppose attempts to change from homosexuality to heterosexuality. If such an argument was to have any rational basis, it would require sufficient knowledge of the origins of homosexual and heterosexual preferences to allow us to recognize which was the innate or constitutional preference in any particular individual. In fact, we have little understanding of why either homosexual or heterosexual preferences develop and the reasons are likely to be many and various. In addition, we know little about the extent to which sexual preferences are stable or immutable. There may be a sub-group in which homosexual preferences are both innate and immutable but as yet we are unable to recognize its members and we certainly have no reason to believe that this would apply to all or even a majority of homosexuals.

These various issues identify areas where caution is needed; whatever the therapist's values, it would seem appropriate for him to consider certain factors before making ethical decisions about treatment. Individuals seeking help with homosexual problems are often under pressure from others to seek a 'cure'. They often *expect* the therapist, unless he is clearly identified as homosexual himself, to hold negative views about homosexuality. Those who are already in contact with other homosexuals, particularly homosexual groups, may have been subjected to considerable pressure to 'conform' homosexually. The therapist should perhaps ask himself if there is any likelihood that he will reinforce these pressures from either direction. And if so should he not refer the patient to someone who can approach his problem from a more neutral standpoint? The paedophiliac highlights this dilemma more starkly. While opinions on homosexuality vary, 'neutral' attitudes to paedophilia are rare. Even so, the almost universal assumption that sexuality between adult and child is ethically unacceptable, if not abhorrent, is being challenged by some professionals.[26] And it has been suggested that current attitudes to paedophilia can be compared to those towards homosexuality in the past.[27]

It is pertinent to consider how acceptability of specific forms of sexuality varies over time. In the nineteenth century, most physicians probably believed that masturbation was harmful to health, even to the extent of causing insanity. They presumably would have had no qualms about warning the patient of these dangers, indeed it may have been regarded as negligent not to do so. In retrospect, those ideas are absurd and whatever their true origin, they cannot have been substantiated by factual evidence. Yet the 'medicalization' of this point of view effectively obscured the real ethical issues involved. The current reaction against paedophilia is likely to be justified on the grounds of 'harm to the child'. Evidence that harm usually or even commonly follows such behaviour is hard to find. The evidence available suggests that harm is more likely to ensue from the social reaction to the event rather than from the event itself. It would therefore appear ethically dubious to justify one's negative feelings about paedophilia on those grounds. And yet most of us, for the time-being at least, will no doubt continue to regard this behaviour as unacceptable. How then should we react to the paedophiliac patient who seeks help? He may be more concerned with avoiding prosecution than stopping his paedophilia *per se*. Should we enter into a professional relationship with him if we find that aspect of his personality unacceptable or even abhorrent? Can we justify a refusal to help if we are unable to suggest a more suitable colleague?

Another clinical example evokes an ethical dilemma which is more insidious perhaps because it is less contentious. This concerns the individual who presents with low sexual interest or drive. Usually this is seen as a problem because of its incompatibility with the greater sexual interest of the partner. The therapist may seek a cause for this 'disability' or recommend treatment, with the implication that diminished sexual interest is wrong or pathological. A parallel may be drawn with low intelligence. Obviously there are circumstances when an individual's intelligence becomes impaired, even occasionally undeveloped because of a pathological process which deserves attention. But usually if problems in a relationship stem from a difference in intellectual capacity, help is given to the couple to come to terms with the difference rather than to try to reduce it. But not so with low sex drive; sex therapists often justify intervention on the grounds that low drive is a consequence of active psychological inhibition. Doubtless that is sometimes the case, but some therapists have difficulty in accepting that a person's low sexual interest may be intrinsic. In such circumstances, we encourage conformity to a norm of sexual activity.

A comparable and perhaps more contentious issue concerns female orgasm. While it is relatively unusual for an adult man to be non-orgasmic, it is far from rare among women. There seems little doubt that many women have become orgasmic with help, realizing the potential that had lain dormant. But a corollary of this has been the growing expectation that every woman should be orgasmic, yet there is no evidence or even likelihood that this is possible. The issue has become confounded by its political implications. An orgasm has become a 'woman's right' of the kind which has often been denied by the self-centred sexual chauvinism of men. A male therapist may now expect feminist censure if he suggests to a woman that she may not have the capacity for orgasm. Obviously it is no more justified to make that assumption than it is to make the opposite, but it is difficult to avoid the process of reinforcing 'norms' and the consequent pressure to conform to them. This is one area in which the therapeutic activities of sex therapists have unwittingly influenced public opinion by generating new expectations. How does one strike the correct balance between encouraging women to realize their sexual potential and creating dissatisfaction with their individual limitations?

Another relevant ethical issue concerns the conflict between the goals of therapy and the cultural or religious norms of the patient. Many sex therapists emphasize the importance of mutual self-assertion and self-protection in the sexual relationship, stressing the need for equality both in the give-and-take of sexual pleasure and in the relationship more generally. In the context of white, Anglo-Saxon, Protestant, or Jewish middle-class culture, from which these therapeutic approaches originate, such principles make sense. But to what extent should they be encouraged in couples from different cultural or religious backgrounds? For the Muslim this may present conflict with Islamic expectations of the sexual roles of men and women. In many societies, particularly those more obviously 'macho-oriented', the sex therapist's principles may conflict with the cultural criteria of masculinity or feminity. By advocating his principles, the therapist may seek harmony within the social environment. When do advantages of the therapist's 'model relationship' outweigh the social dissonance that it may produce? It also, once again, takes us into the realm of sexual politics. The amount of conflict produced tends to vary with the degree of cultural or religious support for the subordination of women. I have to admit to a degree of missionary zeal in this respect. I firmly believe in the social and interpersonal value of equality in sexual relationships as described above, yet I am conscious of the conflict that it may produce in some of my patients. Usually my zeal is overpowered by entrenched social influences. The therapist should not get the extent of his 'power' out of proportion. But the ethical dilemma is there, and it is accentuated by the increasing tendency for women to reject traditional social norms, and hence to be receptive of therapy goals, while their partners prefer the status quo. In such cases, therapy may only reinforce tension that had already developed in the relationship because of the changing expectations of women. It is pertinent to ask when it is helpful to increase tensions in this way.

Informed consent and the acceptability of treatment methods

Having considered the potential influence of the therapist on his patient, what other ethical issues arise in the negotiation of treatment for sexual problems? The need for goals that are acceptable both to patient and therapist has already been stressed. But what about the acceptability of the treatment method itself?

Most forms of sex therapy present no particular problems in this respect, relying on the active co-operation of the patient or couple to carry out 'homework assignments' in the privacy of their own home — tasks which are within their control to do or not to do. Nevertheless, it is desirable from every point of view to give a clear account of what will be involved, such as the type of homework assignment, content of the counselling sessions, and frequency and duration of treatment. When this is done a proportion of patients or couples decline the offer of treatment, either explicitly or by default, and this emphasizes the importance of *informed* consent. If informed consent is not sought, patients may enter a form of therapy which they do not understand or like but from which they cannot escape without loss of face. Such a situation is commonplace in many psychiatric clinics, particularly within the British Health Service, where the patient does not pay for treatment. Treatment proceeds from one session to the next with no clear objective or plan having been stated and no clear opportunities for the patient to say 'yes, I do want to give this a try' or 'no, I don't'. Initial assessment merges imperceptibly into ill-defined treatment; the patient complies or is seen to be unco-operative or 'poorly motivated'.

Most sex therapists recognize the desirability of establishing a clear 'contract' with the patient at the outset. This not only requires him to make a responsible decision whether to accept this particular offer of help, but is also therapeutically beneficial if treatment is accepted. The patient may reject the offer not because he is 'poorly motivated' but because he does not like or trust the therapist or does not feel comfortable with the style of treatment proposed.

There are specific components of treatment that present problems and there may be a need to correct patients' false expectations. They may, for example, incorrectly and apprehensively believe that therapy will require them to 'perform sexually' in front of the therapist. The need for a physical examination and the particular form it takes can create difficulties. Some therapists may be inflexible in following certain procedures, such as having the partner present or involved at this examination. Failure to prepare the patient or couple for this procedure may result in alienation or rejection of treatment. Obviously it is not possible or even desirable for every eventuality to be agreed upon at the outset — but if the therapist is sensitive to possible rejection of a new idea and allows proper and unprejudiced discussion during the course of therapy, these difficulties can often be avoided. A common problem is the unacceptability of masturbation techniques by some patients. When these techniques are rejected by the patients they may feel that they are unreasonably old-fashioned or unco-operative. This can have a destructive effect on treatment and also lower patients' self-esteem unnecessarily.

Measurement of physiological changes, especially genital responses, such as erection or vaginal response, may be used to monitor treatment or even as a form of treatment itself, as with biofeedback techniques.[28,29] Once again, fully informed consent is desirable with continuing sensitivity of the therapist to how acceptable these forms of treatment are to the patient. The patient may not have understood what was involved, in spite of careful description, or may not have anticipated his or her emotional reactions to the procedure.

A form of treatment which has caused particular concern is aversion therapy. In the 1950s and 1960s it was used quite commonly for the treatment of various forms of deviant sexuality including homosexuality. The inefficacy of treatment methods aimed at eliminating existing behaviours rather than establishing new ones has already been mentioned and in the light of clinical experience, as well as theoretical reappraisal, aversive techniques are now seen to have a much more limited role. They may be useful, however, in helping the patient who is in danger of committing a sexual offence to increase his self-control, particularly if combined with other more positive methods of treatment.[1,30] But can the use of noxious stimuli such as electric shock or induced nausea ever be justified on ethical grounds? Much of the criticism of these techniques involves a comparison with 'brain washing'. I have closely examined this assumption elsewhere[1] and pointed out that the similarity between 'thought reform' techniques and aversion therapy, *as generally used*, is negligible, not only because of the differences in noxiousness and duration involved, but also because of the need, in the case of thought reform, for total control of the individual's environment. In the absence of such 'total manipulation', there is little chance of altering a person's reactions or beliefs unless such changes are sought by him. Hence providing that aversive techniques are only used in a setting where the patient is able to reject or withdraw from treatment, the ethical problem is not one of 'Clockwork Orange' control.

Obviously there are ethical considerations in the type of noxious stimuli used. They should be safe and no more unpleasant than they need to be for the purpose. Their intensity should be chosen to suit the tolerance of the individual patient and he should still have control over the level of intensity used. There have been several reports of methods which do not follow these principles and they have consequently received just criticism.[31] But if we ensure the fully informed consent of the patient in the use of safe and tolerable aversive stimuli, do we satisfy ethical requirements? Does aversive treatment differ from other painful forms of treatment such as surgery or dentistry? In my view, the remaining ethical issue involves, once again, the nature of the patient–therapist relationship. At best, an aversive technique should be seen as one particular form of help incorporated into a more broadly-based approach. It should not be seen as a complete or sufficient treatment method in its own right. It should be associated with the same kind of mutually-respecting 'adult–adult' relationship between patient and therapist that I emphasized earlier. Of crucial relevance, is the effect that the aversive procedure has on this relationship. Two consequences are likely; the patient may feel anger towards the therapist, and he may feel humiliated by the experience. In my own assessment of the usefulness of aversion therapy, I found I could only participate by making active efforts to counter both these consequences, usually by discussing the patient's feelings, helping him to express them, and at the same time, attempting to compensate for any negative effects. One could argue that I may have, with this approach, reduced the efficacy of treatment or conversely that benefits that did accrue were more a result of relationship factors than of the aversive technique itself. But in any case, I concluded that the focus on the relationship was an essential ethical condition. It could also be argued that in following this principle, I was more concerned to reduce my own discomfort or guilt about hurting someone and to reassure myself that I was not the sadist that aversive therapists are often accused of being, than to help the patient. I would nevertheless hold the view that by adhering to these principles, one incorporates an ethical safeguard. I would therefore not be prepared to use the aversive approaches advocated recently in which, instead of impersonal noxious stimuli, systematic criticism and humiliation by onlookers is used; so-called 'shame-therapy'.[32] Happily the indications for aversive techniques are now so limited that they are seldom used. But the principles involved may have more general relevance.

The use of aversive techniques to facilitate self-control over unwanted sexual behaviour brings me to the next ethical issue — consent to treatment by the sexual offender, which is not only informed but also free from coercion. It is not unusual for an offender, say a paedophiliac, to be referred by the court for treatment, such treatment to be given as a condition of sentence. How can one establish, at a stage when the sentence has not been passed, what the offender himself wants, other than his understandable desire to placate the court? With psychological methods of treatment, particularly counselling or psychotherapy, the issue is less crucial because treatment is not likely to be effective unless the offender wants it to be. Nevertheless, he may find himself 'trapped' in therapy because of his sentence. The use of aversive techniques in these circumstances is clearly a cause for concern, and even more critical, the prescribing of drugs such as the anti-androgen-cyproterone acetate, oestrogens or benperidol to control sexual drive. Once sentence, which includes the condition for treatment, has been passed, control for what is done passes from the court, with its public safeguards, to the doctor, with probably no external scrutiny at all. The crucial distinction arises between 'therapy', which is usually regarded as in the interest of the recipient, and 'social control' where the aim is primarily to protect society. The use of a penal procedure like imprisonment is straightforward in that it comes unequivocally into the second category and is only administered with the public safeguards of the legal system. But when 'social control' becomes confused with medical treatment, those safeguards disappear and ethical problems ensue because of the possibility that the offender's interests are dealt with at the same time as those of society. The use of drugs to suppress libido in sexual offenders creates a precedent which, with the development of drugs to control other drives such as aggression, may have much wider and more fundamental ethical significance.

Clearly a case can be made for the use of libido-suppressing drugs both to the benefit of the individual and as a means of 'social control'. There may be individuals who have not as yet tangled with the law but who are in danger of doing so and who seek medical help. Drugs may then be useful and the problem of informed consent does not differ substantially from that with other types of drug therapy. There will also be those who following conviction are regarded as a serious threat to public safety and for whom the use of drugs as an alternative 'social control' to imprisonment may be justified; can 'consent free from coercion', normally required before administering medical treatment, ever be obtained with sufficient confidence when the alternative is another method of penal control? In these cases I would argue that treatment should be administered by the court in the same way as any other penal measure and not be labelled euphemistically as medical treatment. Currently, there is no legal machinery for such administration. This is a complex and important ethical issue which urgently needs debate. (There are some similarities here to ethical problems arising in the use of the parole system.[33])

There are other forms of 'treatment' for sexual offenders which deserve separate consideration because of their irreversible nature and potentially far-reaching effects. Both surgical castration and various forms of psycho-surgery (see Chapter 8) have been used, and the ethical question is whether they should be used under any circumstances. Castration is much less commonly used to-day, partly because it has been shown to be relatively ineffective.[34] The value of psychosurgery is not clear from the available evidence. Given the generalized effects that both procedures may have on personality, I would require solid evidence of predictable outcome in each case before I could begin to justify their use. It is difficult to see how such evidence could be obtained.

The management of the transsexual patient

Transsexualism as a clinical problem poses ethical issues that are perhaps unique and which require separate consideration. Transsexuals believe themselves to be, or seek to become, members of the sex opposite to that of their own bodies. The causes for this condition are not understood and even professionals concerned to help these people find it a puzzle. Because of transsexuals' overriding desire to live and be accepted as members of their psychological sex, they seek medical help to change their bodies to conform with their psychological gender identity. Such sex re-assignment may require, apart from an adjustment in behaviour, in the case of a male to female transsexual, electrolysis of facial hair, oestrogenic hormones to feminize the skin and body fat, mammoplasty, penectomy, orchidectomy, and vaginoplasty. For the female to male transsexual, androgenic hormones to increase body and facial hair and muscle bulk, mastectomy, hysterectomy, oophorectomy, and possibly phalloplasty may be sought (as yet the advantages of phalloplasty are dubious and no-one has succeeded in surgically creating a penis that can either transmit urine or become naturally erect). An enormous amount of medical help is likely to be required in the long-term process of sex reassignment which, at best, is always difficult.

The first ethical issue concerns the basic acceptability of the procedure, especially as it involves surgical alteration of the anatomy. It may be regarded as immoral because it is seen to tamper with nature.[35] Some surgeons have been reluctant to involve themselves, or have been discouraged by their legal advisers from doing so, for fear that they may be prosecuted under the archaic Mayhem statutes. These derive from feudal England and were intended to deter men from evading military service by having some part of their body removed (usually fingers or toes). The surgeon responsible for the maiming was liable. Holloway[36] however was able to find only one case in the legal literature in which a surgeon had been convicted under such a statute and this was not for sex re-assignment surgery. He gives the considered legal opinion that, provided fully informed consent is obtained, the surgeon cannot be held liable for sex re-assignment surgery under such laws. But such is the lack of understanding, fear, or revulsion commonly expressed in relation to transsexualism that prosecution is still considered a possibility. According to Hastings[37] the absence of Mayhem from the recently revised statutes of Minnesota was an important factor in allowing one of the earlier sex re-assignment operations in the United States to take place. This concern has not been extended to those cases, such as adreno-genital syndrome or Klinefelter's syndrome, where there is an identifiable physical cause for the incongruity between psychological and physical gender. (It may prove to be relevant that there are a number of reports of endocrine abnormalities in female-to-male transsexuals[38] but no so far in the male-to-female form.) A further objection has come from some psychiatrists who view transsexualism as a form of psychosis and sex re-assignment surgery as a totally unacceptable collusion with the patient's delusional system. The mental state of the transsexual is indeed important in deciding whether he is able to give 'informed consent'. It is usually not possible to justify a diagnosis of psychosis or any other particular psychiatric condition.[39] Transsexuals often have personality problems, perhaps particularly the male-to-female[40] but this is often an understandable consequence of prolonged gender identity confusion and is a likely to be a justification for sex re-assignment as a contraindication.

Transsexualism has been described as an iatrogenic condition; before the first surgical re-assignment there was not the demand for such treatment as now exists. It is perhaps not surprising that before such a procedure is regarded as feasible it is not often requested. In fact, many people with gender identity confusion may resolve much of their confusion once they learn that such a change is possible, even if the prospect is remote. There certainly seems little doubt that apart from the specific request for surgery, the other manifestations of transsexualism have been well-known for centuries.[41]

As the medical profession has become more familiar with the problem, there has been a greater preparedness to seek solutions to the transsexual's problems. With recognition that a proportion of transsexuals are clearly better off after re-assignment surgery than they were before, a number of centres around the world have provided this type of treatment. The professional in such a centre faces a further ethical problem: the conflict between the rights of the patient and the doctor's responsibility for his patient's welfare. The relationship between transsexual patient and doctor is to a considerable extent a game in which the patient has no doubts about his or her wishes and whose primary purpose is to persuade the doctor to accede to them. The doctor in return is conscious of the possibility of an unfavourable outcome — that by no means do all transsexuals fare well following surgery. Failure is of two principal types. First, the patient's expectations of the benefits of surgery may be unrealistic, looking for resolution of most of his problems. In fact, the problem of 'passing' successfully into the new sex will not be affected by genital surgery except indirectly through an increase in self-confidence. Commonly the patient discovers that life is still difficult and he may return for more surgery. The second kind of failure is in surgical technique. Vaginoplasty and phalloplasty pose considerable technical challenges to the surgeon and frequently go wrong. Post-operative complications may be prolonged or serious.

The doctor when confronted with a patient seemingly determined to pursue sex reassignment, naturally wishes to establish that the patient will cope with, and benefit from this major change. Hence, more or less all specialist centres now require a period of one and a half to two years of 'real life testing' in the new role before irreversible surgery is carried out.[42] The patient may go along with this plan, or if he has sufficient money seek a surgeon who will co-operate without a testing period. (This contest between patient and doctor is reminiscent of a request for abortion when psychiatric approval is required, though with rather different stakes).

The dilemma for the doctor in these cases is compounded by a further factor. Given a patient who may be psychologically unstable, the doctor may fear litigation following surgery by the patient or his family, although this has only rarely occurred.[36] This fear is accentuated when the doctor is not confident that he has the support of colleagues in his decision to operate. For this reason, and because of the enormous demands on medical resources that follow, the decision about surgery is a major one. There is now a tendency to rely on specialist gender identity committees to take a corporate clinical decision.[43] Clinical experience that can be properly evaluated is still limited and there is no doubt that we should continue to appraise critically the management of these unhappy and distressed people.

Confidentiality

In most forms of psychiatric treatment information obtained from patients is of a highly confidential nature. This is particularly so where sexual problems are concerned. Special consideration has therefore to be given to the method of keeping records and to the type of information recorded. The use of special files, distinguishable and separate from general medical files, is probably mandatory.

Psychiatrists are usually trained to take a detailed history which is systematic and far ranging. They are less well trained to select crucial information in a particular case, and usually follow the principle that the more information one has, the less likely will some important factor be overlooked. The acquisition of large amounts of confidential and intimate information may also enhance their 'charisma' in the patient's eyes. We need to question seriously the amount of information we obtain (and especially record) in the management of sexual problems. There are two implications. The first is related to the therapeutic consequences: the vulnerability produced in the patient by a one-way exchange of information may reinforce a tendency to take a passive role in therapy rather than the active 'adult' role that is needed. The second implication is more directly ethical. Is the therapist justified in obtaining information which is not clearly relevant to the patient's treatment? In the newer, more behavioural forms of sex therapy, specific behavioural tasks, usually small steps towards the goals of treatment, are set by the therapist. If the patient or couple can carry these out satisfactorily then the next tasks are assigned and so on. Only when difficulty is encountered in achieving the tasks is it necessary to look for explanations, and relevant background information may then be sought. A couple can go through a course of such therapy with little problem and consequently with the therapist knowing very little about their past lives.[18] Obviously a certain amount of information has to be obtained at the outset in order to arrive at a reasonable contract for treatment. Yet many therapists consider that they have failed in their professional duty if they do not find out about important past events. The need to justify requests for confidential information remains an important ethical issue in sex therapy as well as other kinds of psychiatric treatment.

When working with couples, particular problems of confidentiality may arise when one partner gives the therapist information that is to be concealed from the other. With information about past events, it is usually appropriate to accept the patient's request for continued confidentiality. When the confidence concerns a continuing or current aspect of the patient's life, this may pose problems for the therapist. The most obvious example is when one partner reveals an on-going extra-marital relationship and expects the therapist to keep the information from the spouse. This may impose a considerable handicap on therapy and can be considered unacceptable on those grounds. My own policy in these circumstances is to indicate that I am only prepared to work with a couple if they commit themselves to their relationship, at least for the duration of treatment. I explain that the basis of my approach is to facilitate an open, self-assertive, and self-protective relationship, and that to attempt that with the therapist and one partner concealing highly relevant information from the other makes a mockery of that approach. There is however a need for caution. The spouse with current extra-marital activity may not anticipate this response from the therapist. Having made the revelation, the withdrawal of the therapist from a treatment contract may place the patient in a difficult position with his spouse. It may therefore be appropriate, when such circumstances are suspected, to

make a general comment about therapeutic policy before the patient
has revealed anything specific.

Professional qualifications

A prevailing concern among sex therapists at present is the maintenance of satisfactory standards of training and clinical practice. It is
not unusual for people who have no professional training of any kind,
and whose qualifications are based only on their own sexual experiences to designate themselves as expert sex therapists. It may be
argued that the maintenance of professional standards is not an
ethical issue, however desirable it is to foster competent practice. On
the other hand, the point is often made that professional bodies
establish and enforce ethical guidelines. Individual therapists working
outside such organizations have no such guidance or constraints. This
point has even been used to justify the exclusion of all non-medical
professionals (such as clinical psychologists) from involvement in sex
therapy, on the grounds that only medical doctors have a 'Hippocratic oath', which bars them from sexual contact with their patients and
a disciplinary body to enforce it. (The fact that most doctors on
qualifying don't take any such oath is perhaps irrelevant). This issue
is a complex one and I shall only deal with it briefly. Much of the
problem stems from the difficulty in defining what are the requirements for a good sex therapist. In matters of unequivocal pathology, it
is relatively easy to justify the need for medical training. For some
sexual problems, therefore, medical expertise is helpful or even
essential but for many more, perhaps the majority, it is of negligible
relevance. Most sexual problems stem from difficulties in communication, false expectations, and interpersonal insecurity, so that the
doctor is no more likely because of his medical training to be equipped
to deal with these issues than the next person. The ability to inform
about normal sexuality and to make individuals or couples comfortable about their sexual feelings is also shown by people from other
professional backgrounds or with no professional training at all. The
'lay therapist' may be as good as any in this respect. The requirement
of training specifically in sex therapy is easier to justify, but has to be
set against the relatively young and fragmented state of the field.
There is genuine disagreement among professionals about the relative
importance of specific skills (e.g. routine medical examination).

This issue is much more important in private practice where,
usually of necessity, the clinician is working in relative isolation.
Within a multidisciplinary health service, the opportunity for sharing
problems or referring cases to clinicians with other skills is inherent in
the system; it is undoubtedly a matter of ethical responsibility for

professionals who work in this context to be clear about their personal limits of competence and the criteria for involving colleagues. All too often, the medical members of the team see their relationships with other professionals as uni-directional in this respect.

In my view, the field of sexual problems has the particular advantage that a simple educational approach can be used in the first instance, often with good effect and frequently sufficient in itself. In cases where this is not enough, additional help and skills can be introduced at a later stage without disadvantage. The border-line between sex education, simple counselling, and more complex therapy are ill-defined.

This brings us to a key ethical issue: the process by which one professional group may seek to limit the therapeutic activities of other groups. On the grounds of protecting the interests of the patient, such limitations may conceal the protection of 'vested interests'. This problem is not confined to private practice. Within the British National Health Service there are recurring instances of such hypocrisy. Members of the medical profession have a long tradition of curtailing the activities of their fellow professions and hence maintaining their own power and influence. Such a process not surprisingly spreads to other groups. In Britain, some clinical psychologists, possibly with genuine grievances about their treatment by more powerful medical colleagues, have come to regard behavioural methods of treatment as being their own province, and have objected to other professionals, such as doctors or nurses, applying them.

Sex therapy is very much affected by this competitive process, particularly as it is seen as a fashionable and often lucrative form of clinical practice. It is thus an ethical problem in this field, as in others, when professional demarcation disputes are obscured behind the cause of patient care.

It may be agreed, nevertheless, that with the various ethical complexities that have been considered in this chapter, there is a strong need for a special or 'professional' status for the sex therapist. If so, we must seek ethically acceptable ways of meeting that need.

References

1. BANCROFT, J.: *Deviant sexual behaviour: modification and assessment*. Oxford University Press, 1974.
2. TAYLOR, B. J. and WAGNER, N. N.: Sexual contact between therapists and their patients. *British Journal of Sexual Medicine* **6**:35–40, 1979.
3. KARDENER, S. H., FULLER, M., and MENSH, I. N. A survey of physicians' attitudes and practices regarding erotic and non-erotic contact with patients. *American Journal of Psychiatry* **130**:1077–81, 1973.
4. KARDENER, S. H. Sex and the physician–patient relationship. *American Journal of Psychiatry* **131**,1134–6, 1974.

5. BANCROFT, J. Commentary on 'incest' by Noble, M. and Mason, J. R. *Journal of Medical Ethics* 4:69–70, 1978.

6. MARMOR, J. The ethics of sex therapy, in *Ethical issues in sex therapy and research* Eds. Masters, W. H., Johnson, V. E., and Kolodne, R. C. Boston, Little Brown, 1977.

7. TUNNADINE, L. P. D.: *Contraception and sexual life; a therapeutic approach.* London Tavistock, 1970.

8. HARTMAN, W. E. and FITHIAN, M. A.: *Treatment of sexual dysfunction.* California, Centre for Marital and Sexual Studies, 1972.

9. HOCH, Z.: The sensory arm of the female orgasmic reflex. Paper read at 5th Annual Meeting of International Academy of Sex Research, Prague, August, 1979.

10. WILLIAMS, M. H.: Individual sex therapy, in *Handbook of sex therapy.* Ed. LoPiccolo, J., and LoPiccolo, L., Plenum, New York, 1978.

11. SCHRENCK-Notzing, A. VON: *The use of hypnosis in psychopathic sexuality with special reference to contrary sexual instruct.* (Trans. C. L. Chaddock, 1956). The Institute of Research on Hypnosis. Publication Society and Juhan Press, 1895.

12. MASTERS, W. and JOHNSON, V. F.: *Human sexual inadequacy.* Boston, Little Brown, 1970.

13. COLE, M.: Human sex behaviour and sex therapy, in *Sexual problems.* Ed. Jacobson, J., London, Elek, 1975.

14. REDLICH, F.: The ethics of sex therapy, in *Ethical issues in sex therapy and research.* Ed. Masters, E. H., Johnson, V. E., and Kolodny, R. C., Boston, Little Brown, 1977.

15. JACOBS, M. THOMPSON, L. A., and TRUXAW, P.: The use of sexual surrogates in counselling. *Counselling Psychologist* 5,73–7, 1975.

16. MASTERS, W. H., JOHNSON, V. S., and KOLODNY, R.: *Ethical issues in sex therapy and research.* Boston, Little Brown, 1977.

17. BANCROFT, J.: Crisis intervention, in *An introduction to the psychotherapies.* Ed. Bloch, S., London, Oxford University Press, 1979.

18. BANCROFT, J.: Sex therapy, in *An introduction to the psychotherapies.* Ed. Bloch, S., London, Oxford University Press, 1979.

19. BULLOUGH, V. L.: Homosexuality and the medical model. *Journal of Homosexuality* 1:99–110, 1974.

20. BELL, A. P. and WEINBERG, M. S.: *Homosexualities. A study of diversity among men and women.* London, Mitchell Beezley, 1978.

21. DAVISON, G. C.: Homosexuality: the ethical challenge. *Journal of Consulting and Clinical Psychology* 44:157–62, 1976.

22. BANCROFT, J.: Homosexuality and the medical profession: a behaviourist's view. *Journal of Medical Ethics* 1:176–80, 1975.

23. BANCROFT, J.: Treatment of homosexuality: some ethical considerations. Paper given at 3rd Congress of World Association of Sexology, Rome, October, 1978.

24. MASTERS, W. H. AND JOHNSTON, V. E. Homosexuality in perspective. Boston, Little Brown, 1979.

25. HOFFMAN, M.: *The gay world.* New York, Basic Books, 1968.

26. CONSTANTINE, L. L.: The sexual rights of children: Implications of a radical perspective, in *Love and attraction.* Ed. Cook, M. and Wilson, G., Oxford, Pergamon, 1979.

27. PLUMMER, K.: Images of paedophilia, in *Love and attraction.* Ed. Cook, M. and Wilson, G. Oxford, Pergamon, 1979.

28. ROSEN, R. C.: Operant control of sexual responses in man, in *Biofeedback: theory and research.* Ed. Schwartz, E. G., and Beatty, J., Vol. 7. New York, Academic Press, 1979.

29. HOON, P. W. The assessment of sexual arousal in women, in *Progress in behaviour modification*, Vol. 7. New York, Academic Press, 1979.
30. BANCROFT, J.: The behavioural approach to treatment, in *Handbook of sexology.* Ed. Money, J., and Musaph, H., Amsterdam, Excerpta Medica, 1977.
31. CAMPBELL, D., SANDERSON, R. E., and LAVERTY, S. G.: Characteristics of a conditioned response in human subjects during extinction trials following a single traumatic conditioning trial. *Journal of Abnormal and Social Psychology* **68**:627–39, 1963.
32. SERBER, M.: Shame aversion therapy. *Behaviour Therapy and Experimental Psychiatry* **1**:219–21, 1974.
33. HOOD, R.: Some fundamental dilemmas of the English parole system and a suggestion for an alternative structure, in *Parole: its implications for the penal and criminal justice system.* Ed. Thomas. D.A. Cambridge Institute of Criminology, 1974.
34. BREMER, J.: *Asexualisation: a follow-up study of 244 cases.* New York, Macmillan, 1959.
35. GREEN, R.: Attitudes towards transsexualism and sex re-assignment procedures, in *Transsexualism and sex reassignment.* Ed. Green, R., and Money, J., Baltimore, Johns Hopkins Press, 1969.
36. HOLLOWAY, J. P.: Transsexuals: legal considerations. *Archives of Sexual Behaviour* **3**,33–50, 1974.
37. HASTINGS, D. W.: Inauguration of a research project on transsexualism in a University Medical Centre, in *Transsexualism and sex re-assignment.* Ed. Green, R., and Money, J., Baltimore, Johns Hopkins Press, 1969.
38. SEYLER, L. E., CAVALIS, E., SPARE, S., and REICHLIN, S.: Abnormal gonadotrophic secretory responses to LHRH in transsexual women after diethylstilboestrol. *Journal of Clinical Endocrinology and Metabolism* **47**:176–83, 1978.
39. HOENIG, J. and KENNER, J. C.: The nosological position of transsexualism. *Archives of Sexual Behaviour* **3**:273–88, 1974.
40. WALINDER, J.: *Transsexualism: a study of 43 cases.* Gotenburg, Scandinavian University Book, 1967.
41. BULLOUGH, V. L.: Transsexualism in history. *Archives of Sexual Behaviour* **4**:561–72, 1975.
42. MONEY, J. and WALKER, P. A.: Counselling the transsexual, in *Handbook of sexology.* Ed. Money, J., and Musaph, H., Amsterdam, Excerpta Medica, 1977.
43. MONEY, J.: Public opinion and social issues in transsexualism: a case study in medical sociology in *Transsexualism and sex reassignment.* Ed. Green, R., and Money, J., Baltimore, Johns Hopkins Press, 1969.

10

The ethics of suicide

David Heyd and Sidney Bloch

I. The special status of the problem of suicide

SUICIDE presents perhaps the most dramatic and demanding clinical situation psychiatrists have to face. At the annual rate of 5000 successful suicides in England and 20 000–30 000 in the United States, no psychiatrist can deny the gravity of the problem. And as the number of attempted (unsuccessful) suicides is roughly 8 to 10 times the number of fatal suicides, there is but little chance that any psychiatrist is spared the direct and personal experience of treating suicidal patients and their families. While the widespread incidence makes suicide impossible to ignore, its very nature makes it difficult to confront — psychologically, therapeutically, and ethically.

Suicide differs in at least four important respects from other clinical circumstances that involve ethical dilemmas. First, most medical and psychiatric problems are concerned with the adjustment of the right means to a given end that is basically shared by doctor and patient; suicide however focuses on the end itself, about which the two parties may hold polarly opposite views. Suicide is not only a *functional* problem to which therapeutic techniques are applied but also an *existential* one — in both the literal and the philosophical senses of the word. The question is not how to achieve a better, more fruitful life, but whether to live at all. The fact that the starting-point in the treatment of the potentially suicidal person is seen in such radically divergent terms by doctor and patient makes suicide a particularly difficult case: the psychiatrist's task extends beyond technically assisting his patient in attaining his own desired goals; he is required to persuade the patient to change his most basic desires and attitude to life.

Secondly, the conflict between the psychiatrist's values and his patient's goals is deeper than a particular and incidental disagreement. The value of life as an end in itself is not only shared by the great majority of people, but also considered as possibly the most important ethical value. Accordingly, the very phenomenon of suicide is generally regarded as a threat or even as an insult to our deepest convictions about the 'sanctity of life'. To some extent this intolerance of the idea of the cessation of life is manifest in our attitude to death in general, which we find hard to face directly, but it is especially acute in the case of suicide, which expresses a *voluntary* and irreverent repudiation of the value of life.

Thirdly, it is difficult for us to rid ourselves of this sense of insult or threat, because the dilemma of suicide is logically and ethically puzzling. As we shall see in the next section, there are unsolvable problems in supplying a rational justification for the value of life and for the alleged moral duty to go on living. Our belief in the obvious value of life is further offended by the relative failure in preventing suicide, either by means of psychiatric treatment or through some form of social engineering. It seems that whatever we do, the rate of suicide in a particular society will remain fairly constant.[1] And the optimism raised by successful prevention in individual cases is partly offset by the alarming number of people under psychiatric and other medical care who nevertheless succeed in taking their own lives. Psychiatry does not seem (yet) to fare better than the more traditional menacing attempts of moralists, theologians, and legislators at stopping people from killing themselves. Suicide is disturbingly ubiquitous and universal — across cultures and ages.

Finally, it is a well-known fact that the suicide rate among physicians including psychiatrists is substantially higher than that in the general population.[2] This special proneness places the psychiatrist in a vulnerable position when he treats a suicidal patient. In other spheres of treatment (of both mental and physical illness) the doctor can more readily remain detached. But the possibility of suicide is considered by almost every human being at some stage of his life and this makes it harder for the doctor to take a balanced and objective view of his suicidal patient. As a result there is the danger of an unsympathetic or unduly paternalistic attitude replacing rational evaluation and humane understanding of the patient's situation.

So unlike many kinds of psychological dysfunction, suicide is not a *state* which may gradually improve (or deteriorate) with the application of particular forms of treatment. It is rather a radical *event* taking place at a specific moment, often totally unpredictable and always irreversible. Furthermore, the act of suicide is motivated by what seems to us to be an unnatural drive or choice, with results which none of us can easily imagine or experience.

Beyond those very concrete problems facing the clinician, there are certain methodological difficulties which the student and theorist of suicide cannot ignore. Although suicide could be thought to be an easily definable concept, closer examination reveals a wide range of definitions and a plethora of partially synonymous terms ('suicide', 'self-killing', 'self-murder', 'self-poisoning', 'attempted suicide', 'parasuicide' etc.). Not being a case of malfunctioning, suicide cannot be defined in terms of a normal or standard state or behaviour. The fact that the business of suicide is the denial of some value, a normative choice, and not just a physical act of terminating biological life, makes the definition of suicide *value-laden*, that is to say not purely descriptive. The language of suicide reflects this characteristic: for example, the lack of any specific Biblical term for self-killing, the emotive phrase 'self-murder' used by Augustine, the attempt to neutralize the value-laden concept by using a scientific term ('intentionally caused self-destruction'), or the more modern clinical and restricted jargon 'self-poisoning'. 'Suicide' itself is a relatively new (seventeenth century) term whose function was to replace the more incriminatory 'self-homicide'.[3]

On the other hand, ethical analysis, let alone moral judgement, cannot ignore the scientific theories about the nature of suicide, that is to say the *descriptive* studies of psychiatry, psychology, and sociology. Both the way suicide is conceptualized and defined and our approach to the moral question of the right to intervene will depend heavily on these descriptive studies, especially on the questions whether suicide constitutes a mental illness or a rational choice, and whether it is an expression of a pure intention to die or a 'cry for help'. Furthermore, the analysis of the element of voluntariness — one of the conditions of suicide according to many definitions — partly depends on our general theory of mind and human behaviour, including in particular the criteria for distinguishing between an impulsive response to a certain stimulus under conditions of stress and a rational choice based on systematic consideration of alternative courses of action.

The awareness of this inevitably 'circular' nature of all definitions and theories of suicide (the interdependence of descriptive and normative factors) is of both theoretical and day-to-day clinical importance. This interdependence will become especially clear when some major views concerning suicide in the history of Western thought are studied (in section III) and the contemporary clinical scene is discussed (in section IV). In the philosophical discussion (in section II) we will suggest that the difficulties in refuting the 'rationality' of suicide are considerable, but nevertheless leave room for a significant measure of morally justifiable intervention. The ethical basis of such an intervention policy is spelled out in more detail in the final part of the chapter (section V). We hope that our philosophical and historical analysis, by broadening the clinical and ethical perspective, will highlight certain principles in the light of which the psychiatrist's own approach can be critically tested.

II. The philosophical point of view: the value of life

That life has value, or indeed is the most valuable thing we have, is usually taken for granted. Being such an obvious 'good', it requires no theoretical justification. Being so naturally held by human beings as a primary value, it needs no inculcation. The principle of the sanctity of life is invoked (either in theoretical discussion or in moral upbringing) only when the value of *other* people's lives is at stake such as in the context of the prohibition of murder, abortion, involuntary euthanasia, and killing in war. In these cases elaborate argument and reasoning are usually called for. But in the case of one's *own* life, the very questioning of its value is taken by many people as a sign of crisis, or even of 'illness' and abnormality.

Yet, the persistent occurrence of suicide (which apparently is a specifically human phenomenon) constitutes a challenge to the obviousness of life's value. On the one hand, it proves that the basic drive to preserve one's life is not always powerful enough to override other drives and wishes. On the other hand, it casts doubt on the possibility of rationally justifying the value of life because it forces us to admit that most people go on living not as a result of a rational choice or well-grounded conclusion of philosophical reasoning. This may not be a disturbing conclusion as long as we are not confronted by a person's explicit preference for death over life. Besides the tragedy of the person's death itself, the absence of rational justification is perhaps the main cause of the shattering impression suicide leaves on us. It also explains the effort, typical of many cultures, to conceal and suppress the occurrence of suicide, either by linguistic euphemism, or by explaining the resulting death as an 'accident', or by other cover-up methods and taboos. In a more Existentialistic vein we can say that the tragedy of suicide is not only the victim's but also that of the survivors, since the act lays bare the absurdity and meaninglessness of life.[4] This philosophical hypothesis is psychologically substantiated by the feeling of emptiness and despair experienced by many people who have survived an unsuccessful attempt on their lives.

The main source of philosophical difficulty in justifying the value of life lies in the symmetry between the two choices of life and death. The prolongation of life does not mean the shortening of death, and cutting life short does not imply having more of the other state (death).[5] Therefore, even if we could assign 'values' to life and death they would be typically incommensurable. How can we compare the state of conscious experience of an identifiable subject with the complete loss of consciousness and personal identity? We are reminded of the famous Epicurean argument: we should never fear death or regard it as an evil, because as long as we live it is not with us, and when we die we are not there to suffer it. We can show how a certain kind of existence and experience is preferable to another kind of existence or experience, but we have no scale of values, no 'parameter', by which we could choose between existence and non-existence. This intellectual perplexity is reflected in the psychological difficulty of conceiving one's own death. Indeed, Freud was convinced that we can never imagine ourselves dead, and that if we try, we always remain there as spectators.[6] This is evident to psychiatrists dealing with suicidal patients who often have fantasies of retaining some form of identity and experience after their deaths (e.g. enjoying the relief from pain, or the revenge on those whom the act was meant to punish).

A possible attempt to avoid the puzzling logical asymmetry of the respective values of life and death consists in shifting the emphasis from life *as such* to the *good life*. It is often argued that what carries value is the good or meaningful life — pleasant, happy, honourable, virtuous, and so forth — not sheer biological life. Thus, assuming any scale of values of the types just mentioned, not only can we compare the value of different lives, but we can also declare certain lives (especially our own in certain circumstances) as not worth living at all. This line of argument underlies the more 'rational' cases of suicide: King Saul kills himself to avoid shame; the terminally ill patient opts for voluntary euthanasia in order to avoid pain; Socrates refuses to escape from prison and drinks the poison to avoid the immoral life of an outlaw: Captain Oates sees no value in his life if it risks that of his companions; and the religious martyr dies in order to avoid the violation of divine commands. In all these examples, considerations of the quality of life rather than the comparative value of life versus death lead to the suicidal conclusion.

It should however be noted that the logical problem of the incommensurability of the values of life and death is thus circumvented only at the price of introducing other controversial values of a moral or theological nature. Ascribing value to life rather than to life of a certain quality has the advantage of universality and independence of subjective belief. Moreover, the proponents of the quality-of-life theory have to concede that life as such is a necessary condition to the meaningful or worthwhile life, and therefore has some secondary and indirect value. These remarks are highly relevant to our practical approach to suicidal behaviour because they have far-reaching ethical implications. As we shall see in section V, there are good reasons to prevent a person from committing suicide even if he sincerely believes at a certain moment that his life has lost all meaning and value. These reasons appeal to the value of life itself from which a new meaning might be created. In other words, even if philosophically speaking only the good or meaningful life is intrinsically valuable, life should be

morally respected and enhanced as the only way or opportunity to
attain that meaningfulness.

This last point suggests that there is a significant difference between
the point of view of the person considering suicide and that of the
psychiatrist, relative, or any bystander. For the subject himself the
question is that of the meaning of life, the subjective assessment of its
value *for him*. For those who judge his decision to take his life, the
question is whether it is right or wrong to do so, rational or irrational,
permissible or prohibited. Thus far we have considered suicide mainly
from the point of view of the agent. We have examined the abstract
notions relating to the value of life and the grounds for its continua-
tion or termination. On this level suicide has no specifically moral
meaning because morality is concerned with the rules and guiding
principles of 'the game of life', whereas suicide is a decision to opt out
of the game altogether. From the point of view of the agent, the
decision to die lies beyond the reach of moral arguments. But the
point of view of others is the moral and ethical one on which we
should focus — by considering, albeit schematically, the major ethical
approaches to suicide in the history of Western thought and then by
examining the moral dilemma of those who may be in a position of
responsibility in the face of a person's intent to kill himself.

III. Major ethical approaches towards suicide in Western thought

The Biblical approach to suicide is usually mentioned only as a
curious exception and indeed there is no specific term for intentional
self-destruction. Throughout the Old Testament there are only five
cases of self-killing — Saul, his slave, Samson, Achitofel, and Zimri —
and in the stories relating their fate any moral condemnation (or
praise) of the act is conspicuously absent. Death by one's own hand is
described as a natural concomitant to another well-grounded and
legitimate intention such as avoiding torture by the enemy, loyalty to
the King, and wreaking revenge. In the same factual and morally
neutral manner the New Testament describes Judas hanging himself
(only with Augustine is Judas's suicide condemned as doubling his
sin).

Suicide played a more prominent role in Greek and Roman culture.
Under certain conditions it was approved and even praised. Aristotle,[7] however, claims unambiguously that killing oneself is 'contrary to
the right rule of life' and unjust to the State; the State consequently is
justified in taking punitive measures against the suicidal person and
his family. Aristotle seems to appreciate the difference that we
mentioned earlier — between the subjective point of view which is

morally neutral (since suicide is voluntary, it cannot be considered according to Aristotle as 'unjust to oneself') and the objective moral judgement of others (if there is an injustice, it must be to the State). A similar extension of the meaning of suicide beyond the subjective can be traced in Socrates's[8] prohibition on taking one's own life. Again, as with Aristotle, it is argued that self-annihilation may be viewed as unjust towards some 'person' other than the agent (thus making it a *moral* wrong), but it is the gods rather than the State who are wronged by the taking of life. For a person is not the owner but only the custodian of life given to him by the gods.

The Romans, however, considered the question of suicide mainly from the agent's point of view, and concluded that it was not subject to moral censure. In Seneca's words, 'mere living is not a good, but living well. Accordingly, the wise man will live as long as he ought, not as long as he can.'[9] Trouble, lack of peace of mind, or a bad turn of fortune are for Seneca sufficient reasons for suicide. Like other Stoics he also values the ultimate exercise of freedom which characterizes our choice of one of the 'many exits' from life. Dying is typically described as a liberating event. In this kind of freedom, says Pliny, we are superior even to the gods. And indeed the incidence of suicide in Imperial Rome was widespread, with no legal sanction against it.

The rise of Christianity as a persecuted religion of a minority group led to many acts of suicide which were justified as martyrdom. The Church responded to the almost epidemic rate of self-destruction by banning it formally in the sixth century. St Augustine[10] presented the theological argument against suicide by interpreting the sixth commandment prohibiting murder as applicable to self-killing no less than to the killing of others. Countering the thesis that suicide was a legitimate way of avoiding sin, Augustine states that suicide is itself the gravest sin. Suicide should be thus considered as wrong under all circumstances with the exception of the definite command of God (as in Samson's case). The most systematic argument against suicide in medieval Christianity is that of Thomas Aquinas (thirteenth century). Thomas[11] presents three reasons:

1. Suicide is a violation of the natural law according to which 'everything naturally keeps itself in being' and which prescribes self-love.
2. It is a violation of the moral law, being an injury to the community of which the suicide is a part.
3. It is a violation of the divine law, which subjects man to God's power and leaves to God the right to take life.

The first reason is self-regarding; the second and third are other-regarding and typically moral in nature. The second reason is a utilitarian one and accordingly conditioned by the assumption that suicide indeed has bad consequences for society. The first and third reasons are absolutist or deontological, that is to say derived from general rules in an unconditioned and a *a priori* manner. Suicide is declared as a triple sin — against oneself, society, and God.

This severe condemnation of suicide had a long-range effect on European attitudes from the time of the Renaissance to suicide. Despite hints of a more tolerant view from the time of the Renaissance (e.g. Montaigne, the poet John Donne, and Montesquieu), the first bold and systematic challenge to Thomas's reasoning came only after half a millennium. In a posthumously published essay, the Scottish philosopher David Hume[12] critically considers the three reasons against suicide, although in reverse order to that of Thomas:

1. If God is omnipotent and governs the world down to the minutest detail, then the act of suicide must also be seen as conforming to his laws and will, and not as an encroachment upon his power. And if suicide is a disturbance of the natural order of the universe, so must be any act of saving life from natural destruction, and this is absurd.
2. Suicide does no harm to society because death absolves man from all his social duties which are reciprocal and binding only as long as the individual benefits from society. Indeed, sometimes an act of suicide may reduce the burden borne by society and hence be even laudable.
3. Suicide is not necessarily against the agent's interests. Misery, sickness, and misfortune can make life not worth living. The fact that people commit suicide despite the 'natural horror of death' proves that in some cases it is not unnatural.

Kant,[13] however, tried at about the same time to support the absolute moral prohibition of suicide using rational, non-utilitarian, and non-theological arguments. Kant does not appeal to the unnaturalness of the act but to its inherent inconsistency: We cannot attempt to improve our lot — escaping pain, misery and despair — by destroying ourselves altogether; suicide is an egoistic act and therefore is paradoxical and logically self-defeating. We have a duty to ourselves to choose life rather than death. This philosophical argument is especially interesting in the light of modern psychological studies of suicide which note the two incompatible goals often manifest in suicide — the wish to die and the wish to improve one's life.

Both Hume and Kant, although holding opposite ethical views on suicide, reflect the modern tendency, starting from the Renaissance, to discuss it on a purely moral level, and not as a religious sin. This change allowed on the one hand the introduction of State laws in which suicide and attempted suicide came to be regarded as crimes, and on the other hand also paved the way for a growing interest in the scientific study of suicidal behaviour and hence a more tolerant approach in moral judgement. In a seventeenth-century study, Robert Burton suggests a clear causal link between depression ('melancholy') and suicide, and interestingly regards it as a mitigating factor in our moral judgement of those persons who are 'mad, beside themselves for the time . . . deprived of reason, judgement'[14] This attempt at a scientific understanding of suicide was crowned in 1897 by the famous study of the French sociologist Emil Durkheim. This is a purely descriptive account of a social phenomenon which assiduously avoids value judgement either by way of assumption or conclusion. Although Durkheim uses the terms 'altruistic' and 'egoistic' to characterize suicides of different types, he definitely does not mean to praise or condone the first and to condemn the second. He is merely analysing the motives of the agent and his relation to the social environment.[15] If there are any normative implications, they consist of a criticism of society and its institutions rather than any blame of the individual, who is regarded as a victim of a poorly integrated society.

The development of psychiatry and clinical psychology in general and psychoanalysis in particular contributed to the process of 'demoralization' of contemporary attitudes to suicide even to a greater extent than sociology and epidemiology have done. In the light of his belief in the strong life instinct and self-love, Freud found the phenomenon of suicide puzzling. In the earlier stages of his theory he solved 'the riddle' by claiming that thoughts of suicide are 'murderous impulses against others' turned back upon the self — treating the self as an object, of aggression and hostility. This theory of introjected aggression was later supplemented by the concept of 'the death instinct' displayed by the superego against the ego; if ego defences breakdown under the thrust of super-ego attacks, the patient is liable to commit suicide.[16-18] Beyond that theoretical interest of attempting to explain the psychodynamics of suicide, modern psychiatry has sought to develop the most effective treatment of potential suicides and methods to prevent actual attempts. Modern psychiatry is also concerned with the care of survivors of unsuccessful suicide attempts and with the bereaved families of successful cases.

Historically, this is a radical shift in the approach to suicide. Instead of a *post hoc* judgement — whether it is theological, moral or legal — there is an effort to diagnose and prevent: rather than trying to discourage suicide by means of threat (of worldly or divine punishment), there is an attempt to eradicate the causes of suicide. Treating has replaced preaching! Like many other phenomena in our culture (madness is a good example) suicide has undergone a deep process of medicalization. This process has, as we shall see in section V, significant ethical implications, and it is by no means universally agreed that the medicalization of suicide has created a more enlightened and humane moral approach. At this stage it will suffice to point out that in both psychological and sociological attitudes to suicide, the subject is regarded as a victim of external forces or as a patient; he is thus absolved from any moral responsibility for the act. It seems that society can avoid having to make moral judgements about suicide only at the cost of eliminating all moral meaning from the act.

Our more 'liberal' view of suicide in the contemporary era is not only a function of the rise of scientific and medical interest in it. Our whole attitude to the value of life and to the valuable life has changed. With the weakening of religious belief and values there is a growing scepticism about the possibility of justifying the value of life and about the traditional criteria of the valuable life. For example, an increasing proportion of couples are dubious about the morality of bringing children into the world. According to the Existentialists the meaning of life and indeed the value of life itself, are derived, from a purely subjective choice rather than from any objective facts and norms. As with many other issues in current ethics, more value is placed on individual autonomy than in previous times, and as — according to many people — a woman has a right over her body in the case of abortion, and a citizen has a right to emigrate from his country, so must we ascribe to everyone the right to opt out of life.

Of course this liberal view of autonomy is not easily applied to concrete cases in the clinic and is incompatible with views held by the vast majority of psychiatrists. Moreover, the search for scientifically valid causes of suicide, which has replaced the moral judgement of the act, paradoxically leaves us in a more ignorant and hence psychologically vulnerable state. For it is certainly easier for society to declare an act of suicide as moral cowardice, virtuous heroism, mortal sin, or even demonic intervention than to face it as a social or psychological problem whose cause is still largely unclear. It is therefore not surprising that the law's view of suicide has changed only very slowly; for example the criminal offence of suicide was abolished in Britain as recently as 1961.

IV. Clinical aspects

As we suggested in the last section, the clinical and scientific view of suicide is in itself a link in the history of the social evaluation of that ever-present phenomenon. The attempt to strip the concept of its moral overtones is best reflected in modern definitions of suicide, which are a necessary starting point to any consideration of its clinical aspects. According to Durkheim:

The term suicide is applied to all cases of death resulting directly from a positive or negative act of the victim himself, which he knows will produce this result.[19]

This broad definition covers cases that we do not ordinarily label 'suicide' such as religious martyrdom, self-sacrifice of soldiers in war, hunger-strikes and self-immolation as a political protest (e.g. Jan Palach in Czechoslovakia), and even smoking. Durkheim's definition requires only the agent's *knowledge* of his resulting death and only an indirect causal link with his action. Indeed, no specific decision to kill oneself is regarded as a necessary condition. Yet, we usually describe as suicide only cases involving an *intention* or a *wish* to die, carried out *actively* by the agent as the result of a specific *decision*. This is a much more narrow and restrictive definition of the concept.

But philosophers since the Middle Ages have known only too well how difficult it is to assess the intention behind an overt act. As in the Roman Catholic doctrine of the Double Effect, an intentional act may have two effects — one intended, the other unintended, though foreseen. For example, a termination of pregnancy may result both in saving the woman's life and in the death of the foetus: only the first outcome is actually desired whereas the second is seen as a necessary and undesirable means or a concomitant result. But we should be careful in applying this distinction between directly intended result and reluctant acceptance of secondary effects, because on the one hand direct intentions may lie hidden beyond the persons' level of conscious awareness and on the other hand intentions which he explicitly claims as primary may not necessarily be so. For example, there is a 'suicidal' intention behind at least some cases of heavy smoking or drinking, dangerous sports like mountaineering and motor-racing, duelling, and heroic altruistic actions. And no less clear for the psychiatrist is the well-recognized observation that explicit expression of suicidal intention is, in many cases, really a cry for help, a desperate wish to gain sympathy, a desire to take revenge, or a hope to be relieved from pain, and so forth. Thus the distinction between direct and oblique intention is not a subtle academic exercise but of utmost importance to the clinician, who assumes a parallel distinction between the conscious and the unconscious, between overt expression of intention and covert motivating forces. It determines both whether a given case should be classified as 'suicide', and the ethical criteria for the right or even the duty of the psychiatrist to intervene.

Most people are naturally inclined to label as suicide: active rather than passive acts of self-destruction; the egoistically rather than the altruistically motivated; the consciously rather than the subconsciously intended; and the action leading to certain death rather than the risky action of gambling with life. However, the active–passive distinction has been criticized as morally and psychologically irrelevant.[20] Durkheim's inclusion of both egoistic and altruistic forms of suicide seems valid from a psychiatric point of view, at least in some cases; the unconsciously intended death may be more effective in causing death than a consciously-expressed suicidal intention; finally, as Stengel has forcefully claimed, the 'suicidal attempt' is no less meaningful a form of suicidal behaviour than the case of completed suicide, although there are reasons to distinguish between the two.[21] Theoretical and clinical studies therefore cast doubt on the common tendency to view as suicide only the first sort of case in each of the above-mentioned pairs. Yet, it is again interesting to note that our moral intuition about the right to intervene in a potentially suicidal act is still based on that natural tendency rather than on more sophisticated philosophical and clinical views of suicide: we do not usually feel morally bound to intervene in the case of a patient who refuses to comply with essential treatment (passive suicide), or in an extravagant and 'irrational' act of heroism or hunger-strike (altruistic suicide), in the heavy drinker's life-threatening habit (unconscious suicide), or in a game of Russian Roulette ('probable' suicide).

The crucial issue in a clinical context is the relation between suicide and mental illness: is suicide itself a psychiatric disorder? Is it caused by mental illness? Is it always associated with mental illness? We should not be surprised that answers to these questions are inconclusive and agreement among those who have studied them limited. There are serious theoretical difficulties in defining both the concepts of mental illness and suicide, and there are major obstacles to empirical research in the form of unreliable sources of information and the different sorts of data and methodology used in psychological autopsies (reports of failed suicides, of surviving relatives, of doctors, of coroners etc.). Then, of course, suicide is directly linked with other factors such as age, sex, marital status, place of residence, physical condition, family history, social class, and even with 'cosmological' factors such as time of the day or season. Methodologically we should be aware that if we take as our data cases of suicide in a particularly suicide-prone group (elderly men living on their own in big cities), we might end up with different results regarding the weight of mental illness in suicide than if we studied another population in a different social context.

Despite the methodological complexities, the available data are persuasive. Barraclough and his colleagues[22] in their impressively thorough examination of suicide in England found that of 100 cases studied 93 were judged to be mentally ill by a panel of three psychiatrists, each of whom independently reviewed all the available evidence on each case. A similar level of psychiatric disorder (94 per cent) was found in a noted American study of 134 successful suicides.[23]

In the British study the majority of patients (64 per cent) were diagnosed as suffering from a primary depressive illness; the next sizable group were cases of alcoholism (15 per cent). The strong link between suicide and depression has now been found by several investigators. In follow-up studies of patients diagnosed as manic-depressive or endogenous depressive, there is a consistent finding that about 15 per cent of them will die by suicide. In one comprehensive review[24] of 30 follow-up studies of patients with various forms of depression, including neurotic depression, Miles obtained the same average figure of 15 per cent.

Other findings pertinent to the association between mental illness and suicide are that: successful suicide is frequently preceded by one or more attempts at suicide; the risk of suicide is high in patients in the period immediately following their discharge from hospital; suicide occurs among patients who have been admitted to a psychiatric hospital; most suicides give direct or indirect warning signals before realizing their plan; and a substantial proportion of suicides consult a physician, their family doctor, or a psychiatrist in the weeks preceding their death — to a far greater extent than the normal population.

All these data support the assertion[25] that suicide-proneness can be effectively diagnosed, and even predicted with some degree of accuracy in individual cases. This is an important matter in the ethics of suicide prevention because it is a well-known principle that we ought to do only what we can do: intervene only when we know we can both identify those who intend to kill themselves and stand a good chance of preventing them from doing so.

Prevention can assume various forms. The family doctor can play a vital role by being sensitive to early signs of serious depression; the Samaritans and other lay organizations claim to have reduced the suicide rate in Britain;[26] effective treatment in psychiatric hospital, and no less important, efficient care following discharge appear to be basic means of reducing the suicide rate. However, it still remains an open question whether these various measures can succeed in preventing suicide in the long run and on a large scale, or whether the basic cause, and hence also cure, of suicide lies on a social rather than psychological level.

If we believe that the ability to prevent suicide has been demonstrated and an important association between suicide and mental illness confirmed, are there still moral grounds for intervention in cases of potential suicide? Suicide prevention may obviously require involuntary hospitalization and forced drug or electro-convulsive treatment, particularly in the case of psychotically-disturbed depressives; it also involves the serious risk of erroneously imposing treatment on a person who is not in fact contemplating suicide, or on someone who wishes to die but is definitely not mentally ill. The justification to intervene is considerably more complicated if the clinical observations mentioned above are rejected *en bloc*. Thomas Szasz, for example, is known for his strident attack on the conventional psychiatric approach to suicide when he states: 'Successful suicide is generally an expression of an individual's desire for greater autonomy — in particular for self-control over his own death'.[27] He proceeds to argue that intervention in suicidal behaviour is always wrong: it is tantamount to a curtailment of a person's freedom and a reflection of the psychiatrist as oppressor and fraud.

The vast majority of psychiatrists would not subscribe to the views of Szasz but instead operate on the premise that their role is to save the life of a person whose suicidal thoughts are in all likelihood the product of psychological disturbance. But as we shall see in the following section, it is by no means obvious whether intervention is justified, even if we assume that suicide is virtually always an indication of mental illness; or that intervention is always wrong, even if suicide is considered as a rational and voluntary act of a 'healthy' person.

V. The ethics of psychiatric intervention and suicide prevention

For psychiatrists the ethics of suicide primarily centres around the moral justification and limits of an intervention policy; this involves both the general prevention of potential suicidal acts and the life-saving measures applied to a person who has actually made an attempt on his life.

The ethical dilemma of whether to intervene in a suicidal act is intensified by the fact that whatever we do, a price must be paid. This dilemma is presented schematically in Table 10.1:

In the light of this scheme of the ethical dilemma of whether to intervene, let us consider three actual clinical cases.

Case A. A 65-year-old widower has insisted on learning the truth about his prognosis from his physician. Two years have passed since his first symptoms led to the discovery of cancer of the colon. Now, with widespread secondaries, he is fully aware that the prognosis is grave. He has but a few weeks or months left to live. Throughout his life he has been an advocate of voluntary euthanasia, and concludes now, that he does not wish to battle futilely against his impending death; he would rather die 'with dignity' and in his full senses than in excruciating pain which calls for massive doses of narcotic drugs. He is also steadfast in his conviction that it would be grossly unfair to saddle his only daughter with his problems. He knows that he can no longer fend for himself and that his only options are to be hospitalized or to move in with his daughter's family. Both prospects are completely unacceptable to him. He has always been proud of his self-reliance, and will not easily forgo it now. He talks candidly about his wish to die — through his own hand. His only 'need' is to collect a sufficient number of hypnotic pills to enable him to die in what he avows to be a decent fashion.

Table 10.1

Intervention	*Non-intervention*
Taking the *patient's* decision as irrational, impulsive, distorted by mental illness.	Taking the *person's* decision as authentic, deliberate, clear-headed, and rational.
On the assumption that his decision is reversible, certain steps, which are also reversible are taken to prolong his life.	On the assumption that his decision is irreversible, no steps are taken, thus irreversibly letting him commit suicide.
Paternalism: forcing the patient to act rationally as an expression of care for his real interests.	Respect for the person's autonomy and liberty to kill himself as to take any other decision, even if it seem irrational to us.
Care for the patient's family who usually ask for intervention.	Taking the person's side rather than that of his family. Priority of his freedom over the family's interests.
The price: forcing him to act against his will, prolongation of his mental and physical misery, serious loss of liberty.	*The price*: missed opportunities, the infinite loss involved in death, possibility of the most 'tragic mistake.'
Underlying assumption: the instinctive drive to save other people's lives plus the professional duty and practice of doctors to do so.	*Underlying assumption*: 'nothing in life is as much under the direct jurisdiction of each individual as are his own person and life' (Schopenhauer).

Case B. A 35-year-old married woman and mother of three small children has been feeling utter despair since the tragic death in a domestic fire of her youngest child some eight months earlier. During this period, her feeling of loss has increased to the point where she now believes that she must join the 'the kiddy in heaven'. She has always been a devout Roman Catholic, now more so than ever. Her belief is strong that the deceased child needs her whilst the three living children can be cared for by her husband and relatives. She is convinced that she is to blame for the tragedy — she should not have left the child unattended. There is absolutely no point in continuing to live her life as at present when 'Paul needs me elsewhere'. She tried to hang herself on the day of consultation but her husband, close to breaking point because of his wife's insistence on being reunited with Paul, managed to intercede. He has no doubt that she will kill herself unless some help can be provided. On the other hand, as a devout Catholic himself, he can appreciate his wife's wish to 'join Paul in heaven'.

Case C. A 40-year-old housewife and mother of three teenage children presents with apathy, withdrawal, and self-neglect over some weeks. During this time she has lost interest in her family and friends, wakes at about 2 a.m. each morning and cannot return to sleep, and has lost one stone in weight. She has developed the unshakeable belief that she is worthless, has let her husband and children down, and deserves to die. She feels quite helpless and sees no future for herself. She suffered a similar episode three years previously for which she was treated as an in-patient with anti-depressant medication. She made a good recovery then and had felt content and cheerful until the onset of her present state.

Case A can be confidently classified as an example of voluntary euthanasia and can hardly be labelled as 'irrational'. Most doctors would respect the patient's wish 'to die in dignity', although they might find it psychologically (and legally) difficult to co-operate actively in his suicide. No psychiatrist would consider forced hospitalization for such a person. In terms of our scheme, we can assume that the patient's decision to die is deliberate, authentic and, in all likelihood, irreversible. The family might well be relieved rather than distressed by his act. Forcing him to continue to live means the prolongation of despair, pain and loss of dignity.

Case C is a common occurrence in clinical practice and characterizes a large class of suicides caused by depression. Virtually all psychiatrists would suspect that her wish to die is not rational and sincere, but that her thinking has been distorted by certain reversible causes. Previous treatment proved helpful, and it can be assumed that therapy for the present state might be equally effective. Unlike the widower of case A, whose liberty is to all intents and purposes lost until his natural death if life is forced on him, the deprivation of liberty through involuntary hospitalization in the treatment of the depressed woman will be temporary and in all likelihood reasonably short. There is much hope of applying therapy which will relieve her of the sense of helplessness and enable her to see that her interests, and those of her family, are better served by her continuing to live.

It is case B which is puzzling and difficult to decide about. Her wish to die can be labelled as irrational only on the grounds of our rejection of her deep religious convictions. Her suicidal wish is not irrational in the sense of being impulsive, lacking deliberation, ambiguous, or distorted by mental illness. Even her close relatives, who stand to 'lose' from her decision, are basically sympathetic to her reasoning. On the other hand, the psychologically sensitive observer would no doubt be tempted to ascribe her desperate decision to her intense grief over the death of her child, and conclude that her despair can be relieved, at least partially with psychiatric treatment. How far should the psychiatrist intervene in such a case? Note that case B is typical of many suicides, not in the specific circumstances but in that blend of basically sound reasoning (at least from the agent's point of view) and non-rational motives; it is a complex which resists disentanglement. The area in the spectrum of cases lying between type-A and type-C cases is unfortunately 'grey' and ethically indeterminate; and no ready-made recipe for solving the dilemma of intervention can be offered. A methodological remark may however prove useful.

There is an asymmetry between the two horns of the dilemma of intervention, because of the irreversibility of the act of suicide, and correspondingly of the decision not to intervene. This source of asymmetry — being temporal in nature — is not often considered by philosophers, who tend to discuss the ethics of suicide on an abstract, theoretical level. But it is of crucial importance in the practical clinical context, in the process of deciding whether to intervene in a particular case of a person set on a suicidal course. The irreversibility of non-intervention places a particularly heavy burden of moral responsibility on the psychiatrist. By contrast, a decision to intervene can always be reversed, if subsequently shown to be mistaken. The psychiatrist's responsibility for an irreversible act is even more serious because the decision is often taken under conditions of uncertainty: is the suicidal intention final, is it authentic, is it rational, will the person be grateful if saved? The typical situation calling for intervention does not always offer definite guidelines to these questions.

This direct responsibility over a potentially irreversible decision under conditions of uncertainty, suggests a 'policy of postponement'. In our view, we are justified in asking or even forcing potential suicides to reconsider their attitude, to give themselves a second chance, or to defer a final decision lest there be a change in circumstances. This postponement policy is logically sounder than one of non-intervention because the intervention itself is a reversible act. If further study of the case shows that suicide is indeed 'rational' and authentic, or every effort at treatment fails to alter the person's frame of mind, or the person persists in his wish to kill himself regardless of change of circumstances — then there is always the option of letting him carry out his intentions. Although there is no good reason to argue that paternalistic regard for the person's interests, and those of his family, is in principle more important than respect for his autonomy and liberty, it seems that the reversibility of the decision to intervene makes the violation of autonomy less weighty. Only in extreme cases such as, for example, a paraplegic who can be technically prevented from killing himself indefinitely, can we question the moral legitimacy of such an act of prevention. The freedom to terminate one's own life, or at least the capacity to do so, remains one of the most basic consolations to human beings. Beyond those temporary measures we may take to save life, ultimately we must remind ourselves of the need to respect this fundamental freedom.

We may conclude by saying that it is better to err on the side of preserving life than on the side of letting it be lost. Although philosophical considerationns may show that there is no logically valid argumeent for the preference of life over death and that our bias for life is completely irrational, we should always remember that the potential suicide may, deep in his heart, share that irrational preference with us.

References

1. DURKHEIM, E.: *Suicide*. London, Routledge and Kegan Paul, 1952, pp. 46–9.
2. STENGEL, E.: *Suicide and attempted suicide*. Harmondsworth, Penguin, 1964, pp. 29–30.
3. DAUBE D.: The linguistics of suicide. *Philosophy and Public Affairs* 1:415–17, 1972.
4. CAMUS, A.: *The myth of Sisyphus*. Harmondsworth, Penguin, 1975, pp. 11–12.
5. NAGEL, T.: Death. In *Moral problems*. Ed. Rachels, J., New York, Harper & Row, 1975, p. 403.
6. FREUD, S.: *Thoughts on war and death*. Standard edition 14:289–90.
7. ARISTOTLE: *Ethica Nicomachea*. London, Oxford University Press, 1925, p. 1138a.
8. PLATO: Phaedo, in *The dialogues of Plato*. Oxford, Clarendon Press, 1953, Vol. 1, p. 62b–c.
9. SENECA: Epistle 70, in *Epistulae morales*, Loeb Ed. London, Heinemann, 1925, Vol.II.
10. AUGUSTINE: *The city of God*. Harmondsworth, Penguin, 1972, Book I, Chapters 17–27.
11. THOMAS AQUINAS: *Summa Theologica*. New York, Benziger, 1947, II, II, Q. 64, Art. 5.
12. HUME D.: On suicide. In *Essays*. Ed. Green, T. H. and Grose, T. H. London, Longmans, 1882, Vol. 4, pp. 406–14.
13. KANT I.: Groundwork of the metaphysic of morals, in *The moral law*. Ed. Paton, J. London, Hutchinson, 1948, p. 89. Cf. *Lectures on ethics*. New York, Harper & Row, 1963, pp. 148–54.
14. BURTON, R.: *Anatomy of melancholy*. London, The Nonesuch Press, 1925, pp. 224–6.
15. DURKHEIM, E.: *Suicide*. London, Routledge & Kegan Paul, 1952, Chapter 1.
16. FREUD, S.: *Mourning and melancholia*. Standard edition 14:252.
17. FREUD, S.: *Beyond the pleasure principle*. Standard edition **18**.
18. FREUD, S.: *The Ego and the Id*. Standard edition **19**:53.
19. DURKHEIM, E.: *Suicide*. London, Routledge & Kegan Paul, 1952, p. 44.
20. GLOVER, J.: Causing death and saving life. Harmondsworth, Penguin, 1977, pp. 176–81.
21. STENGEL, E.: *Suicide and attempted suicide*. Harmondsworth, Penguin, 1964, pp. 82–3.
22. BARRACLOUGH, B., BUNCH, L., NELSON, B., and SAINSBURY, P.: A hundred cases of suicide: clinical aspects. *British Journal of Psychiatry* 125:355–73, 1974.
23. ROBINS, E., MURPHY, G. E., WILKINSON, R. H., *et al*: Some clinical considerations in the prevention of suicide based on a study of 134 successful suicides. *American Journal of Public Health* 49:888–98, 1959.
24. MILES, C. P.: Conditions predisposing to suicide: a review. *Journal of Nervous and Mental Disease* 16:231–46, 1977.
25. SAINSBURY, P.: Depression and suicide prevention. Paper read at the 10th Anniversary of The Belgian Group for the Study and Prevention of Suicide, 1980.
26. BAGLEY, C.: Social policy and the prevention of suicidal behaviour. *British Journal of Social Work* 3:473–95, 1973.
27. SZASZ, T.: The ethics of suicide. *The Antioch Review* 31:7–17, 1971.

11

The ethics of involuntary hospitalization

Louis McGarry and Paul Chodoff

DOES society, with the help of psychiatrists, have the right to deprive an individual of liberty because of alleged mental illness? If so, what are the grounds on which this action can be taken? Is dangerous behaviour or its threat the only legitimate reason, or can benevolent psychiatrists take such a step for the individual's own good? These are the main ethical issues which underlie the increasingly intense debate now taking place between those who would abolish or severely limit involuntary hospitalization on psychiatric grounds and those who would continue it as a medical and humanitarian necessity.

Nothing is more precious to mankind than freedom say the libertarians. No one would dispute that to be free is a sovereign value or deny that psychiatrists who participate in the physical detention of people particularly the non-criminal, against their will must view their responsibility with great concern. But how 'free' can the mentally ill person really be? It has been said that it is possible 'to die with one's rights on'[1] and also that 'Internal physiological or psychological processes can contribute to a throttling of the human spirit that is as painful as any applied from the outside.'[2] At any rate, it has been longstanding social policy that persons in the grip of mental illness and in need of asylum but lacking the judgement to consent to it, may be involuntarily hospitalized.

Those who espouse the libertarian ideal and would abolish the involuntary hospitalization of the mentally ill often quote John Stuart Mill in his essay *On Liberty*. However, those who actually read the text will find that Mill excluded from his libertarian principles those not 'in the maturity of their faculties', or 'in a state to require being taken care of by others', or whose behaviour was 'incompatible with the full use of the reflecting faculty'.[3] Clearly, Mill made an exception of the mentally ill.

One of the historical roots of the present reaction against mental hospitals and the perjorative connotation of the very word asylum, despite its dictionary meaning of refuge or even sanctuary, is that in the last quarter of the nineteenth and the first half of the twentieth century mental hospitals became vast warehouses for human beings without hope. Typically these institutions were located in rural settings far from the communities of origin of the patients in their wards. An extreme example of such a disposition of the mentally ill occurred in the City of New York.

Until recent years, the mentally ill of that city were hospitalized at three large state institutions two counties and fifty miles away in rural Suffolk County on Long Island. By 1955, 32 000 patients had accumulated within their walls. It took three hours to travel there from the city by public transport. State mental hospitals like these throughout America, where almost 600 000 patients had been gathered by the mid-fifties, were ruled over by superintendents, for the most part benevolent and paternalistic, but no baron ever had greater authority over the lives of his fellow-men.

Over the past 25 years the pendulum has swung spectacularly away from the sprawling and isolated state hospitals. There have been extraordinary changes in the care and treatment of the institutionalized mentally ill. Among the factors contributing to these changes have been the advent of effective anti-psychotic medications, the tremendous growth of in-patient psychiatric wards in general hospitals, the open door rather than the locked ward of the past, and the community mental health movement. The latter movement has advocated the short-term treatment of the mentally ill in facilities within communities of origin, with the least disruption possible to family, community, and work ties. By 1980, in America, the census of hospitalized patients in state and country mental institutions had declined (and continues to decline) to about 200 000. Hospitalization is now usually brief and the development of long-term institutional dependency occurs less often than in the past.

But the large mental hospitals are still with us and so is the warehousing of the mentally ill which has been their legacy and has become a major factor in the upsurge of civil libertarian activism of the late sixties and seventies. Activists made these hospitals a prime target and attacked them particularly through class action law suits in the United States Federal Courts with a vigour which raised a question about the real target of the assault. Indeed, a much respected leader in the cause of civil rights and adequate treatment for the mentally ill, Morton Birnbaum, both an attorney and a physician, accused some of his civil libertarian legal brothers of having as their goal 'to destroy the state hospital system in spite of the fact that there is an insufficient number of adequate alternative community mental health facilities.'[4]

Increasingly voices are being heard saying that the pendulum has swung too far and has resulted in a massive emptying of state hospitals, forcing chronic seriously disabled patients into urban ghettos, where the quality of their lives is, at best, marginal. As Rachlin put it 'will history record that we have once again discovered the ship of fools, this time to anchor it in the inner city ghettos?' And further, 'Indeed it may well be appropriate to declare a moratorium on the involuntary communitization of the mentally ill.'[5]

So sacred is the principle of liberty in Western society that one must be cautious in expressing reservations about its application. But this principle even though based on altruistic motives, may be inappropriately exercised. It is as susceptible to abuse as the paternalistic altruism which governed the management of the institutionalized mentally ill in the past. Even in the cause of liberty extreme measures may have evil results and Draconian solutions of ethical dilemmas are seldom effective.

Legal aspects

Although the problem of involuntary hospitalization has ethical roots, it comes to be expressed in legal forms. Thus, whatever his views, a psychiatrist cannot be truly ethical if he ignores or is unaware of relevant laws and standards. Though true in a general sense, this principle is difficult to adhere to since the laws of the 51 American legal jurisdictions governing involuntary hospitalization are inconsistent and in a state of flux. Similarly the 1959 Mental Health Act for England and Wales is also in the process of revision.

Since 1969 many of the commitment statutes in the United States have been changed. Although in 1979 the Supreme Court upheld both of the two prevailing legal doctrines governing commitment, the police power of the State and *Parens Patriae*, in fact the former is becoming dominant throughout the country. The police power criterion requires a finding that by reason of mental illness there is a likelihood of dangerous behaviour toward the self or others. The doctrine of *Parens Patriae*, although still applicable in many states, is being discarded or downgraded by an increasing number of them. *Parens Patriae* is defined as the state acting to protect its sick who are 'in need of care and treatment' and who do not have the judgment to seek treatment. In addition to the growing reliance on police power for civil involuntary commitment, procedural and substantive standards more applicable to criminal cases and requiring proof beyond a reasonable doubt have been advocated in place of the civil evidentiary standards which require proof by a preponderance of the evidence.[6] (In the *Addington* case,[7] however, the Supreme Court allowed the states to adopt an intermediate standard requiring 'clear and convincing' evidence instead.) To the extent that they are 'criminalizing' the civil commitment process, are these trends also criminalizing psychiatric patients, and is it ethical for psychiatrists to support them?

Let us review briefly and more specifically the history of the applicable mental health law of one state, Massachusetts, and the ethical dilemmas posed for committing physicians. The Massachusetts law, written in 1955, until it was repealed in 1970, provided that:

> Mentally ill person, for the purpose of involuntary commitment . . . shall mean a person subject to a disease, psychosis, psychoneurosis or character disorder which renders him so deficient in judgement or emotional control that he is in danger of causing physical harm to the self or others or the wanton destruction of valuable property or is likely to conduct himself in a manner which clearly violates the established laws or ordinances, conventions or morals of the community.[8]

Read literally, such a standard permitted the involuntary hospitalization of an unconventional neurotic. It is an illustration of an era when commitment was too easy and gave too much power to the psychiatrist, at least theoretically.

Despite the looseness of this standard, Massachusetts physicians during the period when it was in force, sensibly sought commitment in the courts only for psychotic patients. Were these physicians by interpreting the law selectively in this manner, behaving ethically or unethically? In our view their behaviour was ethical judged on the basis that their implementation of the statute had a favourable effect on the quality of people's lives. Conversely and ironically, in the same state a practice which was humanitarian in purpose — the continued detention in a psychiatric hospital of mentally ill citizens awaiting trial in order to spare them the rigors of the criminal justice system — turned out to be destructive of the lives of these patients as they sometimes underwent many years of unnecessary detention.[9] We are a government of laws and not of men, so the proud statement goes, but it is men and women who implement the law, in this case psychiatrists and ultimately judges.

What ethical posture should psychiatrists take when they are required to commit patients to understaffed and inadequate facilities? One might refuse to do so on ethical grounds but would not such action serve only to worsen the plight of the patients? Perhaps a more ethically responsible action would be to attempt to improve laws and programs to the best of our ability within political and fiscal reality.

The 1955 Massachusetts law was superseded by a new, exclusively police power commitment standard, requiring a prior act or threat of physical harm to the self or others for commitment.[10] Research into the effects of this law assessed whether 688 randomly selected involuntary public mental hospital admission applications conformed to the elements required by statute to establish the likelihood of serious physical harm to the self or others.[11] The study compared involuntary admissions during periods before and after the implementation of the new police power commitment statute. The researchers were surprised to find that although there had been a rise in the number of applications which were legally adequate under the police power statutory standard (from 54.2 per cent under the old law to 61.0 per cent under the new) the difference was not statistically significant. Thus 39 per cent of the involuntary applications failed to meet the legally required admission criteria despite the fact that they were printed on the official application form itself. It was concluded that *Parens Patriae* is alive and well in Massachusetts. Changes in the law do not necessarily become changes in practice. Perhaps ethical principles influencing psychiatrist behaviour are more inherently conservative than legal styles.

In England and Wales the Mental Health Act of 1959, which is still in effect, legally permits very broad discretion for physicians in involuntarily committing the mentally ill.[12]. Thus, 'mental disorder' as defined in the English statute for purposes of involuntary commitment:

means mental illness, arrested or incomplete development of mind, psychopathic disorder and any other disorder or disability of mind.

coupled with:

said disorder warrants detention for medical treatment, and that it is necessary in the interests of the patient's health or safety or for the protection of other persons that the patient should be so detained.

In England, the controversy over whether detention and commitment for mental illness is ethical appears to be similar in kind but less intense than in the United States. Possibly reflecting the national genius for compromise and accommodation, great store is set on informal, persuasive measures to effect hospitalization of the mentally ill. Although, of course, praiseworthy in intent, the use of informal procedures beyond a certain point raises an ethical issue in itself since in fact pressure on a patient by relatives and physicians can become coercive. This question along with the issue of voluntarism generally, will be discussed later.

It appears also that the sharp distinction and the conflict between police power and *Parens Patriae* criteria for involuntary hospitalization which is developing in the United States is, at least presently, less prominent in the United Kingdom and in other Western countries.

Within professional psychiatric circles in the United States a vigorous debate on these issues is taking place. A consensus may be forming in opposition to what is felt to be the excesses of the civil liberties approach to mental health with its emphasis on the dangerousness criterion for commitment and consequent adverse effects on patient welfare. The American Psychiatric Association, having rescinded its 1972 statement on involuntary hospitalization[13] (which could be criticized as something less than a ringing affirmation of the ethical nature of the practice), is now engaged on a re-examination of its views. Possibly a new position statement will be forthcoming, stimulated by the work of psychiatrists like Alan Stone[14] and Loren Roth.[15]

However, the other side of the debate about the legitimacy of involuntary hospitalization as put forward by some psychiatrists, but more strongly by civil liberties lawyers and activists, is certainly very active. Thus, the 1970 Platform Statement of the American Association for the Abolition of Involuntary Mental Hospitalization[16] reads in part:

1. Throughout the entire history of psychiatry, involuntary psychiatric interventions, and especially involuntary mental hospitalization, have been regarded as morally and professionally legitimate procedures. No group of physicians, lawyers or social scientists have ever rejected such interventions as contrary to elementary principles of dignity and liberty and hence as morally and professionally illegitimate. The AAAIMH does.
2. Membership in the Association thus offers a means to identify publicly those persons (in the mental health field and outside of it) who oppose psychiatric and psychological practices resting on the use of state-supported force and fraud.

The driving force in this Association is Dr Thomas Szasz. In an earlier work[17] Szasz presents the abolitionist position in a manner which his opponents would describe as simplistic, even naive, and fragmentary. The essence of his view (since reiterated in a rather repetitious manner in other works) is expressed in the following phrases:

Psychiatric emergencies fall into one of two categories. The passive, stuporous is one type. Legally, he should be treated like the unconscious medical patient. The other is the aggressive paranoid person who threatens violence. Legally, he should be treated like a person charged with an offense; psychiatrically, it would be desirable, of course, if he were not incarcerated in an ordinary jail but in a prison-hospital, where he could receive both medical and psychiatric attention.

In the paragraph following, Szasz adds to his categories of psychiatric emergency organic disorders such as 'diabetic hypoglycemia'. Apparently, he does not believe that mania or psychotic depressive illness or catatonic excitement ever present an emergency. Prison-hospitals, indeed! Western society had experience of that way of dealing with the deranged in the eighteenth century and before with tragic results[18] It is difficult to imagine how anyone could seriously suggest that substituting the criminal justice system for civil procedures would improve the plight of the mentally ill but this is what Szasz has, in fact, done. And, as has happened in California under the Lanterman–Petris–Short Act, when civil commitment is made difficult because of onerous procedural and substantive requirements, the criminal justice system comes to be more heavily used.[19] Szasz appears to be sincere in his espousal of this alternative but most psychiatrists believe that it would be disastrous for mentally ill patients for his views to prevail and this is true not only in the United States but throughout the West.[20]

As a concession to the attacks on commitment, it has been suggested that involuntary patients be placed under guardianship. This has been tried in California, since 1969, for the indigent 'gravely disabled' mentally ill in-patients of that State. A recent study of this system was highly critical. It appeared that due process operated only in a *pro forma* manner with little or no protection of the civil rights of patients under guardianship procedures.[21]

Does this not suggest again that issues which are essentially ethical dilemmas are not capable of solution merely by imposing legal remedies?

How voluntary is voluntary?

Whatever position is taken about involuntary hospitalization all parties in the dispute are in agreement that it is better for all concerned — doctor, patient, society — that mental hospital admission be on a voluntary basis. However, true voluntarism, like its close relative, informed consent, is an ideal toward which to strive but it is in fact rarely attained. Most apparently voluntary decisions to enter hospital contain an element of coercion. Thus, family, friends or neighbours, or an employer are likely to apply pressure on patients who ultimately present themselves or are brought by family or police to a mental hospital for admission. Or the mentally disabled person may be coerced less directly by an indifferent or cruel world to seek protection and relief within the hospital. And even within an institution which he has apparently freely entered, some believe that he cannot be considered entirely free to make his own decisions. An American court has even found that an ostensibly civilly committed sex psychopath in a secure institution could not possibly give informed consent to high risk research because such institutions are so inherently coercive.[22]

It seems sensible to think of voluntary mental hospital admissions as representing a spectrum of assent ranging from those who are highly coerced by outside circumstances and are attempting to avoid or palliate criminal prosecution or punishment, to those for whom coercion is minimal or internal and who are seeking true asylum. This is particularly true of the previously hospitalized. Thus to persuade or encourage a mentally ill person to seek needed in-patient care while usually worthwhile is not as simple and unambiguous an endeavour as Dr Szasz would have it. Depending on the nature and style of the persuasion, it can easily become subtle and then direct coercion. Furthermore, the quality as well as the reasons for acceptance of hospitalization may differ. Consent can range from affirmative willingness to the passive, non-protesting acquiescence of a reluctant citizen bending to external pressures.

The complexities and ambiguities of the actual operation of voluntarism is illustrated by some experiences with it as a legislative goal. In Massachusetts law, for example, a person brought to a mental hospital on the strength of an involuntary application for admission has the absolute right, and must be given notice of the right, to elect to be a voluntary patient. Many such patients elect to become voluntary or more accurately 'conditional voluntary' since, if they decide to terminate their hospitalization, they must serve written notice and may be detained for up to three working days while the hospital authorities decide whether to petition for a court-ordered involuntary commitment. Szasz predictably has branded this procedure 'an unacknowledged example of medical fraud'.[23][†] Although there may be grounds for this accusation, it ignores the fact that the patient electing the conditional voluntary alternative can, with the assistance of counsel, force a decision for (or against) release on the hospital authorities within three days whereas an involuntary observation admission lasts ten days before the authorities must decide whether to seek court-ordered involuntary commitment. In research [11] into the Massachusetts Mental Health Reform Act of 1970, it was found that prior to its implementation the ratio of involuntary admissions to voluntary was 3:1. Under the new Act, this ratio was reversed thus indicating at least partial efficacy. Can these statutory provisions and their apparently favourable results be labelled seductive or even coercive? It *is* disquieting to report that a study designed to assess how well they comprehended their rights and options, a large percentage of conditional voluntary Massachusetts patients did not understand

† That such accusations are not confined to one side of the Atlantic is exemplified by the British National Association for Mental Health (MIND) Special Report (1975), written by Larry O. Gostin, a lawyer, which suggests that a large number of supposedly voluntary patients are, in fact, coerced into 'voluntary' admission.[24]

them or only understood them imperfectly.[25] Nevertheless, as mentioned above, conditional voluntary patients have increased autonomy, and at least in contractual terms, are in a better position than involuntary patients. In Massachusetts it was found[11] that among over 3000 conditional voluntary patients, three hospitals petitioned for commitment on only 42 occasions (1.4 per cent) resulting in involuntary commitment for only 21 patients (0.7 per cent). Partial data from the smallest of these hospitals indicate that in 1974 approximately 360 of 1000 conditional voluntary patients exercised their option to give notice of an intention to sign out of the hospital. About 250 of the patients withdrew their letter of intent to leave, approximately 95 were discharged, and there were only 12 petitions for involuntary commitment. In short the right to leave the hospital is frequently exercised by these patients, and is rarely abrogated.

The 1959 Mental Health Act for England and Wales created a form of patient status dubbed 'informal' resembling voluntary admission to general medical hospitals for any medical purpose. Although, under the English law, this status can be changed to involuntary, 'informal' has generally come to mean that no conditions are attached to the admission and that hospitalization is terminable at any time either by the patient or mental hospital authorities. This concept was greeted with great favour in the United States but it has not really caught on in state and county institutions.[26] Two states had statutory provision for immediate release on the request of the patient in 1961 and by 1971 this had risen to only eight. Mental hospital authorities in the United States have been reluctant not to have a means of detaining patients who on admission may appear to be benign, but, like the initially well defended paranoid, with further observation may prove to be a real threat to the community. It should be noted, however, that in the general hospitals, where the majority of psychiatric admissions take place in America today, most are of the informal type. These patients, although generally less disabled than those in state or county hospitals, have a status no different than medical and surgical patients.

The considerable changes in the status of admissions to mental hospitals described in this section raise ethical issues other than the one which has been previously discussed, that is, how really voluntary is voluntary? A troubling issue is whether psychiatrists may actually be doing harm to their patients by acceding too readily to current trends towards quick and easy discharge and short hospital stays. Certainly these practices reflect more adequate treatment measures and they avoid the iniquities of the 'warehousing' of previous times. However, they may also reflect an abrogation, under libertarian pressure, of psychiatric responsibility to assure that patients remain in hospital long enough for treatment to be effective. Are patients shuttling in and out of a revolving door and spending their extramural time in dangerous and uncaring environments very much better off than those consigned to long-term hospitals? Psychiatrists have a responsibility to attempt to improve the less restrictive facilities available to seriously ill mental patients, but they also ought not to succumb to prevailing fashion when they are convinced that it is not always in the best interests of those patients.

From what has been written thus far, it is clear that a profound change has taken place in the United States in the relationship between American psychiatrists and their patients with regard to involuntary hospitalization. Society, principally through the agency of lawyers and courts, is now looking at that relationship with very much more mistrust than formerly existed. Grave abuses were perceived and the supreme value of personal liberty was believed to be threatened. As a result the ability of psychiatrists to arrange for the hospitalization of seriously ill patients has been severely, possibly damagingly, curtailed. Although most apparent in the United States, the currents of opinion responsible for these changes are also being felt in Western Europe and can be expected generally in similarly constituted societies.

As an outgrowth of the ferment taking place in recent years in the United States, there have been two subsidiary developments, both important in their own right and also having major ethical connotations. These developments are the right to treatment and the right to refuse treatment. They go beyond the issue of psychiatrists hospitalizing patients against their will to questions about what ought to be done and is permitted to be done to those patients once hospitalization has been effected.

Before the ethical issues which arise in connection with these concepts are discussed, a brief outline of the relevant legal substrate seems appropriate.

The right to treatment

As mentioned, the legal crusade that it is against due process to commit a mentally ill person involuntarily and not provide him with adequate treatment was inaugurated in 1960 by Dr Morton Birnbaum.[27] It should be noted incidentally that his intent was not to empty the hospitals but to apply pressure for better treatment.[28] At any rate his initiative began what became a deluge of lawsuits, characteristically of the class action, civil rights variety in the Federal Courts. The landmark case is Wyatt v. Stickney in 1972.[29]

In this case the New Orleans Circuit Court accepted the opinion of an Alabama Federal District Court that 'a person who is involuntarily civilly committed to a mental hospital does have a constitutional right to receive such treatment as will give him a realistic opportunity to be cured.' Furthermore, District Court Judge Johnson heard testimony from experts across the United States as to what constituted 'adequate treatment'. The judge developed an extraordinary document describing in great detail what constituted 'Minimum Constitutional Standards for Adequate Treatment of the Mentally Ill'. These standards included the delineation of an adequate staffing plan, the number of square feet per patient for the Day Room, the dining facilities, the requirement of air conditioning and ventilation to ensure that the temperature in the hospital ranged between 68° and 83° Farenheit, provision for diet in accordance with religious requirements, and many other details.

In the important O'Connor v. Donaldson case[30] of 1975 the United States Supreme Court in a divided and rather equivocal decision seems to have at least partially blocked the right to treatment concept. A concurring opinion of Chief Justice Burger states, 'few things would be more fraught with peril than to irrevocably condition a State's power to protect the mentally ill upon the providing of such treatment as will give a realistic opportunity to be cured.' However, the Court also said, 'In short a State cannot constitutionally confine without more [sic]* a non-dangerous individual who is capable of surviving safely in freedom by himself or with the help of willing and responsible family or friends.' The Court did not define 'more' except that it had to exceed 'indefinite simple custodial confinement'.

A dimension of the *Donaldson* case which caused great consternation among American psychiatrists, particularly those in the public sector, was that two of the psychiatrists responsible for Donaldson's care and treatment were found by the jury to have acted 'malevolently' toward Donaldson; he was awarded $38 500 in both compensatory and punitive damages against the two doctors. The 'spectre' arose of state hospital psychiatrists, acting in good faith, becoming scapegoats for the inadequacies of public mental health facilities. This fear may be exaggerated. The jury found malevolent bad faith in the two doctors. Ethically and legally none of us should be above the consequences of such behaviour if it can be proved before a court of law. Whatever standards are set for ethics in psychiatry they cannot be so low as to countenance malevolence towards patients.

The legal fate of the right to treatment concept in the United States is still very much unresolved as a number of cases continue to find

---

* The essence of the judgement is that mere custodial treatment is insufficient constitutionally.

214   *Psychiatric Ethics*

their way through the courts seeking final Supreme Court resolution. What is apparent, however, is that legal activism and judicial control of psychiatric facilities are coming up against limitations and contradictions. Legislatures continue to be recalcitrant about appropriating money, administrative problems are stupefying, vast amounts of time (costing money) are consumed, clinical problems refuse to disappear before judicial fiat. And yet there is reason to believe that the overall effect of right to treatment pressure has been positive, not dramatically but significantly, as the public, legislature and psychiatrists have been forced to look at, and take some action about, intolerable conditions they could previously ignore.

Thus, at an ethical level, psychiatrists need to be careful to avoid acting on the irritation and sense of injury they may feel as they see their well intentioned efforts slighted and sneered at, and themselves blamed by eager legal reformers for conditions beyond their control. In 1958, Dr Harry Solomon, then President of the American Psychiatric Association, stated, 'I do not see how any reasonably objective view of our mental hospitals today can fail to conclude that they are bankrupt beyond remedy.'[31] Can we, in the 1980s, afford to look with a sanguine eye on the situation today? While standing firm against and trying to moderate some of the excesses of right to treatment, psychiatrists everywhere need to rise above wounded professional pride and support the ultimate aim of the movement to improve conditions and facilities which determine the care available to their seriously ill patients.

What if we cannot promise adequate treatment for prospective involuntary patients? Does this mean that we should then cease our efforts to hospitalize them against their will? Alan Stone[14] advocates this course of action, taking the position that deprivation of liberty can be justified only if good treatment can be offered in exchange. On the other hand, as has previously been pointed out in this chapter, this may be a gospel of perfection not necessarily in the interests of patients who may be better off in even substandard institutions than 'wandering the streets'. Those who take the latter point of view, of course, are even more obligated to bend all efforts to improve the inadequate facilities.

A particular prickly ethical problem is the attitude to be taken with regard to patients whose mental disorders are not susceptible to current treatment methods. Are we to abandon them possibly to degradation, possibly to prisons, if we cannot offer to 'cure' them? Surely care, as in the era of moral treatment, is in the best tradition of medicine, and asylum, in spite of its present implications, can be humane. Other physicians are not expected to cease trying to help terminal cancer patients they cannot cure, nor should the fact that our care may have to involve an element of compulsion deter us from similar goals.

By concentrating on the right to treatment of involuntary patients, are we thereby shortchanging the much more numerous voluntary ones who require a wider and more varied range of services than hospitalized psychotics and victims of brain disease? This argument may be extended as suggested by Roth to the dictum 'that not only psychiatric patients but all persons who are incompetent to seek medical treatment should, as a matter of ethics and policy, be provided treatment.'[28]

The right to refuse treatment

Succeeding an era when the courts looked with disfavour on mental hospital physicians who did *not* enforce treatment (particularly drug treatment) on involuntary patients, we have now entered on one where the situation is almost completely reversed. As a culmination of the civil liberties approach to mental patients, and with the doctrine of informed consent as a model, the United States courts in the 1970s have moved to uphold the committed patient's right to refuse customary treatment (drugs, ECT).[32] Two recent cases, one in New Jersey (Rennie v. Klein),[33] the other in Massachusetts (Rogers v. Okin)[34] carry this trend to a very far point indeed. Both decisions make it clear that commitment *per se* does not give permission to treat.

Because of its far-reaching effects and its very critical attitude towards psychiatry, it is instructive to go into some detail about the New Jersey case. The opinion states that except for emergency situations, involuntary mental patients have the qualified right to refuse psychotropic medication. The opinion was highly critical of medication practices in New Jersey state hospitals. Based upon outside expert testimony, the court cites five 'representative' cases where the use of psychotropic medication is described variously as 'unjustified polypharmacy', 'force or intimidation', being 'grossly irresponsible', having 'little medical justification', 'side effects were blatantly ignored by doctors', and so on. The court was much concerned about such side effects of neuroleptic drugs as tardive dyskinesia. Although conceding the usefulness of the neuroleptics, the court cited psychiatric authorities and its own witnesses' contention that such drugs are not necessarily always indicated in psychosis and, furthermore, 'Testimony also indicated that the drugs may inhibit a patient's ability to learn social skills needed to fully recover from psychosis, and might even cause cancer.' In any case, the judge was persuaded that patients, whether voluntary or involuntary, had a qualified right to refuse treatment based upon the constitutional rights to due process and privacy. The remedies the judge ordered in this case will surely be repugnant to the psychiatrists of the New Jersey Department of Mental Health. He required that special patient advocates be appointed in each New Jersey State Mental Hospital with the specific responsibility to implement the right of patients to refuse treatment. These advocates may be social workers or psychologists but also may be people with paralegal experience and not necessarily lawyers. The New Jersey State Commissioner is enjoined to see to it that the advocates are autonomous. The court order further requires that a listing of all the side-effects of all neuroleptic drugs used on a particular ward of a hospital either be posted on the walls or be available on the ward. Furthermore, consent forms for all neuroleptic medications are required to include a description of all side effects 'in plain language'. The advocates can refer decisions to medicate involuntary patients forcibly to independent psychiatrists who shall be hired and payed for by the New Jersey Department of Mental Health. Such an independent psychiatrist has the authority to override decisions to medicate even those involuntary patients found to be 'functionally' or 'legally incompetent'. The court has retained jurisdiction in the matter and requires monthly reports detailing the implementation of its intermittent order until a final order is promulgated.

In the Massachusetts case,[34] it is reported[35] that even before the decision was handed down, the effect of a temporary restraining order permitting refusal of treatment was highly disruptive of patient care. 'Widespread periodic medication refusals were observed by staff'; 'The episodic and contagious quality of refusals and manifestly more disturbed behaviours' were observed. Over a two-year period 'Eighty-nine patients deteriorated in their clinical state, fifty others had prolonged hospital stays and fourteen others were refused admission.' This information, when presented to the court had little effect on its ultimate decision.

Hospital psychiatrists confronted with the strictures of the right to refuse treatment decisions feel that unless they are reversed or modified by the Supreme Court, their overall effect on treatment of involuntary patients will be devastating. Such patients will no longer be dealt with under a treatment model but rather under a segregation model[28] whose purpose is to protect society and themselves against their dangerous tendencies. As has already been bitterly pointed out it will be difficult to institute adequate treatment under the essentially custodial conditions which will then prevail.[36]

Obviously the purposes of the lawyers and judges responsible for the right-to-refuse-treatment doctrine are not evil nor do they intend chaos and anarchy. They see disconcerting side-effects from drugs and other modalities of treatment and even their abuse; they believe in the rightness of informed consent before any clinical procedure or treatment and that it can be applied to all patients, including involuntary psychiatric ones; they believe the relationship between people should be based on equality and therefore contractual rather than on benevolence and thus hierarchial; they may even believe that they have only introduced procedural safeguards rather than road-blocks in the way of compelled treatment.

Most psychiatrists on the other hand believe that the theory and the reality of permitting involuntary and often incompetent patients to make their own decisions about treatment will be damaging to the patients and destructive in general of treatment planning. These psychiatrists contend that judges and lawyers simply do not under-stand what goes on in psychiatric wards among seriously disturbed patients. A particular error will be to take at face value the verbal statements of such patients rather than also taking into account other communications which may convey a different message from those uttered: the psychiatrists also are likely to believe that an attitude of benevolence is an acceptable model for some human relationships even between adults.

As the authors of this chapter we agree wholeheartedly with the psychiatric position enunciated above. We believe that all psychiatric patients ought to have the best treatment available even if this is not always effective. This should be true not only for those who can assent to treatment but also for those who, hopefully temporarily, are unable to do so by reason of mental defect which seriously impairs their judgement. We acknowledge that this latter belief, while ethically correct is susceptible to abuse and that all reasonable safeguards against human error or malevolence should be incorporated in relevant statutes as long as these are not crippling of care and treatment. Surely the cardinal ethical principle sacred to medicine of *primum non nocere* applies here as it does to involuntary hospitalization generally. The following section from the Hippocratic Corpus is still relevant:[37]

As to diseases, make a habit of two things — to help, or at least to do no harm. The art has three factors, the disease, the patient, the physician. The physician is the servant of the art. The patient must co-operate with the physician in combating the disease.

Finally, and of great importance with regard to all the issues which we have discussed in this chapter is the current troubled relationship between psychiatrists and lawyers. It can be taken that both groups intend good for those disturbed human beings who come into the psychiatric orbit without positively asking to do so. But the vantage point from which they view the problem and their ways of dealing with it are often very different for doctors and lawyers.[2] Perhaps it would be well to remind both parties that when being free from external restraint comes into conflict with being free from dehumanizing disease, the conflict should not be seen in terms of drama (right against wrong or black against white) but rather as tragedy (one right against another right).

References

1. TREFFERT, D. A.: Dying with your rights on. Presented at the 12th Annual Meeting of the American Psychiatric Association, Detroit, Mich., 6–10 May, 1974.
2. CHODOFF, P.: The case for involuntary hospitalization of the mentally ill. *American Journal of Psychiatry* **133**:496–501, 1976.
3. MONAHAN, J.: John Stuart Mill on the liberty of the mentally ill. *American Journal of Psychiatry* **134**:1428–9, 1977.
4. BIRNBAUM, M.: The right to treatment: some comments on its development. In *Medical, moral and legal issues in mental health care*. Ed. Ayd, F. J., Baltimore, Williams and Wilkins, 1974, pp. 97–141.
5. RACHLIN, S.: When schizophrenia comes marching home. *Psychiatric Quarterly* **50**:202–10, 1978.
6. Lessard v. Schmitt, 349 F. Supp. 1078 (Ed. Wis. 1972).
7. Addington v. Texas, Supreme Court Opinion, 47 LW 4437 (1979).
8. Mass. General Laws, Chapter 123, Section 1. (Repealed Nov. 1, 1970).
9. McGARRY, A. L.: The fate of psychotic offenders returned for trial. *American Journal of Psychiatry* **127**:1181–7, 1971.
10. Mass. General Laws, Chapter 123, Section 1.
11. McGARRY, A. L., SCHWITZGEBEL, R. K., LIPSITT, P. D., and LELOS, D.: Final Report, Civil Commitment and Social Policy, Grant No. MH 25955 Centre for Studies in Crime and Delinquency, 1978. (In press.)
12. Halsbury, Earl: *Statutes of England* 2nd edn., Vol. 39, Chapter 72, London, Butterworths, 1959.
13. Position statement on involuntary hospitalization of the mentally ill of the American Psychiatric Association (revised). *American Journal of Psychiatry* **130**:392, 1973.
14. STONE, A. A.: *Mental health and law: a system in transition*. National Institute of Mental Health, Centre for Studies in Crime and Delinquency, Department of Health, Education, and Welfare Publications No. (ADM) 75–176, US Government Printing Office, Washington, DC, 1975.
15. ROTH, LOREN, H.: Mental health commitment: the state of the debate, 1980. *Hospital and Community Psychiatry* **31**:385–96, 1980.
16. BROOKS, A. D.: *Law, psychiatry and the mental health system*. Little, Brown, Boston 1974 pp. 608–9.
17. SZASZ, T. S.: *Law, liberty and psychiatry: an inquiry into the social uses of mental health practices*. Macmillan, New York, 1963, p. 226.
18. FOUCAULT, M.: *Madness and civilization, a history of insanity in the age of reason*. Random House, New York, 1973.
19. URMER, A. H. *et al.*: *The burden of the mentally disordered offender on law enforcement*. ENKI Research Institute, Chatsworth, California, 1973.

20. ROTH, M.: Schizophrenia and the theories of Szasz. *British Journal of Psychiatry* **129**:317–62, 1976.
21. MORRIS, G. H.: Conservatorship for the "gravely disabled": California's non-declaration of non-independence. *San Diego Law Review* **15**:201–37, 1978.
22. Kaimowitz v. Michigan Department of Mental Health, Civil No. 73–19434, Circuit Court, Wayne County, Mich. 10 July, 1973).
23. SZASZ, T. S.: Voluntary mental hospital admission: an unacknowledged example of medical fraud. *New England Journal of Medicine* **287**:277–8, 1972.
24. GOSTIN, L. O.: *The Mental Health Act from 1959 to 1975: observations, analysis and proposals for reform*, Vol. 1. A MIND Special Report. London: MIND (National Association for Mental Health), 1975.
25. OLIN, G. B. and OLIN, H. S.: Informed consent in voluntary mental hospital admissions. *American Journal of Psychiatry* **132**:838–41, 1974.
26. CURRAN, W. J. and HARDING, T. W.: *The law and mental health: harmonizing objectives*. World Health Organization, Geneva, 1978, p. 80.
27. BIRNBAUM, M.: The right to treatment. *American Bar Association Journal* **46**:499–505, 1960.
28. ROTH, L.: Involuntary civil commitment: the right to treatment and the right to refuse treatment. *Psychiatric Annals* **7**:50–76, 1977.
29. Wyatt v. Stickney, 344 F. Supp. 373 (M.D. Ala. 1972).
30. O'Connor v. Donaldson, 422 US 563, 1975.
31. SOLOMON, H. C.: Cited in *Action for mental health, final report of the joint commision in Mental Illness and Health*. New York, Basic Books, 1961, pp. 267–8.
32. Mental disabilities. *Law Reporter*, Vol. 2, No. 1, July – August, 1977, p. 44.
33. Rennie v. Klein, Civil Action No. 77–2624, Federal District Court of New Jersey, 14 Sept., 1979.
34. ROGERS V. OKIN, 478F. Supp. 1342 I.D. Mass. 1979.
35. GILL, MICHAEL Personal communication, September 1979.
36. APPELBAUM, P. S., and GUTHEIL, T. G.: Rotting with their rights on: constitution theory and clinical reality in drug refusal by psychiatric patients. *Bulletin of the American Journal of Psychiatry and the Law* **7**,308–17, 1979.
37. *Hippocrates*. Trans. Jones, W.H.S., The Loeb Classical Library, Cambridge, Harvard University Press, 1923.

12
Psychiatric confidentiality and the American legal system: an ethical conflict

Jerome Beigler

This chapter is not intended as a general discussion of the ethical issues which arise as a consequence of the psychiatrist's obligation not to divulge his patient's communications. Rather it is a case study account of the ethical problems engendered by legal demands for information about patients which the psychiatrist may believe to threaten the confidentiality of the therapeutic relationship. Conflict of this kind is more likely to occur in a highly adversarial legal system such as that operative in the United States today. However, since the tendency to replace subjective ethical judgements by codified contractual arrangements covering every contingency seems to be gaining currency, the chapter will serve a cautionary role for psychiatrists throughout the West. [editors].

THE ethics of confidential communications between patient and physician has been codified since the fourth century BC in that part of the Hippocratic Oath which states: 'All that may come to my knowledge in the exercise of my profession or in daily commerce with men, which ought not to be spread abroad, I will keep secret and will never reveal'.[1]

In England, although no formal privilege law for medical communications has been enacted, it is quite possible to live up to the spirit of the Hippocratic Oath because of an informal understanding and respect in the British courts for medical confidentiality. An informal doctrine of confidentiality, while giving no absolute protection in the law, gives 'a certain amount of confidence to professionals' regarding the privacy of communications with patients.[2]

The situation is considerably different in the United States where the adversarial judicial system has evolved into a complex fabric of detailed statutes and policies. Each of the states has its own laws, and superimposed is the federal legal system. Psychiatrists in ordinary practice need give little attention to such matters, but once the first subpoena arrives 'commanding' disclosure of private professional communications, one realizes how much the application of fundamental constitutional rights to patient–physician privacy is taken for granted.

The psychiatrist, by the nature of his work, becomes privy to sensitive information of high potential value to, among others, employers, creditors, legal adversaries, law-enforcement agencies, and insurance carriers. Yet he cannot perform his work properly unless he can assure his patient of real confidentiality. Society is faced with a continuing struggle between two countervailing rights: the right to privacy, which enables a distressed citizen to avail himself freely of psychiatric help, versus the right of an information-hungry society to cope with the problems of law enforcement, insurance management, computerized credit systems, and equitable employment and education practices.

As I have said, in England (and I understand in France also), these problems are ameliorated by a high degree of legal regard for medical privacy. In the United States, however, matters are otherwise. It is a lawyer's ethical responsibility to exploit all sources of information in order to represent his client within the limits of the law. Except for the privilege which adheres to lawyer–client communications, an American lawyer regards discovery of evidence as supraordinate to most other social values. The practice of law requires a high order of legal, juristic, legislative, and political expertise. It is troublesome and expensive, yet it provides a system of inter-professional tension that tests and develops the fabric of democracy.

Also characteristic of an adversarial legal system is that by its nature it leads to definition of the subliminal elements in the jurisprudential and ethical atmosphere in which we practice. In the United States the psychiatrist's responsibility to maintain confidentiality requires that he become aware and competent in areas ordinarily taken for granted.

But before continuing, the definition of three interrelated terms is relevant:

'Privilege' is a narrow and technical term, pertaining to litigious and judicial situations of discovery or testimony in which communications are protected from disclosure by statute or public policy. The word 'privilege' comes from the Latin *privilegium*, derived from *privus*, private, peculiar; and from *lex*, the law; thus private law, meaning laws providing special prerogative or exemption, originally obtained as the result of position, power, and/or influence.[3,4]

'Confidentiality' is a broader term with both legal and ethical implications. It applies to the non-disclosure of communications in many social and professional relationships in the spheres of health, insurance, employment, education, credit, and business.

'Privacy' is the broadest term and has been defined by Justice Brandeis as the 'right to be left alone'.

The ethics of confidentiality

Section 9 of the Principles of Medical Ethics of the American Medical Association states, 'A physician may not reveal the confidences entrusted to him in the course of medical attendance, or the deficiencies he may observe in the character of patients, unless he is required to do so by law or unless it becomes necessary in order to protect the welfare of the individual or of the community.' The American Psychiatric Association elaborated the American Medical Association's 'with annotations especially applicable to psychiatry'[5,6] and Section 9 is expanded to specify:

1. Protection of medical records.
2. Release of confidential information only with the informed consent of the patient or under 'proper legal compulsion'.
3. Adequate disguise of clinical material for teaching or publishing.
4. Maintenance of confidentiality in consultations.
5. Only immediately relevant material may be disclosed (no speculations).
6. Patients must be advised of the lack of confidentiality and the nature of an examination when it is for purposes of security, employment, or determination of legal competence.
7. Discretionary breach of confidentiality to protect patient or community from imminent danger.
8. A judicious balance between protecting confidentiality for a minor and yet making available necessary information to parent or guardian.
9. A psychiatrist may 'dissent within the framework of the law' when ordered by a court to reveal confidences; a patient's right to confidentiality and unimpaired treatment must be given priority; the psychiatrist may request limitation of court-ordered disclosure only to that which is relevant.
10. A patient may be presented to a scientific group only with the patient's informed consent and with the audience acceptance of the obligation to maintain confidentiality.

Most of these specifications are self-explanatory and readily acceptable. 'Proper legal compulsion' of Subsection 2 requires clarification as does the permission to 'dissent within the framework of the law' of Subsection 9. Both stipulations reflect the results of many legal battles. Psychiatrists have learned that passive compliance with a subpoena or other legal demands for confidential information can be challenged and to comply to a subpoena is not necessarily ethical. The right of a patient to confidentiality and to unimpaired treatment may take precedence within broad legal limits. Unfortunately in most American states there are no statutory protections of confidentiality and privilege. Only about ten states have effective psychotherapist--patient privilege laws; and most physician--patient privilege laws are ineffective owing to the many exceptions. Experience has proved, however, that active political and legislative intervention by psychiatrists can improve the legal ambience in which psychiatry is practised. In my view the psychiatric ethics of confidentiality includes the responsibility to achieve the enactment of proper legislation to protect confidentiality and privilege.

To arrive at a perspective on how the unique history of privilege law in the United States has shaped the ethics of confidentiality, briefly let us examine the following:

The history of privilege law and the patient as litigant

Privilege law applied to communications first became part of English common law with regard to the lawyer–client relationship, when it became clear that for the administration of justice communications between lawyer and client must be immune from discovery.

A bid for priest–penitent privilege was made unsuccessfully by an English Jesuit priest, Father Henry Garnet, in 1606; he was accused of complicity in the Guy Fawkes Gunpowder Plot because he had not disclosed to the authorities his prior knowledge of the plan learned in the confessional. There was no priest–penitent privilege and he was sentenced to be hanged.[7]

In England confidentiality was considered an attribute of the professional gentleman until 1776 when the English courts set a precedent by coercing a surgeon, Mr Caesar Hawkins, to testify in a famous trial against the Duchess of Kingston for bigamy.[7]

There was no English or United States statute providing privilege in the physician–patient relationship until 1828 when the State of New York passed an absolute privilege law.[7] Other states adopted similar statutes but with an increasing number of exceptions so that today there is only limited physician–patient privilege,[8] and in most jurisdictions physicians can be coerced to testify.

The first American case involving psychiatrist–patient privilege occurred in 1952 when Dr Roy R. Grinker, Sr., refused out of his own convictions, as well as on his patient's request, to testify in an alienation of affection case brought by her husband.[7,9,10] Risking citation for contempt of court, Grinker claimed privilege on the basis that confidentiality was a prerequisite to the therapeutic relationship. The judge found that the psychiatrist–patient relationship required protection more than even that between physician and patient and ruled in Grinker's favour. Although the case was not appealed and hence did not become a formal legal precedent, it was cited in much subsequent litigation.[10]

As the need for statutory protection of the psychiatrist–patient relationship became more apparent, organized action by professional groups began. At first privilege equivalent to that between client and lawyer was sought.[11] However, the requirement that a lawyer must breach privilege should his client be contemplating a future crime or if the client waives his privilege would in some situations prevent a psychiatrist from discharging his ethical responsibility to his patient. Often the establishment of a working relationship with a trustworthy therapist can help a potentially aggressive patient control his criminal tendencies. Also, a patient may not be able to waive his privilege intelligently because he does not remember details of his communications or does not realize the significance of his disclosures.[10] In addition a few patients are self-injurious and provision should be made to protect their interests, at times even against their will. There is a conflict here between some authorities who argue that privilege belongs only to the patient and others who believe that some psychiatric patients must be protected from themselves. In Illinois and Wisconsin, such clinical realities have been recognized legislatively by the inclusion of a psychiatrist's or physician's privilege to be used in the patient's interest.

The priest–penitent privilege also is not an adequate model for privilege in patient–psychiatrist relationships. The former was established historically to separate church and state. Furthermore United States case law has defined that this privilege applies only to the religious functions of the cleric; his role as counselor, adviser, or therapist is not protected.

A further perspective on the effects on the ethics of confidentiality by legal factors is seen in the review of the criteria for privilege, as defined by the legal scholar, J. H. Wigmore.[12] He presents four criteria to warrant the judicial or legislative establishment of privileged communications:

1. The communications must originate in a confidence.
2. The maintenance of that confidence is vital to achieving the purposes of the relationship.
3. The relationship is one that should be fostered.
4. The expected injury to the relationship through fear of later disclosure is greater than the expected benefit of judicial administration forcing breach of confidence.

Using these criteria it seems that the characteristics of psychiatric treatment, particularly psychotherapy, conform precisely to the requirements for privilege of communications.

In practice such privilege has been established in the United States for the relationships between lawyer and client, physician and patient, priest and penitent, and spouses. More recently privilege has evolved for the patient and his psychotherapist including in some jurisdictions the psychologist who has established privilege independent of and supraordinate to that of his client.

The exceptions to the psychiatrist–patient privilege are:
1. In order to protect patient and society the psychiatrist may breach confidentiality should the patient require involuntary hospitalization.
2. When the judge orders a psychiatric examination. The patient is informed that communications will not be privileged, but that testimony will be limited to issues involving the patient's mental condition and will not include evidence from the patient regarding the facts of a civil or criminal charge.
3. When the patient introduces his mental condition as a claim or defence in a civil proceeding. This is the patient–litigant exception. It would be unfair to raise mental condition as an issue, for example, in a personal-injury case, and not have appropriate *relevant* testimony. In most states the testimony of a treating psychiatrist in a criminal case is not required, but relevant evidence could be provided by a court-appointed examining psychiatrist.[9,10]

As experience with the patient–psychotherapist statutes has accumulated, it has become apparent that the patient–litigant exception is troublesome.[7] For example, a California woman, who had been in psychoanalysis sued for divorce on grounds of mental cruelty. She was subpoenaed along with her psychoanalyst for depositions on the basis that she had brought her mental condition into issue when claiming mental cruelty. The husband contested her fitness to have custody of their children because she had required psychiatric treatment.[7] Although the courts denied the husband's arguments, it became apparent that the law caused an ethical dilemma for the psychiatrists concerned.

The Illinois legislature saw the patient–litigant exception as a hazard in that a couple with a marital problem could be deterred from seeking counselling lest their confidential disclosures be revealed in court if a contested divorce eventually were sought on the basis of mental cruelty. Since this would tend to promote divorce, the legislature passed an exception to the patient–litigant exception in divorce or custody cases.[10]

Another ethical dilemma confronts the psychiatrist when a patient claims 'pain and suffering' as part of a personal-injury suit. Defendants have exploited such a claim on the basis that having brought mental condition into issue, privilege is thereby waived and all communications are therefore discoverable. The psychiatrist must decide how vigorously to protect his patient's privacy and how much he is willing 'to dissent within the law'. But there is a broader ethical question. To prevent disclosures irrelevant to the points in issue, but embarrassing, the patient might have to withdraw his complaint of pain and suffering. In this regard a patient seeking psychiatric treatment may jeopardize rights to legal redress otherwise available to those who are untreated. Although some psychiatrists maintain that a person suing for personal injury must accomodate to the provisions of law, most would claim that this situation is not tolerable to the profession or to society. The remedy is to initiate legislation which specifically provides that pain and suffering does not constitute a mental condition in the legal sense. To date such a stipulation has been enacted in Illinois[10,13] and the District of Columbia[14] and is included in the model state confidentiality law of the American Psychiatric Association[15–17].

These ethical problems confronting psychiatrists when their patients become litigants make it apparent that when a person becomes a psychiatric patient he potentially impairs his prior legal rights. Accordingly the ethics of his profession requires that a psychiatrist should be aware of unusual legal complications imping-ing on his patients and of his responsibility to protect them. The problems of confidentiality in divorce and personal-injury litigation can best be remedied by appropriate legislation.

Another complicated ethical problem involving litigation occurs when a patient brings into issue his mental condition as a part of a legal claim, for example, in suing for damages for a traumatic neurosis. In a series of well-publicized California cases[18–24] two psychiatrists went to jail rather than testify even though their patients had waived privilege by bringing mental condition into issue. The psychiatrists believed that such a waiver would allow discovery of all communications between psychiatrist and patient, including those not relevant to the suit. It was apparent that such disclosures would have a chilling effect on accessibility to psychiatric treatment. Patients would be reluctant to enter treatment lest their confidential disclo-sures might be forcibly exposed in future litigation. Again it became clear that a patient potentially jeopardized his legal rights simply by seeking psychiatric treatment.

As the result of intense litigation supported by various psychiatric groups, the California courts found that although privilege had been technically waived, disclosures should be limited to a few facts because society's interest lay in enabling the conduct of psychotherapy. But subsequent cases[24] illustrated that more specific judicial and legislative guidelines were necessary. In one case, a prestigious judge advised that the court appoint an examining psychiatrist on a non-privileged basis to assess the patient regarding the issues in contest and that only if this proved inadequate should the treating psychiatrist be asked to testify.[25]

Arguments have been made that the psychiatrists who entered jail did so for masochistic and exhibitionistic reasons, but most psychiatrists would accept the necessity to protect confidentiality in the interests of patient, profession, and society. 'As asepsis is to surgery, so is confidentiality to psychiatry'.[26]

The problems of the patient–litigant exception are far from resolved, but progress has been made as evidenced by the passage of laws in Illinois and the District of Columbia which weave a net of legal strictures against breach of confidentiality and enable a psychiatrist to honour his obligation to protect his patient's interests.[13,14]

A further ethical and legal issue is whether a psychiatrist's privilege should be separate from that of the patient, thus enabling a psychiatrist to protect his patient from himself should this be necessary. Legal scholars differ in their views on this problem. Most argue that the privilege belongs only to the patient as is true of lawyer–client privilege. In some jurisdictions the priest has privilege separate from his penitent. Except in Wisconsin,[27] a physician's privilege is waived at the patient's request. In the California cases the psychiatrists went to jail to protect their patients from uninformed waivers. Grossman[28] has argued convincingly in favour of a psychiatrist's separate privilege. The Illinois statute provides privilege to the psychiatrist in order to protect the patient from an uninformed waiver, but also to protect the psychiatrist's communications to the patient.[29] Civil libertarians, antipaternalists, and others argue against such a privilege on the basis of the patient's right to self-determination whatever the consequences. Some legal scholars have expressed concern that the psychiatrist's privilege could be used as a shield for malpractice; hence the Illinois law stipulates that the psychotherapist's privilege can be applied only 'on behalf of and in the interest of' a patient;[13] this is similar to the Wisconsin physician–patient privilege statute.[27]

A problem has surfaced recently with regard to privilege in group therapy. A Virginia judge found that privilege did not apply in marital therapy because the presence of a third party (the spouse) did not allow for privacy.[30,31] In contrast, the Illinois and District of Columbia statutes impose a duty of confidentiality on all participants in group therapy; unauthorized disclosures are subject to legal penalties.[13,14] Thus again the therapist's ethical responsibilities are shaped by legal precedent. We need to keep in mind, however, that legal precedent can in turn, be shaped by our own interventions.

In summary, the ethical behaviour of a psychiatrist with regard to legal privilege becomes an issue when a patient is a litigant. On the one hand a disabled person has the right to obtain psychiatric help, for which an assurance of confidentiality is a prerequisite; on the other hand the meting of justice in the course of litigation requires discovery of information. The problem is where to draw an optimal line between these countervailing rights. In England a judicial high regard for confidentiality enables the ethical obligation of the psychiatrist to maintain privacy. In the United States the balance is in favour of discovery, requiring that a psychiatrist be cognizant of legal matters and avail himself of legal help to protect patient and profession; and also that he help to modify the law by active intervention in legislation and litigation.

Psychiatry and law enforcement agencies

The relationship between psychiatry and law enforcement agencies in the United States also involves important ethical issues about confidentiality. Again it is a matter of countervailing rights. On the one hand it is in the interests of society, as discussed above, that psychiatric treatment be readily available; on the other hand society requires the enabling of law enforcement, and psychiatrists may be in possession of information useful to law enforcement agents. But if such information should be disclosed without a patient's consent, the ability of a psychiatrist to help a specific patient would be negated and his ability to help other patients lessened to the degree he has proved himself unable to maintain a confidence.

Another problem involving a difficult ethical judgement is whether a patient with a law enforcement problem (such as drug abuse) should be allowed to stay in treatment, without the police being notified, thus affording the patient an opportunity for rehabilitation. Similarly a potentially dangerous patient has a better chance of re-establishing control over his aggression if he is able to maintain a working relationship with a therapist whom he can trust not to betray him. And yet those with a problem of drug abuse or aggression are crime-prone, often have poor prognoses, and seldom respond to legal intervention or rehabilitation.

In view of the above realities: the surge of drug-abuse problems with the Vietnam war, the development of Methadone as a potentially effective treatment, and the awareness that privacy would be prerequisite to the success of therapeutic interventions, a set of federal laws and regulations was passed to enable the operation of alcohol and drug abuse treatment programmes.[32] The confidentiality of patient records was reasonably protected by law, but the implementation of the programme was marred by so many police incursions that Dr Nyswander, who originated the Methadone programme, commented in her ten-year summary report that much of the failure of the programme could be attributed to 'politically-inspired (police) control'.[33]

In accordance with a public health model, should psychiatric records be used in the assessment of driver's license applicants, drug abusers, gun-permit applicants, and child abusers?

A convincing case has been made for the breach of confidentiality in the reporting of child-abuse cases. But experience demonstrates that because of limited social resources and funds, family problems causing child abuse cannot be resolved by simple reporting, and the treatment of abusing parents is complicated by the necessity of reporting.

A particularly complex law enforcement problem was crystallized in the 1976 California case known as *Tarasoff*.[34] The commentaries by judges, lawyers, scholars, and psychiatrists have been voluminous.[35] The decision imposes on the psychiatrist a limited duty to warn a presumed intended victim of a patient's aggression. Because of the incompatibilities with other California laws and with clinical realities, it presents psychiatrists with a very difficult legal, ethical, and clinical dilemma. The parents of a murdered student (Tarasoff) sued the therapists and the university for not having warned them of the dangerousness of the homicidal patient–student who had been in treatment. The courts found the parents had an actionable complaint which was later settled out of court. The therapist had alerted campus police to the patient's dangerousness and they arrested him but found him harmless and released him. California law makes involuntary hospitalization difficult. The therapist had ruptured the therapeutic alliance by his warning, thus losing his therapeutic leverage, and on her return from a vacation Ms. Tarasoff was murdered by the patient. The judicial decision has resulted in many legal and clinical uncertainties. Many psychiatrists concluded there is now a general duty to warn supposed intended victims, but this has proved impractical because the ability to predict dangerousness is quite limited. Experience demonstrated that most intended victims already were aware of the danger and were helpless to protect themselves. Also false-positive warnings could expose the therapist to legal action should the 'victim' have changed his life unnecessarily or become ill because of the warning. Further, if the warned victim also proved to be dangerous, the original patient might be exposed to danger and could sue the psychiatrist for breach of confidentiality and endangerment.

It was learned that after the *Tarasoff* decision many patients with problems of aggression avoided treatment, interrupted their treatment, or could not use it effectively out of fear of being betrayed.[35] Thus, ironically, a judicial mandate to use psychiatrists as agents of social control resulted in the impairment of the therapeutic relationship, the one avenue of intervention most likely to help a patient establish control over his aggression. In addition there was erosion of public confidence in the ability of a psychiatrist to assure confidentiality.

One remedy to the problem is to make warnings discretionary rather than mandatory, thus allowing the psychiatrist first to use his clinical resources, then to seek help if necessary from the patient's family and friends, and from relevant authorities so as to institute involuntary hospitalization, and only after all this has failed, to consider warning a specific victim. Again the wisdom of stressing confidentiality to enable treatment is illustrated.

A further step in the erosion of the doctor–patient relationship from law enforcement agencies occurred in the case of *Zurcher v. Stanford Daily*.[36] In 1978 the United States Supreme Court upheld the validity of a warrant obtained by Sheriff Zurcher to search the premises of the student newspaper of Stanford University for photographs of a student incident in which police had been injured. He could have had a subpoena issued, but feared this would bring delay during which evidence might be destroyed and he also wanted immediate results. The newspaper itself was not suspected of a crime although search warrants are usually issued for good cause against those suspected of having committed an offence. Simply posting the warrant on the door legalizes forcible entry and entitles search of whatever premises and objects are listed on the warrant. A subpoena is the more usual and orderly process; it allows a citizen to use his constitutional guarantees against unreasonable search should he see fit. Only if there is reasonable concern that evidence will be destroyed if a subpoena is issued, should a search warrant be sought. The press reacted vigorously to the case protesting the threat to its freedom of such surprise searches.[37] Several bills were introduced in Congress to reverse the impact of the decision.[38]

Less well understood is that the *Zurcher* decision set a precedent for a surprise search of any innocent third party suspected of having evidence of a crime. Hence the office of a doctor, lawyer, clergyman, or any other citizen could be searched. Shortly after the *Stanford Daily* episode Zurcher obtained a warrant to search the premises of a psychiatrist in possession of evidence relevant to the investigation of a former patient who had complained to the police of a sexual attack. The investigator, rather than wait for the routine response to his request for information, insisted on searching the doctor's premises. Not only was the patient's file exposed to unreasonable search and seizure, but also those of the psychiatrist's other patients. If Nixon's 'plumbers' had been able to avail themselves of a search warrant, they need not have unlawfully entered Dr Fielding's office for the psychiatric records of Daniel Ellsberg[39,40] (who earlier had released the Pentagon Papers)!

To add to the seriousness of this problem, warrants were also issued to search the public defender's office in the same county.[40] At about this time a warrant was also issued to search the files of a San Francisco drug-abuse clinic, even though this was against federal regulations.[41] When the clinic's director resisted access to his files lest the disclosures wreck the whole programme, he was detained.[33] This was a major breach of confidentiality in which protective federal regulations were not honoured, and a suit to seek redress was subsequently filed.[41]

In 1978 Hawaii passed its Act 105 authorizing the use of search warrants in the 'public interest' to monitor the Medicaid programme. This law was interpreted to mean that a warrant to search a provider's office and/or home could be obtained on only an affidavit stating that the provider participated in the Medicaid programme and the public interest justified a search. Police invaded the office of a Honolulu psychologist and seized records not only of his Medicaid patients, but also of his private patients.[42] Although the act was soon declared unconstitutional, its passage has had disturbing implications for patient–psychiatrist confidentiality.

These examples further illustrate the creation of ethical dilemmas for psychiatrists by legal and legislative developments. It is noteworthy that the court decision declaring the Hawaii Act unconstitutional was implemented through the vigorous intervention of the Hawaii Psychiatric Society as *amicus curiae*, illustrating the relevance of the stipulation in the American Psychiatric Association code of ethics regarding 'dissent within the law'.[6] A series of proposed laws introduced in the United States Congress in 1978 and 1979 under the guise of 'medical records privacy acts' poses a new threat to the doctor–patient relationship by law enforcement agencies. Heralded by President Carter and the Congress as laws to protect medical privacy, the proposed legislation actually provides detailed guidelines for access by law enforcement agencies to medical records, and mandates compliance with 'administrative or judicial summons or subpoena'[43] and with a ' search warrant or formal written request' from law enforcement agencies without notification of the patient.[44] Furthermore, protective state laws would be superseded by this federal legislation.[44,45]

This disconcerting pattern is also reflected in three other legislative developments: (1) Senator Edward Kennedy introduced the FBI Charter Act of 1979, which contains a 'physician-informant' provision (This Act purports to restrict the use by the FBI of physicians as informants but could be used to coerce confidential information); (2) In his 1980 State of the Union address President Carter recommended that the strictures on CIA access to confidential information be loosened;[46,47] and (3) the Federal Register of 2 January 1980 contains a notice of intent to make 15 changes in the Alcohol and

Drug Abuse Confidentiality regulations which would effectively eliminate confidentiality and provide for the use of psychiatric records to
initiate criminal prosecution.[48]

Conclusion

The issues raised here pose ethical problems for the psychiatrist which
are both difficult and delicate. Faced with what he regards as heavy-
handed intrusion by courts and law enforcement agencies on confidentiality which is paramount in his work, he must plot a course of
action. He can passively acquiesce with events as legally mandated
and which are thus beyond his control or he can vigorously attempt to
influence legislatures and courts and 'dissent within the law' to the
fullest extent possible. In my view the latter alternative seems to be in
the best ethical traditions of our profession.

References

1. *Stedman's medical dictionary*, 23rd edn., New York, Williams and Wilkins, 1976.
2. GUNN, J. personal communication, 1980.
3. *Webster's new international dictionary*, 2nd edn., Springfield Mass., Merriam 1952.
4. *Oxford English Dictionary*, Compact edn., Clarendon Press 1971.
5. *Judicial council opinions and reports*. Chicago, American Medical Association, 1977.
6. The principles of medical ethics with annotations especially applicable to psychiatry. *American Journal of Psychiatry* **130**:1058–64, 1973.
7. SLAWSON, P. F.: Patient–litigant exception. A hazard to psychotherapy. *Archives of General Psychiatry* **21**: 347–52, 1969.
8. CROSSMAN, M.: Confidentiality: The right to privacy versus the right to know, in *Law and the mental health professions*. Ed. Barton, W. E. and Sanborn, C. J. New York: International Universities Press, 1978, pp. 137–84.
9. GOLDSTEIN, A. S. and KATZ J.: Psychiatrist–patient privilege: The GAP proposal and the Connecticut statute. *American Journal of Psychiatry* **118**: 733–9, 1962.
10. BEIGLER, J. S.: The 1971 amendment of the Illinois statute on confidentiality: a new development in privilege law. *American Journal of Psychiatry* **129**:311–15, 1972.
11. *Confidentiality and privileged communications in the practice of psychiatry*, Report No. 45. New York: Group for the Advancement of Psychiatry, 1960.
12. WIGMORE, J. H.: *Evidence in trials at common law*. Vol. 8. Boston, Little Brown, 1961, sec. 2285, p. 527.
13. *State of Illinois Mental health and Developmental Disabilities Confidentiality Act*, Section 10(a) (1), p. 6. Department of Mental Health and Developmental Disabilities, 1979.
14. *District of Columbia Mental Health Information Act*, Title V, Section 501–4, 1978.
15. Official Actions of the American Psychiatric Association. Model law on confidentiality of health and social service records. *American Journal of Psychiatry* **136**: 138–44, 1979.
16. NYE, S.: Commentary on model law on confidentiality of health and social service records. *American Journal of Psychiatry* **136**:145–7, 1979.

17. BEIGLER, J. S.: The APA model law on confidentiality. *American Journal of Psychiatry* **136**:71–3, 1979.
18. LIFSCHUTZ, J. E.: A summary of my court experience. Read at the Panel on levels of confidentiality in the psychoanalytic situation, 58th annual meeting, American Psychoanalytic Association, Washington, DC, April 1971.
19. Privacy and the psychiatrist. *Time*, 27 April, 1970.
20. TURNER, W.: Legal right goal for psychiatrist. *New York Times*, 14 Dec. 1969.
21. *Caesar v. Mountanos*. U.S. Ct. Appeal, 9th, No. 74–2271.
22. M. D. gets jail sentence in privilege challenge. *Psychiatric News* 17 April 1974.
23. George Caesar jailed, CPA protests quickly. *Northern California Psychiatric Society Newsletter*. August, 1977.
24. *Robertson, Murphy v. Penny*, Sup. Ct. Cal. Calender No. 385947.
25. HUFSTEDLER, S.: Concurring and dissenting opinion in *Caesar v. Mountanos*. Calif. Appeals Ct., 74–2271, 1976. 542 F 2d 1064 (9th Cir 1976).
26. BEIGLER, J. S.: Psychiatry and confidentiality. *American Journal of Forensic Psychiatry* **1**:7–19, 1978. Also: in *Hearings before the Sub-committee on the Constitution of the Committee on the Judiciary, U. S. Senate Ninety-fifth Congress second session on S.3162. A bill to secure and protect the freedom of individuals from unwarranted intrusions by persons acting under color of law.* Washington, DC, US Government Printing Office, 1979 pp. 254–61.
27. *Wisconsin Statutes* 905.04 Physician–patient Privilege (3), pp. 196–7.
28. GROSSMAN, M.: Confidentiality and third parties. A report of the APA Task Force on Confidentiality as it relates to third parties. Task Force Report 9, June, 1975, Washington, DC, American Psychiatric Association.
29. VISOTSKY H. and SACHNOFF L., personal communication, 1977.
30. Privilege denied in joint therapy. *Psychiatric News*, 4 May, 1979.
31. Patient–physician privilege may be lost through group session. *Clinical Psychiatry*, June, 1979.
32. PL 93–282, The Federal Alcohol and Drug Abuse Treatment Programs; 42 US Code 4582, pp. 29–30; 40 Federal Register 27802 EE, 1 July, 1975.
33. DOLE, V. P. and NYSWANDER, M. E.: Methadone maintenance treatment: a ten-year perspective. *Journal of the American Medical Association* **235**: 2117–19, 1976.
34. *Tarasoff v. Regents of Univ. of Cal.*, 529 P. 2d 55, 118 Cal. Rprtr. 129 (1974) (Tarasoff I); 17 Cal. 3d 425, 551 P. 2d 334, 331 Cal. Rprtr. 14 (1976) (Tarasoff II).
35. WISE, T. P.: Where the public peril begins. A survey of psychotherapists to determine the effects of *Tarasoff*. *Stanford Law Review* **31**: 165–90, 1978.
36. *Zurcher V. Stanford Daily*, 46 LW 4546, US Supreme Court, 31 May 1978.
37. High court's threat to freedom. Editorial, *Chicago Sun-Times*, 8 July, 1979; Surprise raids a threat to all. Editorial, *Chicago Sun-Times*, 10 July, 1979. Walter Cronkite: A supreme threat to freedom of press. *Chicago Sun-Times*, 20 March, 1979 Media tell fear of muzzle on criticism from new ruling. *Chicago Sun-Times*, 19 April, 1979.
38. S.31562, S.3164, 95th Congress, 1978; H.R.3486, 96th Congress, 1979.
39. BEIGLER J. S. and CROSSMAN, M.: *Hearings before the Subcommittee on the Constitution of the Committee on the Judiciary, US Senate, 95th Congress, second session on S.3162, a bill to secure and protect the freedom of individuals from unwarranted intrusions by persons acting under color of law.* Washington, DC US Government Printing Office, 1979, pp. 223–77, p. 225.
40. BEIGLER J. S.: Testimony of the American Psychiatric Association before the Subcommittee on Courts, Civil Liberties and the Administration of Justice of the House Committee on the Judiciary, US House of Representatives, on H.R.3486 and the implications of *Zurcher v. Stanford Daily*, 1 June, 1979.

41. ZANE, M.: Suit filed over drug clinic raid. *San Francisco Chronicle*, 29 August, 1979.
42. Court stops state seizure of records. *Psychiatric News*, 1 February 1980.
43. JAVITS, J.: *Congressional Record*. Proceedings and debates of the 95th Congress, second session, Aug. 23, 1978, pp. S14203–S14207. Washington, DC, Government Printing Office. Sec. 206 (n).
44. JAVITS, J.: *Congressional Record*. Proceedings and Debates of the 96th Congress, first session: 125 No. 24, pp. S1845–S1853, 1 March, 1979. Sec. 206 (b) (10), p. 1848.
45. RIBICOFF, A.: S. 865 Privacy of Medical Information Act, pp. 3874–82; S.867 Privacy of Research Records Act, pp. 3883–8, *Congressional Record* **125,** 4 April, 1979.
46. Text of the President's State of the Union Address to a Joint Session of Congress *New York Times*, 24 January, 1980.
47. Congress Moves to Relax Curbs on CIA. *Science, New York* **207**: 965–6, 1980.
48. Public Health Service, HEW, 42 CFR Part 2, Confidentiality of Alcohol and Drug Abuse Patient Records. *Federal Register* **45**: No. 1, 2 January 1980, pp. 53–4.

13
Ethics and child psychiatry
Philip Graham

THE child holds a special position in psychiatric issues requiring ethical judgement because his actions are regarded as the responsibility of his parents; consequently any intervention in preventing, diagnosing, and treating psychiatric disorders in the child inevitably involves people other than the child. Whether the responsibility of the professional lies in meeting the interests of the parent or those of the child is not a matter of controversy when these interests coincide; but when they conflict the issues raised are obviously complex.

It has been pointed out[1] that although parents are usually effective protectors and advocates of their children this is not always the case; a child will in some situations need an advocate other than his parents. In disputes over custody, for example, and in other legal procedures, such as those involving hospital commitment, parents have an overwhelmingly powerful voice and may indeed be professionally represented. The child, except in unusual circumstances, such as when responsibility for his care has been assumed by a welfare or social services department, will not have an independent advocate. Paediatricians, general practitioners, psychologists, and psychiatrists may decide, on the basis of evidence made available to them in their clinical work, that they need to act as advocate of the child. If these clinicians do assume this role they are often aware of the risk of losing the parents' goodwill and that in the long run, their power to promote the child's interests may be reduced.

Further complexities in ethical issues concerning children stem from the fact that the child's own moral judgement is not fully developed and consequently his capacity to be involved in decision-making is limited. Moreover, the child's increasing capacity for moral judgement as he matures means that those concerned need continually to reappraise this capacity when decisions affecting his welfare are required. In the mentally handicapped child (and adult) a prolonged, sometimes permanent state of immaturity of understanding and moral judgement exists. Here it seems appropriate to take account of mental rather than chronological age when deciding how much weight should be given to the child's own contribution.

Children are subject to different constraints from those experienced by adults. Compulsory schooling and the prohibition of full-time paid employment are examples. Such rules and regulations are seen by adults as necessary for the process of socialization, but it is important for us to acknowledge not only that children themselves may think and feel very differently about these matters, but also that many adults are ambivalent about the values to which children are directed. These broader issues relating to status of the child, socialization, and values will not be discussed further in this chapter. Instead attention will be given to ethical questions which may arise in three areas: (1) the clinical processes — especially diagnosis and treatment — in which psychiatrists are involved; (2) research and teaching; and (3) situations in which psychiatrists may be expected to provide advice though not a clinical service.

Diagnosis

Various aspects of the diagnostic process in child psychiatry (and indeed in psychiatry generally) have been called into question over the last two decades both from a practical and ethical point of view. Concerns have been expressed over the negative effect of specific diagnostic labels and over the value and justification of screening programmes to identify disturbed and slow-learning children.

The diagnostic process

Although diagnosis has long been accepted by many psychiatrists as a central feature of medical and psychiatric procedure in childhood, opinion has differed regarding the proper nature of the diagnostic process and the value attributed to it. The need to classify disorders is clearly necessary as a form of shorthand communication between professionals and as a pointer to particular treatment, but there has been increasing dissatisfaction with the notion that a diagnostic label is anything like an adequate guide to management. Thus Rutter[2] comments: 'The decision regarding care or placement must take into account social impairment, persistence of problems and availability of suitable treatments as well as the diagnosis of type of disorder. Not all people with a particular disorder require the same action and individual differences must be taken into account so that services are tailored to individual needs (rather than slotting individuals into pigeon holes which offer a diagnosis cum treatment package)'. One may assume that a diagnostic process which does not entail obtaining information along these lines is incomplete and unsatisfactory as a basis for action.

Diagnostic labelling

Ethical concerns about the effects of diagnostic labelling revolve around two main issues — the use of inaccurate, inappropriate, or misleading labels, and the potential negative effect of a label on the quality of the child's life.

The debate about inappropriate labelling has centred mainly around the use of the terms 'minimal brain dysfunction syndrome', 'hyperkinetic child syndrome', and 'conduct disorder', to describe states in children whose 'disability' can arguably be seen as unwillingness to conform to the norms of behaviour regarded as desirable by their parents and teachers.[3] Inability to concentrate, overactivity, impersistence, and disruptive behaviour are indeed statistically somewhat loosely associated with minor electroencephalographic abnormalities and other signs of neurophysiological dysfunction, but in many cases the causal nature of this association has not been adequately established. Strong criticisms have been mounted[4-5] over the alleged use of medical labels to describe social problems and of the consequent tendency, to be discussed below, to prescribe medication as a form of social control. Box,[5] for example, refers to the 'increasing employment of medical solutions to school problems which are essentially moral, legal and social', and accuses the school medical system of attempting to screen, prevent, and treat 'non-organic behaviour disagreements'.

The ethical position of the child psychiatrist involved in the diagnosis of behaviour problems which largely revolve around deviant and troublesome behaviour is certainly fraught with difficulty. It is probably easier if the psychiatrist limits his attention to those severe disorders which, one might assume, would result in maladaptation even to a better than average if not optimal domestic or school environment. Many would also argue that the psychiatrist's task when faced with non-conformity and deviance involves not only adequate assessment of the child but also a full appraisal of the environment in which the child is apparently, and perhaps only apparently, creating the difficulties. Assessment of a child who shows disruptive school behaviour should therefore include a consideration of the teaching methods used and of the means applied to achieve classroom control. These issues are further discussed later in relation to treatment.

The negative effects of the application of labels are fully discussed by Hobbs[6-7] who forcefully makes the point that a diagnostic tag like 'mental retardation' can stick to a child for life and adversely affect his opportunities. However labels can obviously exert positive as well as negative effects. A child upon whom inappropriate and unhelpful pressure has been placed may be given a learning programme much *more* suited to his needs and abilities once a label of 'brain damage' has been attached to his disorder. Excellent facilities for autistic children may only open their doors to a child once this label has been assigned to him. Further, the use of labels can be viewed as a pragmatic as well as an ethical issue. Is there good evidence that labels act to the detriment of children? Findings are not clear-cut. In a frequently quoted study conducted by Rosenthal and Jacobson,[8] children were given randomly assigned intelligence scores which were then passed on to their teachers. At the end of an academic year children who had been allocated low scores were achieving significantly less well than those allocated high scores. However various attempts to replicate the study[9] have not obtained such clear-cut findings and even in the original study the results held for younger but not for older children. Research has also been done on the effects of labelling children as offenders by comparing the outcome of boys charged and found guilty of certain offences with that of boys who had shown equally serious antisocial behaviour but who had not been involved in criminal proceedings. Here the evidence[10] tends to support the negative effect of labelling.

Most psychiatrists would be appropriately wary of the use of diagnostic labels when communicating with people whose attitude to such labels was uncertain or unknown. In an interview with a parent or teacher, a psychiatrist should regard it as an essential part of his job to explain the terms he uses and to ensure that these are understood, at least at the time of the interview. I must admit however that this is a counsel of perfection; in practice once a report has been dispatched the psychiatrist often has little control over the way his words are interpreted. The issue of confidentiality is, of course, of considerable relevance in this context.

Screening

With improved resources and better screening instruments there has been an increased tendency to screen groups of children for the presence of developmental delay and behaviour disturbance. Again there is a danger both that children will be inappropriately labelled and that expectations of services may be raised in parents' minds when in fact none are available. I would regard it as necessary to ensure that those involved in screening programmes, including parents, are made aware of the limitations of screening methods. Moreover it is unethical to institute such programmes unless services are adequate to treat children who are identified as having some problem.

Treatment

Ethical questions in the provision of treatment in child psychiatry are of major importance because most forms of treatment currently offered have uncertain benefits.[11] Where existing therapy is clearly beneficial, as, for example, in the use of the bell and pad in nocturnal enuresis, consideration of ethical issues is limited to the adequate explanation of side-effects and the need for the psychiatrist's awareness of the dangers of symptom suppression or symptom substitution. When, as in the case of the example given, these aspects have been investigated and it has been concluded that the issues are straightforward, ethical factors will have been adequately dealt with. Unfortunately most treatment in child psychiatry does not fall into this desirable category and a careful assessment is necessary of the risks and benefits involved.

Many psychiatrists believe — though their belief is regrettably little acted upon — that the application of treatment of unproved efficacy brings with it an ethical obligation to conduct evaluative research. Certainly it can be convincingly argued that the lack of this research is morally less defensible than the conduct of research using untreated control subjects, and this issue is further discussed in Chapter 15. As the situation exists at present, the use of various forms of treatment in children produces problems of their own, and these different forms will therefore be considered separately.

Medication

The use of stimulant medication in children presenting with overactivity, distractibility, impersistence, learning disabilities and other behavioural or cognitive deficits is partly a result and partly a cause of the delineation of the hyperkinetic syndrome, the nature of which has already been mentioned in this chapter. It is well established that methylphenidate and dexamphetamine-sulphate can produce improved performance in learning tasks in laboratory research and that they can also reduce distractibility, impersistence, and disruptive behaviour in the classroom.[12-13] This effectiveness is not limited to children diagnosed as hyperactive but has been shown, at least in the laboratory situation, to enhance performance in normal children.

The widespread use of stimulant drugs has nevertheless been criticized, especially by Schrag and Divoky[4] in the United States, and by Box[5] in Britain. Their arguments are similar to those they have been employed against the use of the hyperkinetic syndrome label, and as these have been discussed earlier they will not be rehearsed now. However the objections to the label are clearly reinforced if, as has been contended, one result is that children are inappropriately drugged into mindless conformity by the use of medication. Thus, according to Box, 'school children by the million in America, and by tens of thousands in this country (the United Kingdom) are being put on long-term programmes of drug therapy simply because their behaviour does not fit in with the requirements of schools'. Although the figures quoted are in all likelihood grossly exaggerated there is no doubt that a very large number of American children and a small but not insignificant number in Britain are treated with stimulant drugs in order to reduce behaviour which, *interalia*, is creating difficulties for teachers and other pupils.

Sedgwick[14] has pointed out, in a thoughtful reply to Box, that the question of the number of children on medication is largely irrelevant. If the treatment *is* effective, the smaller number of children being treated in Britain may be due not to any praiseworthy concern for children, but to the neglect of the needs of the poorly achieving child. The first issue to determine is whether, for the individual child, the disadvantages of medication are clearly outweighed by the benefits. Further, the possible change in attitude of other children, parents, and teachers if the behaviour of the treated child is improved cannot be regarded as unimportant. Especially if behavioural change can be achieved in no other way, the diminution of rejection by teachers and peers as a result of reduced disruptiveness on the part of the child could be seen as a clear benefit to him. If this benefit however was not accompanied by improved learning ability or was achieved only at the cost of the child's becoming depressed and apathetic on the drug (a not infrequent occurrence) the use of medication might well be regarded as unjustified.

The criticism levelled most ferociously against the use of stimulants is less pertinent than other points that should be made. The first of these relates to the efficacy of alternative forms of treatment. Wolraich and his colleagues[15] have demonstrated that for certain types of behaviour associated with the 'hyperactive child' syndrome, behaviour modification can be as effective and in some cases superior to drug therapy. Obviously dangers of stimulant medication such as medicalization of social problems, side-effects, and dependence should lead to cautious and judicious use of drugs, and only after other less harmful measures have failed. The second issue concerns the possibility that the use of medication may discourage the therapist from trying to understand the child's feelings and behaviour. Finally, there is the question of what degree of severity of the problem justifies the prescribing of stimulants. Differences of opinion on this last point probably account for the hitherto much more widespread use of stimulants in the United States compared to Britain. Most British child psychiatrists reserve medication for severely over-active disruptive children even in the knowledge that stimulants improve concentration and performance in less severe cases and in normal children. In so far as this policy has been rationally considered by British psychiatrists it is probably the result of a calculation that the known and unknown risks of medication outweigh potential benefits in all but the seriously handicapped child. The view is also taken that it is no part of the psychiatrist's job to smooth out normal variations in learning ability especially when a lower level of concentration is often accompanied by greater vivacity, curiosity, and explorativeness, all of which have their own appeal and may be lost with exposure to medication. Failure to demonstrate[16] long-term improvement in learning ability or behaviour by drugs is a further discouragement to their application in less severely affected children.

Before leaving the subject of physical methods of treatment, it is worth mentioning the use of more drastic procedures such as electro-convulsive therapy and temporal lobectomy. Again the questions of efficacy and risk require much thought, particularly in the light of the possibility of long-term and perhaps permanent damage resulting from these physical manipulations of the brain. If a child's psychiatric condition however is very severe, it is unreasonable to place these measures out of his reach merely because of age. On a visit to the Soviet Union I was assured that the use of electro-convulsive therapy was illegal in children under the age of 16; if this is the case, the admittedly extremely rare but not unknown case of a pubescent child with a prolonged catatonic illness would be deprived of the most effective available treatment. Although the presence of seriously aggressive behaviour in a child with intractable temporal lobe epilepsy may be appropriately regarded as an additional reason for considering temporal lobectomy, the use of psychosurgery in aggressive teenagers without evidence of brain dysfunction must surely be regarded as a highly questionable procedure. Aggression as an indication for psychosurgery is discussed further in Chapter 8.

Surgical sterilization of promiscuous mentally handicapped teenagers has also been the subject of controversy. In Britain the Department of Health and Social Security has recommended a consultation procedure before sterilization is undertaken in a child under the age of 16.[17] A more recent report of a working group on contemporary medical/ethical problems[18] suggests that this recommendation should also apply to mentally handicapped people over the age of 16. The working group concluded that, in a female, only 'proven parental incapacity' (a woman has had a child and signally failed to provide adequate parental care) coupled with an inability to manage contraceptives constitutes sufficient justification for sterilization. It suggests that male promiscuity be controlled by appropriate drugs rather than surgery.

Psychotherapy

Individual and family psychotherapy are probably the most common forms of treatment used in child psychiatry and there is modest evidence for their efficacy in a range of emotional disorders and certain psychosomatic conditions.[11,19] Ethical problems facing the psychotherapist include their uncertain benefits, the danger of the subtle indoctrinating nature of the techniques used, and the potential neglect of, and lack of respect for, parental concerns (in individual child therapy) or individual development (in family therapy).

The uncertainty of psychotherapy's benefit provokes the question of the degree to which parents and their children should be informed about the chance of being helped by this treatment. Honest disclosure is advantageous in that it enables parents to decide whether they are prepared to accept treatment in the light of the costs involved (e.g. therapist fees, time out of work, child's time out of school). The issue may prove more complicated since parents sometimes opt out of therapy ostensibly for these material reasons, but in fact because they suspect, perhaps justifiably, that therapy will be painful to them and to the child. There are advantages in the therapist's pointing to the likelihood of such pain occurring at the onset of treatment. The usefulness of relatively brief, focused treatment embarked upon on a 'contract' basis for a specified number of sessions is attractive but the view of many therapists is that not all psychiatric conditions in childhood are likely to respond to such brief measures. The issue is clearer where it has been reasonably established, as in the case of interpretative psycho-analytic therapy for childhood autism, that a treatment is probably of no benefit.[20]

In this case it is obligatory for the therapist to point out the evidence explicitly and, if he undertakes such intervention, to indicate its experimental and non-therapeutic nature.

The indoctrinating quality of different forms of psychotherapy — the overt or covert process in which the therapist imposes his values on his patient — has been frequently discussed (e.g. in relation to child guidance work by Blumenfeld[21]). The issues in the therapy of children and families are scarcely different compared to those in the treatment of adults (see Chapter 6). In so far as family therapy — especially in work with disturbed children — is becoming increasingly popular, it is worth examining some of the specific ethical problems associated with this form of treatment. It is, for example, common practice for family therapists to insist that the father attends treatment sessions. His participation may lead to an alteration in family functioning whereby his paternal role and authority are undermined; this is especially the case in working-class families in which division of responsibilities between parents tends to be clearly defined. Most family therapists are well aware of this danger but a danger it remains. Many parents are reluctant to divulge criticism of their children to the therapist in front of them, and hesitate to do so. The practice of family therapists however is to encourage expression of such negative feelings in the reasonable belief that the child knows what the parent feels anyway, and that unless there is an honest acknowledgement of these aspects of communication little progress in improving family relationships is likely. The risk exists that parents will develop a habit of negative thinking about their children which they would otherwise not have adopted. Another issue concerns the therapist's use of certain potent procedures. Techniques such as family sculpting and paradoxical injunction in family therapy may sometimes be practised without the therapist's awareness of the degree to which he is engaged in paternalistic manipulation.

I do not need to emphasize the importance of clinical research in contributing to a greater understanding of the risks and benefits of family therapy which in turn will no doubt clarify the ethical problems mentioned.

Finally, the limiting nature of each form of psychotherapy when practised in an exclusive manner warrants comment. In individual therapy with children it is common practice for material disclosed by the child to be kept secret from the parents on the grounds that the child will not produce this material once he knows his parents will be informed. This exclusion raises anxieties in them, and it is arguable whether therapy of this type should be undertaken unless concomitant discussion occurs with parents and they are fully agreeable. There is a danger that parents are persuaded to consent when they may be exercising accurate judgement in their concern that their child's individual therapy will be associated with an undermining of their own authority. A converse problem arises in family therapy when, because the child is not given an opportunity to express his feelings privately to the therapist, he may not disclose his concerns about, for example, physical violence to himself or between his parents, which may be at the root of his problems. Many practitioners who have a preference for either individual or family therapy acknowledge the advantages in providing an opportunity for both individual and family sessions to occur, at least during the phase of assessment.

Behaviour modification

Ethical aspects of behaviour modification have been usefully discussed[22] in the context of its application in treating problems in gender identity; Rosen and his colleagues make the point that parents and mental health professionals often have to decide whether a particular outcome can really be regarded as beneficial. In general the element of manipulation involved in behaviour modification is more overt than in psychotherapy and may therefore, paradoxically, be less open to unconscious abuse. On the other hand, the very effectiveness of the procedures involved, as, for example, in the achievement of classroom control with disruptive and aggressive pupils, raises additional questions similar to those I have discussed when considering medication. Achieving an atmosphere of tranquility in the classroom through behavioural methods (or with drugs), can hardly be regarded as justified unless, as a result, improved opportunities are created for learning, which enable children who are the target of these therapeutic measures to benefit as well as their classroom colleagues. Intervention which leads to behaviour control without positive effects on the children towards whom it is directed, is clearly open to objection.

Special educational and hospital in-patient provision

While until recently the availability of separate educational provision for disturbed and slow-learning children was seen as advantageous to such children, and indeed as a form of positive discrimination, attitudes have swung noticeably. It is now thought preferable to educate children with exceptional needs as far as possible alongside ordinary children in order to ensure minimal stigmatization and as a much normal school experience as is feasible. In the United States, this changed attitude is reflected in various State and Federal laws (e.g. Public Law 94/142) and in Britain in similar legislation (e.g. Section 10 of the 1976 Education Act), and in official government documents such as the Warnock Report.[23] Nevertheless there is almost universal agreement that *some* special and separate provision continues to be necessary and desirable, at least for severely handicapped children. In so far as psychiatrists have responsibility for advising on educational needs, they are involved in decisions which have a distinctly ethical component, regarding, for example, the desirability of a separate school placement for a disruptive child who is benefiting from his current education but is disturbing others, or the wisdom of placing a child in a special residential school because, while special schooling is necessary, limited resources of the education authority have led to no suitable day placements being available.

There is often considerable and, I would say, highly understandable pressure from teachers on psychiatrists for them to use their influence to facilitate the removal of extremely difficult children and adolescents to special educational or even hospital institutions. In this situation the psychiatrist needs to ask a number of questions and to ensure that they are being honestly answered by all concerned including, of course, himself! Have all possible measures been tried in order to keep the child in an ordinary school? For example, has the employment of additional staff been envisaged? If this possibility has been rejected as too costly an alternative, has the local authority concerned made realistic comparisons between the actual costs and a special school placement? Will placement outside the ordinary school really help the child? If not, has this been stated openly to the parents and teachers concerned so that there is no doubt in anyone's mind for whose benefit removal from the ordinary environment is planned? How aware is the child himself of the real reasons for the proposed placement? Bruggen and his co-workers[24] have shown that posing these sort of questions, in relation to proposed admission to an adolescent psychiatric unit, can actually form a focus for therapeutic work. Although many psychiatrists will feel that this approach is inappropriate in some clinical situations there is no doubt that it can in others shed light on the real reasons for parents requesting admission for their child or adolescent.

The question of involuntary commitment of children to hospital on grounds of mental illness has been discussed by Black[25] in relation to British procedure, by Roth[26] in the United States, and more generally by Tooley.[27] In Britain, unless the child's parents have legally forfeited their parental rights, their consent to commitment cannot be overridden by the contrary wishes of their child if he is under the age of 16. In the case of Parham v. F. R., discussed in detail by Roth,[26] a similar position was taken by the United States Supreme Court. The Court rejected the need for separate representation of the child in the absence of evidence of clear-cut abuse and neglect by the parents, or evidence that the psychiatrists involved had acted in bad faith. It is of interest, however, that various relevant professional organizations had advised in their submissions that adolescents, younger children not living in an intact family, and all children admitted for a period longer than 45 days, should have the right to a due process hearing presumably with independent advocacy.

Research

The lack of established knowledge about the cause, prevention, and effective treatment of child psychiatric disorders highlights the need for research to be vigorously pursued. Indeed some psychiatrists have argued that with current knowlege so slender, the conduct of research is ethically more justified than clinical practice. Some practitioners who participate in both research and clinical work are more comfortable in their research activities than in applying treatment of dubious validity in possibly spurious attempts to alleviate suffering.

Most ethical issues affecting research in children are similar to those which occur in adults, and are dealt with elsewhere in this book (see Chapter 15). However there are special problems in children concerning ethical principles that researchers would consider as well as different issues in relation to informed consent. Helpful ethical guidelines in the conduct of research involving children have been recommended by a Working Party of the British Paediatric Association.[28] Although the Committee mainly concerned itself with research on physical disorders and physical methods of investigation, the principles it set forth are readily applicable to the study of psychiatric conditions and to the use of psychological techniques.

The chief principle, the report advocates, which should underlie ethical judgements in research entails the risk — benefit ratio. Risks — of causing 'physical disturbance, discomfort or pain or psychological disturbance for the child or his parents' — are classified as negligible (less than those occurring in everyday life), minimal, more than minimal but not definitely harmful, and harmful. The main problem in psychological research is that it is extraordinarily difficult to assess risks in advance. A psychiatric interview, for example, in an epidemiological survey in which a child is asked among other items about his concerns, anxieties, and fantasies could be seen, and indeed has been seen, either as a non-intrusive benign procedure involving negligible risk (compared for example to the everyday experience of exposure to insensitive criticism from parents, teachers, and peers), or as a potentially highly disturbing event leading to prolonged distress because previously suppressed material is now exposed with little or no attempt to make it meaningful for the child. The determination of risk in child psychiatric research can be evaluated systematically. Thus a follow-up of investigated children and their parents can do much to clarify the question of degree of disturbance caused. In general, follow-up studies suggest that research interviews with children are either experienced as trivial events or as pleasurable or as helpful, but it would be surprising if the occasional child was not seriously upset.

Another risk of research especially pertinent to children is the possibility that a treatment offered, which in normal clinical practice would not have been made available, might become associated with maladaptive behaviour which would not otherwise have occurred. Thus, an investigation involving the use of medication may lead to an habitual pattern of tablet-taking to solve problems of living. This particular problem has arisen in studies of the use of stimulants for over-activity and of hypnotics for sleep disorders in infancy. The investigator has an obligation, when offering treatment that is not requested, to ensure that it is undertaken only where there is a strong likelihood of its being efficacious (unfortunately a rare event in child psychiatry), or where the parents (and the child if he is of sufficient age) are highly motivated to accept treatment. Thus, in one study of the value of hypnotics for severe sleep disorder, only children whose parents were unambiguously motivated were entered in the trial.

The benefits of research can be considered in terms of whether they involve the child or family studied, or only other children. Research offering no benefit to the child — non-therapeutic research — is legal in English law[29,30] and indeed without this type of work it would be impossible to establish norms on physiological and psychological parameters in children without problems. Knowledge which accrues from the investigation of normal children should not be underestimated; many a child with a temporary disturbance such as nocturnal enuresis has been saved intrusive and even harmful treatment by a knowledge of the wide prevalence of the condition in the general population and its good prognosis without intervention.

We face a major problem in applying the principle of risk – benefit ratio because the magnitude of the benefit is always uncertain. Thus, a hypothesis regarding the aetiology of childhood autism might involve the examination of cerebrospinal fluid. The likelihood of a positive finding might be exceedingly small, but, if such a result were obtained understanding of the nature of the condition could be significantly advanced. The people most qualified to evaluate the chance of benefit are the investigators and their colleagues working in allied fields, but for understandable reasons they may be influenced by their enthusiasm for their work to overestimate likely benefit and underestimate potential risk. It is for this reason, among others, that the establishment of ethical committees or similar bodies, whose task is to adjudicate as impartially as possible on the basis of the risk – benefit principle, is so essential. It is clearly important that, when ethical committees consider research involving children, at least some of their members should be aware of the special problems inherent in research in this age group. The committee's considered judgements are of particular relevance in the case of institutionalized mentally handicapped or mentally ill children who may lack an independent advocate. An investigation, for example, of the administration of hepatitis virus to mentally handicapped children at Willowbrook State School was heavily criticized[31] on the grounds that the procedure was of no possible benefit to these children. The procedures adopted in the Willowbrook study would probably not have gained the acceptance of an independent scrutiny; the lesson learned is that investigators, with the best possible motivation to increase knowledge and improve preventive measures, can be helped by independent guidance when their procedures appear even slightly questionable.

There is general agreement that parental consent should be obtained before any research procedure is carried out in children and adolescents under the age of 18. Consent should only be sought after a full explanation of what the research will entail and this should involve an honest disclosure of both likely risk and potential benefit. No specific age has been established in Britain at which the child himself must provide consent in addition to his parents but it seems an increasingly popular view that the child should participate in the consent procedure to the limits of his understanding. It is for example perfectly possible for a 10-year-old child to appreciate that a venepuncture will not be of benefit to him but possibly benefit other children who also suffer from his condition.

While the risk exists that children's altruistic motivations might be inappropriately 'played upon', there is perhaps an even greater danger that children may be debarred from altruistic activity because of the overprotective attitudes of adults. Moreover, where altruistic behaviour has occurred it may also be considered ethically desirable for public acknowledgement of this fact. For example, I am currently collaborating in an investigation involving the donation of deciduous teeth for estimation of their lead content; the six or seven year old children donors are given a badge depicting a child with a large dental gap and the message 'I gave a tooth'. I would regard as ethically undesirable the situation in parts of the United States where clinical research involving children is virtually impossible because of an overriding concern for their rights. Advances in knowledge for the ultimate benefit of the afflicted necessitates inconvenience to be experienced by individuals who do not themselves suffer; and the privilege of participating in such activity should, I believe, not be denied to children who will benefit from the socialisation and other aspects of the experience.

Teaching

Clinical instruction to be effective sometimes requires live demonstration of diagnostic and treatment techniques. However most psychiatrists would argue that situations in which children are interviewed about the nature of their feelings and problems in front of an audience of medical or other students are not ethically appropriate. The introduction of one-way screens and video recording has made the demonstration of clinical skills and clinical phenomena less intrusive but has brought its own ethical difficulties.

Clinical teaching should involve the minimum of interference and parents (as well as children, to the limits of their understanding) should be informed of the status of observers and the degree of confidentiality that will be exercised. The opportunity to meet observers behind one-way screens is important when there is a possibility that a student is personally acquainted with the child and family, especially if it is not clearly understood that acquaintances should not observe. Similarly, presentation of video material requires special concern in the case of children since they may outgrow their problem while a record of their abnormality is retained. Parents' consent to preservation of video recordings should not be allowed to override the right of the child to decide the fate of the material, when he reaches an age at which he is capable of appreciating its nature. Automatic destruction of video recordings after a defined period, say five years, is another, perhaps, more feasible and preferable alternative.

One controversial aspect of teaching is the degree to which parents should be informed of the trainee status of doctors, social workers, psychologists, and psychotherapists who participate in the diagnosis or treatment of their children. It could, paradoxically, be argued that because some research findings indicate that trainees have greater success in certain conditions than their trained counterparts, parents should be warned if their children are to be seen by experienced professionals! Most child psychiatrists would agree that, as in other fields, where an establishment is used for training purposes parents should be informed of this fact and assured that if their children are to be seen by trainees, adequate supervision will be provided by experienced staff. The quality of this supervision is of course an issue in itself which has ethical implications.

Providing a psychiatric opinion

The child and the law

Since ethical aspects of forensic psychiatry are covered elsewhere in this book (see Chapter 14), mention will be made here only of issues which relate specifically to children. I should first note that responsibility accorded to children for criminal offences they have committed varies with age. Thus, in England and Wales a child under the age of ten cannot be charged with any criminal offence, although over the age of eight suspicion of an offence can be grounds for instituting proceedings which may result in the child's removal from parental care. Betwen ten and 13 years children can be charged with a criminal offence but it must be proved that they knew their actions were wrong. From the age of 14 a child is assumed to be responsible for his acts, and from 17 years he is subject to the full processes of the law.

Psychiatrists who advise the court on how to deal with a child offender are of course likely to be less concerned with the retributive and deterrent element of the judicial decision than in the question of whether the court is acting in the interests of the child and his family. It is a matter of argument whether the psychiatric report should be limited to information relevant to the making of this decision or whether the psychiatrist should impart his knowledge (assuming he has it) of the nature of the offence which might lead the court to alter its view of its gravity. Most psychiatrists would feel that in order to provide a report which will prove helpful to the court and to the child, they need to interview the parents as well as the child, and also to have access to any reports from his school. In circumstances where information from parents is obtained by social workers or probation officers, the psychiatrist's view will be limited by lack of direct contact. The status of his report based on such partial material might be regarded as dubious and it is therefore essential for the psychiatrist to indicate the basis on which he is providing his opinion.

It is often unclear to child and family, and regrettably to the psychiatrist, for whose benefit a psychiatric report is being prepared. If the court's question is whether the child is or was suffering at the time the offence was committed from some form of mental disorder, the report may well be seen as serving the court. If on the other hand the need is for information to enable the court to understand the nature of the circumstances leading to the offence and the family background, the report is more likely to be of benefit to the child. Most psychiatrists who prepare reports appreciate that their submissions may serve both purposes and make this explicit to the child and his family. In the case of a conflict of interests the interests of the child should take priority over those of the court, as long as this does not involve untruthfulness or any danger to society.

An interesting issue which may involve the court and is specific to childhood is school truancy. Truancy in general is the business of the school welfare officer and the court but school refusal stemming from neurosis lies within the province of the child psychiatrist, school psychologist, and social worker. A situation does arise in school refusal in which collusion between parents and child is so great and prospects of successful treatment by conventional psychiatric means so small that the psychiatrist may wish to institute legal action in order to achieve an enforced separation. The ethical basis for bringing legal action is fragile; the psychiatrist should therefore limit his actions to a clear statement that he can see no objection on psychiatric grounds why legal measures should not be adopted.

Adequacy of parental care

The paramount requirement for normal emotional and intellectual development in children is parental care of high quality. Many ethical questions face the psychiatrist when, for a variety of reasons, care has become or threatens to become of a kind which ranges from sub-optimal to deplorable.

The psychiatrist may be consulted by a couple, one of whom has had a psychiatric problem, who are seeking advice about embarking on parenthood. More commonly he may not be consulted by them but find himself uncertain as whether to discourage, for example, a husband and wife whose severe personality disorders, in all likelihood, disqualify them from competent parenthood. Most psychiatrists are reluctant to accept as part of their job the provision of such unsolicited advice. I regard it as reasonable to promote discussion about parenthood since inevitably those couples most in need of discouragement are least likely to seek or heed advice.

A related ethical dilemma occurs when a psychiatric opinion is sought in a decision about termination of pregnancy. Psychiatrists opposed to termination on religious grounds may regard it as necessary to disclose their views before examining the patient but this is unfortunately not always the case. Since psychiatric grounds for termination are open to wide interpretation it is worthwhile from a child psychiatrist's point of view to indicate the dismal social and psychological outcome of children whose mothers requested termination and were refused it.[32]

Serious psychiatric disorders in the post-partum period pose ethical problems when the interests of mother and newborn conflict. Close contact between the two may benefit the mother but place the child at risk, resulting in a most difficult situation. A knowledge of the bonding process may assist the psychiatrist who faces this problem. A realistic appraisal of the mother's capacity to provide adequate parenting in the future is also important. A large body of psychiatric opinion holds that the child's interests are paramount. Thus, if a mother suffering from chronic schizophrenia or a severe personality disorder is judged as probably unfit to provide adequate parental care, the child's interests will be served best by a prompt move towards permanent substitute care involving long-term fostering or, preferably, adoption. An ethical problem is associated with the possibility, however slight, that the mother will cope and wishes to keep the child. Should she be encouraged? There is in these circum-stances an understandable tendency for a doctor who has known the mother for some time, and become identified with her interests, to overlook the likely fate of the child.

Psychiatrists now frequently participate in decisions regarding the care of children subject to non-accidental injury (child abuse), either in appraising the mental state of the parents or, more generally, in determining the adequacy of parental care in relation to the child's interests emotional development. Again most psychiatrists believe that the child's interests are paramount although those of the parents should obviously be considered too. The decision is often a difficult one, and particularly when the quality of available substitute care falls well short of adequacy. Decisions made in these cases, at least in Britain, are the responsibility of Social Service Departments, and the psychiatrist's role is limited to the provision of factual information and advice.

In other circumstances a difficult ethical decision may have to be made by the psychiatrist as whether to initiate action by a social welfare department. A psychiatrist treating a child and family may become aware of neglect or rejection of such magnitude that he feels impelled to act. In this situation, as Eisenberg[33] has pointed out, not to act is to act, and a failure to take initiative may result in a deplorable outcome.

This dilemma can be at least partially resolved by including as a member of the treatment team a social worker with statutory responsibility to ensure adequacy of parental care. It is then necessary to make explicit at the outset the different roles and responsibilities of the professional staff who are involved.

Finally, the ethical position of the psychiatrist requested to offer an opinion on the issue of child custody in divorce proceedings requires mention. Increasingly, psychiatrists regard it as inappropriate to provide an opinion in these circumstances without interviewing both parents as well as the child. If the psychiatrist sees his role as primarily, though not exclusively, serving the best interests of the child, he should stipulate in advance that, regardless of whether his report is favourable to the parent whose lawyer has requested it, it should be made available in full to both parties. The general development of the family court as has occurred in some American states with its avoidance of the adversary procedure in custody cases, would do much to reduce the inherent ethical complications which face the psychiatrist.

Conclusion

The needs of children are undoubtedly best met by providing support to parents who are regarded as likely to act in the child's interests. However, as evidenced by the current interest in child advocacy and in children's rights, there is a growing social concern for children whose parents fail to act favourably for them. This issue is well illustrated in the case of child abuse and custody disputes. There is a natural tendency to deny that parents can be cruel to their children, a phenomenon which resulted in much delay before the wide prevalence of child abuse was recognized. A similar situation now applies to the sexual abuse of children. It would be particularly unfortunate if resistance to belief in the occurrence of sexual abuse arose because psychiatrists, as a result of their training, were unrealistically disposed to regard children's complaints as fantasy. In this, as in all other aspects of the practice of child psychiatry that I have dealt with in this chapter, awareness of the ethical issues involved together with intimate knowledge of relevant scientific evidence, will help to ensure that the psychiatrist acts in ethically desirable ways.

References

1. DUNCAN, A. S., DUNSTAN, G. R., and WELBOURN, R. B. (ed.): *Dictionary of medical ethics*. London, Darton, Longman, and Todd, 1977, pp. 40–2.
2. RUTTER, M. (1976): Classification, in *Child psychiatry, modern approaches*. Ed. M. Rutter and L. Hersov. Oxford, Blackwell, pp. 359–84.
3. BOSCO, J. J. and ROBIN, S. S. (ed.) *The hyperactive child and stimulant drugs*. Chicago, University of Chicago Press, 1976.
4. SCHRAG, P. and DIVOKY, D.: *The myth of the hyperactive child*. New York: Pantheon, 1975.
5. Box S.: Hyperactivity: the scandalous silence. *New Society* 1 December 1977, pp. 458–60.
6. HOBBS, N.: *The futures of children*. San Francisco, Jossey-Bass, 1975.
7. HOBBS, N.: *Issues in the classification of children*. San Francisco, Jossey-Bass, 1975.
8. ROSENTHAL, R. and JACOBSON, J.: *Pygmalion in the classroom: Teacher expectation and pupils' intellectual development*. New York, Holt, Rinehart, and Winston, 1968.
9. BROPHY, J. E. and GOOD, T. L. *Teacher–student relationships: causes and consequences*. New York, Holt, Rinehart, and Winston, 1974.
10. GOLD, M. and WILLIAMS, J. R.: National study of the aftermath of apprehension. *Prospectus* **3**:3–12, 1969.
11. GRAHAM, P.: Management in child psychiatry: recent trends. *British Journal of Psychiatry* **129**:97–108, 1976.
12. CANTWELL, D. and CARLSON, G.: Stimulants, in *Pediatric psychopharmacology: the use of behaviour modifying drugs in children*. Ed. Werry, J. S., New York, Brunner/Mazel, 1978.
13. CONNERS, C. and WERRY, J. S.: Pharmacotherapy, in *Psychopathological disorders of childhood* Ed. Quay, H., and Werry, J. S., New York, Wiley, 1979, pp. 336–86.
14. SEDGWICK, P. *New Society*, 5 January 1978, p. 31.
15. WOLRAICH, M., DRUMMOND, T., SALOMON, M., O'BRIEN, M., and SIVAGE C.: Effects of methylphenidate alone and in combination with behaviour modification procedures on the behaviour and academic performance of hyperactive children. *Journal of Abnormal Child Psychology* **6**:149–61, 1978.
16. QUINN, P. and RAPOPORT, J.: One-year followup of hyperactive boys treated with imipramine and methylphenidate. *American Journal of Psychiatry* **132**:241–5, 1977.

17. DEPARTMENT OF HEALTH AND SOCIAL SECURITY Sterilisation of children. DS 333/75 London, 1975.
18. WORKING GROUP ON CURRENT MEDICAL/ETHICAL PROBLEMS. Sterilisation of the mentally handicapped. *Lancet* ii:685–6, 1979.
19. LASK, B.: Family therapy outcome research 1972–8. *Journal of Family Therapy* 1:87–91, 1979.
20. RUTTER, M., GREENFELD, D., and LOCKYER, L.: A five- to fifteen-year followup study of infantile psychosis II. Social and behavioural outcome. *British Journal of Psychiatry* 113:1183–99, 1967.
21. BLUMENFELD A.: Ethical problems in child guidance. *British Journal of Medical Psychology* 47:17–26, 1974.
22. ROSEN, A. C., REKERS, G. A., and BENTLER, P. M.: Ethical issues in the treatment of children. *Journal of Social Issues* 34:122–36, 1978.
23. DEPARTMENT OF EDUCATION AND SCIENCE: *Special educational needs*. Report of the Committee of Enquiry into the Education of Handicapped Children and Young People. London, HMSO, 1978.
24. BRUGGEN, P., BYNG-HALL, J., and PITT-AIKENS, T.: The reason for admission as a focus of work on an adolescent unit. *British Journal of Psychiatry* 122:319–29, 1973.
25. BLACK D.: Age of consent. *Health and Social Services Journal* 89:286, 1979.
26. ROTH, L. H.: Mental health commitment: the state of the debate 1980. *Hospital and Community Psychiatry* 31,385–96, 1980.
27. TOOLEY, K.: Ethical considerations in the involuntary commitment of children and in psychological testing as a part of legal procedures. *Mental Hygiene* 54,484–9, 1970.
28. WORKING PARTY ON ETHICS OF RESEARCH IN CHILDREN. Guidelines to aid ethical committees considering research involving children. *British Medical Journal* 280:229–31, 1980.
29. SKEGG, P. D. G.: English law relating to experimentation on children. *Lancet* ii:754–5, 1977.
30. DWORKIN, G.: Legality of consent to non-therapeutic medical research on infants and young children. *Archives of Diseases in Childhood* 53:443–6, 1978.
31. Editorial. Ethics in research. *British Journal of Hospital Medicine* 2:759, 1968.
32. FORSSMAN, H. and THUWE, I.: One hundred and twenty children born after application for therapeutic abortion refused. *Acta psychiatrica scandinavica* 42:71–88, 1966.
33. EISENBERG, L.: The ethics of intervention: acting amidst ambiguity. *Journal of Child Psychology and Psychiatry and Allied Disciplines* 16:93–104, 1975.

14
Ethics and forensic psychiatry
Jonas R. Rappeport

What is forensic psychiatry?

Pollack, who has discussed this issue at length, distinguishes two distinct areas in which the professions of psychiatry and law interact.[1] The broader one involves legal issues touching upon the practice of psychiatry. These include commitment, guardianship, the right to treatment, and the right to refuse treatment. The term 'forensic psychiatry' should be limited to the actions of psychiatrists in assisting the law to carry out some of its responsibilities. Included are what Pollack calls 'psychiatry for legal purposes', covering issues like criminal responsibility, competency at the time of a crime, testamentary capacity, child custody, and others where psychiatric opinions are sought by the law to arrive at decisions. Many psychiatrists do not make this distinction and are likely to designate as forensic psychiatry all facets of psychiatric legal involvement. This chapter will focus on ethical problems that arise mainly in Pollack's narrower definition of forensic psychiatry.

The word 'forensic' comes from the Latin *forum* and in the context of forensic psychiatry refers to the fact that the psychiatrist's report is made public, that the relationship between psychiatrist and client is not private and therapeutic but open to the scrutiny of others. The ancient forums have today become the legislature and the courtroom. They furnish psychiatry an opportunity to assist the law in maintaining a safe and orderly society.

Because the psychiatrist's forensic role is quite different from his usual medical one of serving an individual patient, questions have been raised as to whether it is ethical for a psychiatrist to serve a third party, the law. Who is being helped — the patient, the lawyer, or the court? This question has been pertinent only after it began to be accepted that physicians specializing in mental disorders had something to offer the law in cases in which insanity or criminal responsibility were at issue. Before this time such cases were decided with such aid as in the McNaughton case of 1843. Gradually psychiatric

The author gratefully acknowledges the help of Melvin G. Goldzband, MD who gave detailed suggestions for rewriting an earlier draft.

specialists were introduced into court proceedings as experts, a trend which became established early in the twentieth century.

The early forensic psychiatrists were aware of the ethical issues that faced them in their efforts to assist the law. They expressed concern about using the physician's role to obtain information for non-therapeutic purposes as well as other ethical problems inherent in forensic work. These concerns have been voiced more recently by, among others, Szasz, Bazelon, Robitscher, and Halleck.[2,3,4,12] Robitscher, for instance, has stated 'The psychiatrist is the most important non-governmental decision-maker in modern life, and he has much more power than most government officials.'[2] The psychiatrist has power to recommend to the court that a defendant be given a life sentence or even the death penalty; that a defendant be considered not guilty by reason of insanity or incompetent to stand trial; or that a deceased's will be invalidated. He can recommend the annulment of a marriage, or who should have custody of the children of a disrupted family. True, the psychiatrist only renders an opinion, and the final decision is that of judge or jury. Nevertheless, we should not underestimate the importance sometimes given to his opinions. To accept these grave responsibilities without careful adherence to ethical guidelines would represent a serious departure from the physician's usual ethical posture. The role of psychiatrists in working with the court and the law has been challenged by Thomas Szasz who asserts that we abuse our power regularly, and, in fact, that we have no place in assisting the law.[3] Judge David Bazelon believes that such a role is legitimate but that it requires real expertise; he accuses psychiatrists at times of pretending to have expert knowledge when in fact they do not.[4] It is quite clear that the danger of abusing this power is so great that it requires constant vigilance lest we cause harm.[5] Because our society is increasingly concerned about human rights, the law is more involved with mental health abuses. Psychiatrists need to become more knowledgeable about legal theories and concepts. Most psychiatric testimony is presented to courts not by individuals who consider themselves specialists in forensic psychiatry but by general psychiatrists who are called upon from time to time for this purpose. Therefore it is becoming urgent that guidelines about ethical issues should be established.

Many ideas expressed in this chapter are my own judgements about ethics, and they may not suit others. They have been influenced by my teachers and colleagues, particularly Drs Robert Sadoff and Irwin Perr, who have worked with me in studying the need for the development of forensic psychiatry guidelines at the request of the American Academy of Psychiatry and the Law. I hope that this chapter will contribute to a discussion on the ethics of forensic psychiatry. Because of my lack of experience of the British and other legal systems, my discussion will focus mainly on the American scene but I hope that the points made and the issues discussed will be of enough general significance to merit the attention of psychiatrists everywhere.

One question requiring attention is who should establish ethical guidelines for any professional group? Should it be done in an evolutionary manner, by fiat, or by majority vote? Perhaps only general guidelines are required which would allow each person to evolve his own ethics, to be judged by his peers when challenged (see Chapter 3) Or, after such guidelines were formulated, those more knowledgeable about ethical principles might develop operational ethical standards. The latter could then be used by peer review and ethics committees in their deliberations concerning specific forensic problems. Many psychiatrists give little consideration to ethical principles when testifying despite the fact that they are sensitive to problems of confidentiality in their relationship with patients. Nevertheless, it is clear that, with increasing involvement in forensic matters, their behaviour in specific situations may be challenged on ethical grounds and they may be brought to account.

Do we qualify as experts?

Before examining specific areas, we should discuss the issue of how expert are our opinions. What gives us the right to testify in so many forensic areas? Are we capable of informing the court about the degree of our expertise and the true level of our knowledge, or are we sometimes not honest about this so that the court is not cognizant of what we do, and do not know? Judge Bazelon has stated with reference to the criminal justice system. 'it is essential that the decision-maker not have the issues of state power and individual liberty obscured by testimony which over-reaches the bounds of the witness's legitimate expertise ... it is essential not only that the decision-maker confront what relevant information is known but that it also be aware of what is unknown. ... Lastly, in evaluating the psychiatric and other information provided, the decision-maker must be able to see clearly the extent to which such information may be coloured by individual and institutional bias.'[6]

Similarly, in a recent article on ethics in mental health care Roth states: 'Expert testimony by mental health professionals may fail to distinguish fact from opinion, e.g. abuse of psychiatric testimony concerning the prediction of violence and application of the death penalty; problems of conclusory testimony and double agentry in the handling of sex offenders.'[7]

Psychiatrists have, on occasion, claimed expertise when their training and experience were minimal. While rules of evidence are so constructed that witnesses must be qualified as experts in court before they can render opinions, some who may be inadequately qualified are still accepted as experts. Standards for determining the qualifications of an expert witness differ in medicine and in law. Of course, if a doctor consciously misrepresents his training or experience, it is a serious matter, not only unethical but fraudulent.

Psychiatric expertise has also been criticized by Ziskin, a psychologist, who argues: 'that psychiatric evidence for almost all purposes and almost all issues is worthless and does not meet the stated requirements of the law on expert testimony'.[8,9] Other critics — Ennis and Litwach among them — have also raised questions about whether psychiatric testimony meets the standards of expert testimony[10] which alone should determine if it is ethical for psychiatrists to testify in the courtroom. These positions opposing psychiatric testimony have not been generally accepted, and psychiatrists continue to be called upon to assist the court. Judge Bazelon calls on psychiatrists not to desert the courtroom[4] and feels that whatever scientific evidence they can offer is helpful. His only plea is that we clarify what we know scientifically and distinguish this knowledge from what may be personal bias.

The issue, in my view, is not whether we should testify, but how we should testify; how honest we are in the adversarial process and how clearly we mark out our legitimate area of expertise in Bazelon's terms. If we cannot do this in an adversarial system, we do not belong in the courtroom. If, however, within the constraints of that system, we can present evidence which fits the requirements of expert opinion, we belong there.

I believe that we can testify honestly and effectively. Although lawyers find it disturbing, it does not bother me that studies indicate our ability to make accurate diagnoses is limited. It is our job to make clear to the judge or jury that our expertise encompasses a more complete understanding of a person and that this goes beyond mere diagnosis. We must make this clear, even to the point of insistence on direct examination, and, certainly, on cross-examination. Since we cannot control the questions we are asked on cross-examination, some of our opinions will not be challenged to the extent that they should be in an adversarial system; the judge or jury will therefore not have a true picture of the limitation of our knowledge. What should we do if the cross-examining lawyer does not do a good job? Is it our responsibility to clarify? Most would say that we are acting ethically as long as our replies do not imply knowledge that we do in fact lack, and as long as we do not purposely try to confuse the issue. If we answer honestly, our doubts or the limits of our knowledge should be evident.

Menninger, Halleck, and Halpern all believe that psychiatrists do not have the expertise specifically to evaluate competency or responsibility.[11,12,13] They argue that participation in this part of the criminal justice protocol represents an unethical role for psychiatrists; furthermore it is embarrassing and degrading to participate in it. Why should we be embarrassed by differing opinions? Orthopaedic surgeons and other specialists disagree in their testimony in personal injury and malpractice cases. Perhaps the greater publicity given to 'insanity' cases means greater exposure to scrutiny? Are we embarrassed to let the public know that the state of our art is such that we do not know everything and that there are different schools and theories in psychiatry?

Even if our opinions amount to no more than an educated guess, the law needs whatever expertise we can furnish. Although some may object to the educated guess concept, we have no insanity tests of our own, only those of the law. Like any other experts called on by the law for assistance, we can refer to a body of knowledge. However, as Bazelon again emphasizes, it is imperative that psychiatrists go only as far as that knowledge will allow: 'The danger . . . is that psychiatric participation in these decisional processes may slide by imperceptible degrees into psychiatric assumption of responsibility for the ultimate decisions themselves.' Rather than confining themselves to those aspects of the problem for which they have expertise, psychiatrists may be seduced into taking responsibility for making judgements or assessing facts about which they have no special competence. As a result, not only does psychiatry become over-extended, but society is deluded into believing that scientific, 'medical' answers exist to a problem and that social, moral, and other determinants of the problem may therefore be ignored.[14]

If our opinions are educated guesses, we face an ethical problem similar to that discussed previously with regard to our responsibility to make clear the limits of our diagnostic ability. Who is responsible for making this clear, the psychiatrist, or the lawyer who cross-examines us? If we function solely as a consultant to those who employ us, what is our ethical duty? If the opposing lawyer does a poor job of ferreting out the weaknesses of our opinions via cross examination, should we do his job for him? I am unable to offer an opinion about this very complex inter-professional problem, but later I do take a stand with reference to testimony in custody cases.

Unfortunately, psychiatrists sometimes transgress the limits of psychiatric knowledge. I have heard such statements in staff conferences as 'I don't like that guy, therefore he is responsible'. Or, 'that blankety-blank committed such a horrible offence, he's got to be responsible. I don't care how crazy he is'. Obviously, conclusions based on such personal bias represent no scientific opinion whatsoever. A psychiatrist is understandably not insulated against having strong personal feelings; however, if such feelings exist, can they justify an opinion supposedly 'scientific'? Is it not unethical to participate in a case when these feelings are generated? Should not a psychiatrist in this situation disqualify himself?

Opinions without examination

What should a psychiatrist do when he is asked to render an opinion about an individual he has not examined, as when a will or life insurance policy is challenged. The patient is dead; only those who knew him remain. The information they offer may enable the psychiatrist to form an opinion as to the deceased's mental state when he wrote his will. In some situations, such as following suicide, psychological autopsy may help clarify the preceding mental state. Sometimes the psychiatrist may not be permitted by law (or legal manoeuvre) to examine a living person but must instead render an opinion from data based on other sources. Generally, a physician does not give his opinion unless he has examined the patient. In other branches of medicine it is easier to interpret such hard data as X-rays and laboratory reports for diagnostic purposes; the interpretation of previous psychiatric hospital records and tests is much more difficult. It has been suggested that a diagnosis should result only from a personal examination and that we should apply the term 'clinical impression' when we offer an opinion in other circumstances. I think this is a useful differentiation but the question remains; if a diagnosis without object examination is not ethical, can a 'clinical impression' be so?

A case in point occurred in the Whitaker Chambers – Alger Hiss case. Carl Binger, a renowned psychiatrist, undertook to observe Chambers in the courtroom in order to give an opinion on his competence as a witness.[15] Dr Binger's testimony that Chambers was a psychopath did not stand up well under cross-examination. While his diagnosis may have been correct, he stated that in reaching his conclusion he had counted the number of times Chambers had looked at the ceiling. Unfortunately for Binger, the prosecuting lawyer also made a count of the doctor's glances at the ceiling while on the witness stand. Dr Binger's testimony thus was discredited. Those familiar with the case have told me that Binger's opinions were based on other observations, but that his anxiety led him to present himself in a foolish light. Was his behaviour unethical? Was he wrong to try to arrive at a diagnosis under difficult circumstances? Would it have been better for him to have stated a clinical impression rather than a specific diagnosis? Perhaps Dr Binger's politics interfered with his expert judgement.

In regard generally to the ethics of psychiatrists rendering opinions about public figures whom they have not examined, one of the American Psychiatric Association's ethical standards states: 'On occasion psychiatrists are asked for an opinion about an individual who is in the light of public attention, or who has disclosed information about himself through public media. It is unethical for a psychiatrist to offer a professional opinion unless he/she has conducted an examination and has been granted proper authorization for such a statement.'[16]

I do not believe that this dictum interdicts the rendering of clinical impressions (not a diagnosis) without examination when requested by the courts. However when speaking to the press caution certainly is advisable. When involved in a notorious forensic case, it is tempting to seek self-aggrandizement and publicity by openly discussing the case. In some cases, however, the public has a genuine need for information and understanding which may reduce anxiety in the face of stories about horrible and frightening crimes. The ethical line here is a narrow one.

A related ethical issue involves a psychiatrist's statements about a dead patient. In a recent paper Robert Moore has stated: 'When we speak of the dead . . . our ethical principles are less clear. Privilege disappears with death so that the psychiatrist is not compelled legally to maintain confidences after the death of his patient or examinee. However, what is ethical may be beyond what is legal . . . lacking absolute guidelines, the psychiatrist should ask himelf some questions before he makes public statements about deceased patients or examinees: Who will be harmed? Who will benefit? Are the benefits to society and my profession great enough value to justify the balance of the two questions above? Why do I really want to do this?'[17]

While Moore is referring to dead patients and incidentally to the problem of the psychohistorian, similar considerations apply to a notorious criminal defendant.

It is ethical to render an opinion (clinical impression and prognosis) based on a review of records, reports, and letters, under certain conditions, but *such opinions should never be rendered if it is at all possible to examine a person directly.* As thorough as records might be, personal examination is far better. Secondly, in those situations where a personal examination is not possible, it must be made completely clear that the opinions expressed are based only on a review of records and other information. When submitting a report in such circumstances, I use a 'rule of three': I mention at the outset that the person was not interviewed, I repeat this when I provide the diagnosis (or clinical impression), and again in the summary and recommendations. Although possibly excessive, this caution is necessary to avoid misunderstanding. Is it the responsibility of the psychiatrist to see that the judge or jury understands these limitations when he testifies, or can he let the responsibility rest with the cross-examiner? It would be unusual for the witness to state spontaneously that the patient was not examined unless asked by the lawyer. Goldzband's[18] policy is to inform the lawyer who requested his evaluation that he must reveal this fact on direct examination. I agree with this position because this particular circumstance is so fraught with the possibility of misunderstanding that it may be the one clear exception to the usual procedure of offering no information unless asked. I believe it is the witness's responsibility to bring it out on direct examination in order to avoid the possible impression of hiding something so important. Complaints have been made to ethics committees against psychiatrists who gave diagnostic and forensic opinions without examination. Because miscarriages of justice can so easily occur, it should be the psychiatrist's primary responsibility to inform the court that he did not examine the individual concerned.

Confidentiality

Perhaps the most important problem in forensic psychiatry as in psychiatry generally, is the issue of confidentiality. It appears evident that in court cases, information obtained from a patient by a physician could be used against the patient's 'best interests'. A number of troubling questions immediately arise. What are the best interests of a murderer? Has the psychiatrist obtained information without the former's full understanding that it might be used to his detriment? Has the interviewee given truly informed consent? Is informed consent possible under the circumstances and is it our responsibility or that of the patient's lawyer? Will the psychiatrist be able to obtain information he needs and still have a fully informed and consenting patient? Is the examinee a 'patient' or an 'individual being examined' when we interview him for his lawyer or the court?

A serious potential for abuse of the relationship between doctor and patient exists whenever a forensic interview is conducted. It is imperative that the patient be informed clearly whose servant the interviewer is. The latter should advise the examinee: 'I represent the prosecutor, the court, or your lawyer (whichever is appropriate); I am here to examine you in order to determine your competency to stand trial; if I report that you are so mentally ill that you cannot stand trial, you will go to a hospital; I may need to report to the court, anything that you tell me; if there is something you don't want me to report, call this to my attention, and I will then have to use my judgement.' This makes the forensic interview totally different from the usual therapeutic relationship where confidentiality is the rule. Although we may try to help the patient to deal with the law, our help is different from that we give in our more usual role. Therefore, it is imperative that the interviewer knows just what are the limits of confidentiality and these must be conveyed to the individual examined.

In some situations however and contrary to what I stated above, it is possible to guarantee the patient full confidentiality (under the lawyer's 'work product rule'). This varies in different jurisdictions and should be promised only under the assurance of the patient's lawyer. Such exceptions, however, do not invalidate the usual rule — that to pretend that the usual doctor–patient role is in effect during a forensic examination, is patently dishonest and unethical.

How can we obtain the information needed to form a well-grounded opinion, yet at the same time protect the individual from revealing information which might be used against him? The late Dr Hoffman[19] offered several solutions, none of them perfect. The examinee's lawyer could be present, but this might interfere with an effective evaluation. The examinee might be warned that he should refuse to discuss the crime. It is exceedingly difficult however to help someone to develop an insanity plea unless his mental processes during the time of the crime are known. The problem remains — how can we obtain information we need in order to help a person without invading his privacy and risking him harm?

Goldzband raises the key question of whose agent we are in forensic practice.[18] If we are not the patient's agent, but a consultant for someone else (defence or prosecuting lawyer or the court), once we have given a warning it is not our responsibility to protect the communications. I cannot offer a clear-cut ethical position about this difficult question; however, I can say that everyone who hears our testimony should know the position we are taking so that it can be evaluated adequately. To expect that we will be allowed to select only what we want to present in forming our conclusions flies in the face of the law's absolute need to know upon what we have based those conclusions.

Special problems may arise when the psychiatrist is engaged by the prosecutor. Has the psychiatrist's 'medical presence' seduced a defendant to confess or reveal evidence previously unknown to the prosecutor? What is the proper use of such information? Is it unethical to tell the prosecutor? What if the patient was not adequately warned? Should the doctor testify about information he obtained in this fashion? In a recent instance, a forensic psychiatrist examined an offender in the belief that under the law his notes were totally confidential and privileged. Upon reading the report, the prosecutor subpoenaed his voluminous notes. The psychiatrist resisted the subpoena but was advised that his interpretation of privileged communications law might be incorrect, and that the notes might have to be submitted. He went to court to fight. The judge insisted on his statutory right to review the notes and, after doing so, decided that the material was too inflammatory and that the prosecutor did not have the right to it. If this doctor had misinterpreted the law, it is possible that his notes could have been turned over to the prosecutor. Most important here is that the examinee had divulged information in the belief that it would be held in complete confidence, but this was something the doctor could not guarantee. (In many American states the notes would be subpoenable.) Was the doctor unethical, implying a guarantee when not absolutely sure? It is imperative that we act most cautiously, even if the result is a less thorough evaluation. If this becomes a problem, the examinee's lawyer is the one to determine the best course.

Our professional cloak sometimes produces confessional material the prosecution might not otherwise obtain. A basic argument of critics who believe that we should not participate in the pre-trial matters is based on problems of confidentiality and the advantage of the 'doctor's cloak'. This begs the question as similar problems arise in pre-sentence work, which is approved of by these same critics. Perhaps the best we can do is to recognize the potential for a serious erosion of the ethics of confidentiality and always inform the patient adequately.

The pre-arraignment evaluation

The ethics of the pre-arraignment psychiatric examination are a matter for concern. A particular instance recently caused a furore in Southern California when it was discovered that a district attorney routinely arranged for a psychiatrist to interview suspected offenders as part of the interrogation procedure, prior to arraignment.[20] Many believed that this violated the rights of the alleged offenders and constituted unethical psychiatric practice.

Was the prosecutor using the psychiatrist's humanitarian role in order to obtain information for prosecutory purposes, or to use at trial to counter an insanity plea? Was the psychiatrist relying on the police (or prosecutor) to inform the defendant that he had a right not to speak to the doctor? Was the defendant competently and knowingly waiving that right?

The issue was considered by various committees of the American Psychiatric Association, each group rendering a different opinion.

When the problem was considered by a task force of the San Diego Psychiatric Society, it was decided that the ethical behaviour in such a situation was to insure that stringent informed consent be obtained in all forensic psychiatric interviews. When the Committee on Law and Psychiatry of the American Psychiatric Association was apprised of the stance that the San Diego group had taken, it responded not with acknowledgement of a needed advance, as anticipated, but with marked disapproval and noted, . . . '(any) examination and evaluation for prosecutory purposes of a suspect before arraignment and before counsel has been obtained raises serious issues as to constitutional rights and privileges against self-incrimination and the ethics and professional roles of the psychiatrist . . . From the standpoint of the privilege against self-incrimination, as a practical matter the suspect may be in more urgent need of counsel before participating in a psychiatric examination and evaluation. From the standpoint of the ethics and his professional role, the psychiatrist, by participation in such an examination and evaluation, engages in a potential conflict of interest situation which clearly should be avoided'[21]

Finally, the Association adopted the policy that psychiatric evaluation of a suspect offender requires approval of the suspect's lawyer.

Section 9 of the American Medical Association Principles of Medical Ethics with Annotations Especially Applicable to Psychiatry reads: 'Ethical considerations in medical practice preclude the psychiatric evaluation of any adult charged with criminal acts prior to access to, or availability of, legal counsel. The only exception is the rendering of care to the person for the sole purpose of medical treatment.'[16]

Why is this such a problem? A person is arrested, read his rights, and is interrogated. In walks the friendly psychiatrist (sent by the prosecutor). He introduces himself as a doctor and sits down to talk to the person in order to discover his mental state now and at the time of the crime. The individual having been interrogated (an experience which probably would make most people anxious) may wish to share his innermost feelings with the psychiatrist; it may be to his benefit to reveal what is going on in his mind now and what was going on in his mind at the time of the crime. Such information may be most useful in a defence of not guilty by reason of insanity. On the other hand, the information could be damaging. Another option for the psychiatrist is to examine the suspect, only after his arraignment and on request of his lawyer. While arraignment occurs promptly, defence counsel's request for an examination may be delayed weeks, possibly months, allowing the development of secondary defences, and elaboration of thoughts and feelings, which may obscure the original condition.

Might not a psychiatric interview be better done at the outset? The answer to this question may depend on the conditions under which the prosecutor's psychiatrist operates. Does he always relay to the defence lawyer everything the individual has told him? Is his orientation prosecutory, defence, or non-adversarial? Does the defence lawyer always know that such an evaluation was conducted? Does the evaluation protect society in any way? By delay, the defendant could be coached to fabricate a psychosis. On the other hand, he might recover completely from an acute psychosis and have genuine amnesia for the episode, thus seriously impairing his ability to convince the court of his insanity at the time of the crime. Had he been examined earlier, the psychiatrist could have reported on his condition at the time of arrest. This is a complicated issue. While pre-arraignment examination before the defendant has obtained a lawyer, may benefit the defendant, and also the public by assisting the prosecution, its potential for abuse is so great that it cannot be condoned. Instead, we should encourage the defence lawyer to request an evaluation as soon after arrest as possible. Under no circumstances should the examination be done without his knowledge. Of course, this position does not preclude any necessary *treatment* prior to appointment of counsel.

The insanity plea

Involvement in the insanity plea is considered the hallmark of forensic psychiatry. Psychiatry receives most exposure through media coverage of sensational trials. Whenever a horrible crime is committed, the insanity plea is considered by the defence. Of those examined to determine criminal responsibility, almost 90 per cent are considered responsible. Of the remaining 10 per cent, probably less than two per cent are found 'not guilty by reason of insanity'[22] Nevertheless, our participation at this stage of the criminal justice process serves an important role.[23, 24]

The ethical issue of concern with regard to psychiatric participation in the insanity plea is how to formulate the opinions which determine our evaluation. Should we testify precisely as we see it, or within the bounds of medical propriety are we permitted to do our best for the side that employs us? My own approach is to do my best for the side which employs me, while still meeting honest medical standards. The ideas I present may be weak and I am willing to admit this under cross-examination.

When evaluating the defendant for the court (supposedly as an unbiased expert), I readily admit that in the case of doubt, I am inclined to find him not responsible. Similarly, I am inclined to rule out malingering since I believe that very few people actually attempt this manoeuvre, and I suspect too many are accused of it. Another troublesome question in evaluating defendants is whether the sole determinant of responsibility is the presence or absence of psychosis. In my view, such a diagnosis alone is inadequate to determine the question of responsibility; the defendant's thought processes and their relationship to the crime must be also considered.

Testifying

A prominent American forensic psychiatrist, Bernard Diamond,[25] refuses to testify if his testimony will harm an individual he has examined; therefore he is never called upon by the prosecution, a situation which he gladly accepts. When he testifies for the defence, his attitude is brought to the jury's attention, as it should be. Is it proper for a psychiatrist to participate in a procedure where he might cause harm? An important dictum in medicine in *Primum non nocere* — 'First do no harm'. A psychiatrist who testifies that a defendant is dangerous, cannot be helped by treatment and will always be a danger to society, is, by such testimony, encouraging the jury to request the most severe sentence, even the death penalty (if this is applicable) and certainly he is doing harm to the defendant. If the latter is not considered mentally ill, and if the psychiatrist is consultant to a lawyer or to the court, and not a physician helping a patient, then the dictum does not apply. A psychiatrist may testify for the prosecution that a defendant is responsible for his behaviour, and with the jury's agreement, he may be sentenced. In a sense, this is doing an individual harm (it is a matter of opinion whether incarceration can be beneficial). Is this a role for the psychiatrist? What about his responsibility to the community? Should society not also receive his help? After all, we do not make a decision but only render a scientific opinion. The decision is that of the court. We only present our understanding of an individual and his behaviour for the court's consideration. It could be argued that good citizens — judges and jurors — should have expert assistance in reaching their decision. Judge Bazelon believes the psychiatrist should stay in the courtroom: 'Total retreat, to my mind, is neither a desirable nor a viable option. Psychiatry today, more than ever before, offers critical insights for our understanding of the mind and human behaviour . . . Unquestionably, inclusion of the psychiatric perspective often enhances the sophistication with which such public and private decisions may be reached.'[4] If we have a role, then we must render the best opinion that we can, recognizing that the opinion may be used in a way that the defendant does not regard as beneficial to him.

How strongly should we press our opinion when testifying? Should we conceal our limitations or take the opportunity to inform the court about them? A wishy-washy witness is not useful but one who is so self-assured that he admits to no possibility of bias, error, or limitation is not credible. A witness who attempts honestly to present his opinion without either exaggeration or self-depreciation is likely to be the most effective.

Pre-trial

Once we have made the decision to testify, other problems arise. In order to present convincing scientific evidence it is necessary to discuss in detail the past history, current reactions, and some psychodynamic understanding of what was going on in the defendant at the time of the crime. Is it proper for him to hear the testimony about the examination? If he were a person evaluated for treatment, one might not discuss these matters with him, but the law states appropriately that the defendant has a right to hear the testimony of all witnesses; he must be able to instruct his lawyer about the accuracy of the information presented. Is it unethical for us to participate under such conditions? We present a formulation which we believe correct but which the defendant may totally reject or find frightening, confusing, or disorganizing to himself or to his family. I do not believe that such testimony is unethical. In a situation where the law must prevail, the defendant has to choose. Does he want psychiatric testimony or not? If he does, then he risks hearing unpleasant things. Experience indicates that most defendants can deal with such testimony.

How far should the psychiatrist go in order to help a defendant? As stated earlier, the role of the forensic psychiatrist, when he is retained by one side, is to do his best to assist that side by meeting the highest ethical and medical standards. Both defendant and lawyer will try to influence the psychiatrist's judgement in the former's favour. In his effort to conform to their needs, can his testimony be biased but still remain within ethical bounds? Is he going too far when he suggests a rare or unusual theory as the basis for a forensic opinion? Sometimes testimony supporting an absence of criminal responsibility sounds incredible. In a recent case[26] in Florida for example, a 14 year old re-enacted a scene he had seen on television via a 'shoot out' with a .22 pistol and killed his 11 year old brother; a psychiatrist witness claimed that the young murderer was not responsible because he had been somehow mesmerized by the television show. The same questions apply to the testimony of a psychiatrist that the behaviour of Lt. Calley, of Vietnam illfame, had been affected by inhaling marijuana fumes in his barracks.[27] Are psychiatrists for the defence in such cases exceeding ethical limits in their efforts to develop an insanity plea? Certainly it is not improper to suggest a novel idea or theory but only if it meets high medical standards and can be tested?

Pre-sentence

When undergoing a pre-sentence psychiatric examination, the defendant may admit guilt for crimes for which he has never been charged. Can this information be used by the prosecution as the basis for new charges? Probably not; however, the prosecutor could start a new investigation. Is it ethical to include such information in his report considering the influence it might have on the judge? What about the psychiatrist's responsibility to the judge and the community? What about the expert's professional integrity if he 'covers up'? Did the patient fully understand the relationship and know what use would be made of the information he divulged? I cannot offer specific answers to these thorny questions; solutions depend on the many variables peculiar to each case. Perhaps, with apologies to Shakespeare, 'To thine own self (and thy profession) be true' is the best we can do until clearer guidelines are established.

Are we acting unethically when our pre-sentence recommendations are not based on firm data? Our ability to predict future behaviour and the effectiveness of treatment may be based on very limited knowledge. It is important to convey the reasons for our opinions and to eliminate personal bias. We also have responsibility to be well-acquainted with the professional literature. As an example, before new data about exhibitionists became available, it was thought that they tended to become rapists; now there is evidence to the contrary.[28]

Probably the greatest danger that personal bias and an exaggerated response to human behaviour will motivate our judgements occurs in the examination of sex offenders accused of actions totally unacceptable to our moral standards. Such 'counter-transference' reactions can arise especially in the case of offences in which adults take sexual advantage of children. Compounding these attitude-induced problems is the tendency for psychiatrist to recommend individual psychotherapy for certain compulsive sex offenders when it is known that they rarely continue with treatment once the legal issue is settled. The law justifiably looks upon our acceptance of the patient's good intentions as at least naive and possibly even as an improper attempt to obtain referrals for therapy.

Death penalty

After conviction for a capital crime, some jurisdictions require an immediate hearing before the same jury to determine whether the sentence should be life imprisonment or death. In Texas, for example, the psychiatrist is asked about the defendant's propensity to commit violent crimes and also about his treatability. The case of Dr James

Grigson is particularly illuminating in this regard. Note his testimony: 'It's my opinion that really Mr. Smith does not have any regard for another human being's property or for his life, regardless of who it may be'. He stated further, 'we don't have anything in medicine or psychiatry that in any way at all modifies or changes their behaviour'[29] The defendant had only one previous conviction — for possession of a small quantity of marijuana. The psychiatrist's testimony was based on an examination of Smith for competency at the judge's request prior to his murder trial. Smith had co-operated but was not told that the assessment was for any reason other than to determine competency; his lawyers were not aware of the examination. After conviction the case was appealed and the appellate court ruled, 'A defendant may not be compelled to speak to a psychiatrist who can use his statements against him at the sentencing phase of a capital trial'[30]. If prosecution desired such an examination, the court added, the defendant should be warned about the use of the findings and have the 'guiding hand of counsel'.

Could Dr Grigson's opinion be considered a breach of ethical principles? He rendered an opinion on data obtained under the guise of another purpose, without informing the patient and his opinion had little or no scientific validity. In any event, the case should serve as a warning how easily one can become involved in questionable activities. In forensic work, it is imperative always to bear in mind the circumstances under which information is obtained. Death penalty testimony also raises, in bold relief, the previously discussed issue of 'doing harm'.

Ethical issues in civil law

Ethical issues arise not only in connection with psychiatrists' participation in criminal cases. Many situations in civil litigation need careful scrutiny for the presence of ethical problems. The one which has caused me most concern involves custody evaluations. Often the psychiatrist is only able to examine one party to the custody suit. Perhaps he is called upon to examine the child's mother who, in fact, may be his patient. He is asked to report on whether she is psychologically sound enough to have or retain custody of her children. Her lawyer, of course, would like the psychiatrist to include a negative opinion about the competing spouse, whom the doctor has not examined or perhaps has seen only briefly in connection with the wife's therapy. Any definite reference by the psychiatrist to the husband's capacity as a father is unethical. It is proper to indicate that, on the basis of experience with the mother, he finds nothing about her which would cause questions about her competence as a mother, but he certainly does not offer an opinion on the father based on statements made by his wife. Her statements are very likely to be self-serving.

Suppose the father displayed sick or inappropriate behaviour during the limited therapeutic contacts described above. Should the psychiatrist mention these and indicate that such behaviour indicates that this man is not an adequate father? If he does this it is his responsibility to make clear that his impressions do not constitute a complete and thorough examination. Statements contained in psychiatric reports may be given exaggerated significance by advocates in an adversarial procedure; opinions should therefore be based only on solid data. Judges have told me about their experience of reports and testimony based on no direct examination or only on a 'passing glance'. They believe such opinions should be considered unethical. Goldzband discusses this issue in greater detail in his recent book *Custody cases and expert witnesses*.[31]

Personal injury

Personal injury or tort cases can lead to ethical problems particularly because money is involved. What should be included in a psychiatric report after examining an allegedly injured individual? What should the psychiatrist do when the patient, claiming that his back was hurt during a fall in a restaurant, relates that he also injured his back two years prior to the restaurant fall while painting at home? If such a statement is included, the patient's lawyer may ask to have it deleted. Is it unethical to do so? If the patient has understood the purpose of the examination, then all his disclosures must be reported. Although the psychiatrist functions in an adversarial role, that does not mean condoning dishonesty. His role is to assist the lawyer as best he can, but only within the requirements of medical ethics. Keeping such information secret, in my opinion, represents collusion. It is therefore unethical, and probably illegal. Irrelevant personal data can be eliminated; however even here careful judgement is required.

A similar problem arises when the patient lies and does not furnish pertinent information in the examination. On the witness stand the psychiatrist may then be presented with the missing facts, e.g. 'Doctor did you know that Mr Jones also injured his back two years prior to the current accident when he fell off a ladder while painting his house?' Indicating unawareness of such an occurrence, the expert witness would be shown proof that it occurred, and then would be asked, 'Doctor, would knowledge of this change your opinion as to the causal relationship of the recent accident to his back problems? ' The answer would then have to be 'Yes, it certainly might'.

Another problem is the possibility that pejorative or 'undesirable' information in a report might be used to coerce a patient into settling a case. One example is a statement that the patient previously was treated for syphilis contracted while on an excursion to the red light district, a matter totally unrelated to the issue at hand. The patient may have willingly spoken of this, despite his knowledge of what it could be used for, because he wanted the psychiatrist to have a full understanding of his medical history. Or it might have been obtained from other medical records. The patient may have asked the examiner not to mention the information. Perhaps he holds an important public position and would not want such information to become public, especially in the courtroom. If it were included in the report he might be forced to settle the case to keep it from being revealed. The psychiatrist has a responsibility even in the forensic setting to protect the patient when ethically permissable. I suspect that at times we do this by unconscious selection of what we recall. Again, this is an issue that must be decided on a case-by-base basis as illustrated by the examples I have given here : not to include the patient's statement that he had previously fallen off a ladder would represent omission of a significant fact; omission of the information about previous syphilis would not.

In the United States, unlike Britain, lawyers operate on a contingency basis in personal injury cases. Since the lawyer is usually responsible for the charges of the psychiatric examination and report, he might prefer that the examining psychiatrist accept such an arrangement. However, participation in any contingency fee arrangement is prohibited by ethical tenets of both the American Medical and Psychiatric Associations. It should be made clear at the outset therefore that the lawyer is responsible for the psychiatrist's fee upon receipt of the report. Some psychiatrists are willing to agree to hold the litigant responsible for charges, but this could be a veiled type of contingency.

Is it proper for the psychiatrists employed by opposing sides in litigation to confer with each other? Most lawyers oppose 'collaboration' or discussion unless prior arrangements have been made. Although informal discussion between colleagues is a standard procedure in medicine, it is not in law. Here the psychiatrist's duty is to the lawyer and he should abide by his wishes. Legal practice is totally different from medical practice. Law is both adversarial and proprietary and opinions are guarded whereas the essence of medicine is its openness and its free communication among colleagues.

A psychiatrist may occasionaly find himself briefly involved in consultation with a lawyer and discover that he cannot be of help. If later he is called upon by the other side to participate in the case, it would be improper for him to do so unless the first lawyer releases him, a highly unlikely prospect.

Forensic hospital practice

Many ethical questions arise in forensic hospital practice. While non-criminal patients may be confined involuntarily in ordinary mental hospitals, patients treated in forensic psychiatric institutions are there on an even stronger involuntary basis. They are there by court order, either having been found not guilty by reason of insanity, being evaluated for this plea, or because they have been transferred from a less secure hospital.

The inadequate treatment offered in many forensic psychiatric hospitals is a pressing ethical issue for all psychiatrists (see Chapter 17). If a patient is to be exposed to adverse conditions beyond a certain limit should we refuse to co-operate in procedures which might result in his confinement in such sub-standard institutions? If we note these poor standards, should we not speak out? One of my colleagues no longer evaluates for competency and responsibility; he believes conditions in his state's forensic hospitals are so bad that he does not wish to contribute to a patient's hospitalization in them.[18]

Strong community or political pressure may be exerted on a forensic psychiatrist not to release a patient because of the community's unreasonable fear. In a study of the staff's decisions to release or not to release forensic patients, Thornberry and Jacoby[32] found evidence of 'political predictions'. They believed that the medical opinions were affected by socio-political considerations. Is it not unethical and a dereliction of responsibility to capitulate to such pressure when the psychiatrist has concluded that the patient is no longer dangerous? A hospital superintendent once confided to me that he had obtained a job and accommodation for one such patient and engineered an 'escape' for him. Several superintendents have obtained releases by arranging a hearing with a judge more receptive to professional opinion than another judge who said, 'I don't care how well he is, he is going to stay in the hospital as long as I hear the case'. Whether or not such efforts are justifiable or ethical, I cannot say. Medicine has an honourable tradition of not responding to social or political pressure in making judgements. The same tradition should apply in these forensic situations, unless we wish to follow the example of certain Soviet practices. (see Chapter 18).

The treatment of those who have been found not guilty by reason of insanity and who have been committed may cause problems if the hospital personnel disagree with the verdict. For example, the hospital psychiatrist may believe the patient was responsible for his behaviour and may have testified to that effect. How does this doctor now treat a patient for an illness that he does not believe exists? Does he merely 'warehouse' the patient because he views him as a malingerer, or does he attempt to treat him responsibly and with as open a mind as he can? It is obvious that any course but the latter would be unethical. A recent case in New York raised such an issue both for the hospital and the courts.[27] A policeman shot and killed a boy whom he thought was about to shoot him. No gun was found on the boy. The policeman was found not guilty by reason of insanity based on testimony by defence psychiatrists that he suffered from an epileptic disorder. The hospital staff, having found no such disorder, and in fact no evidence of mental illness, wanted to release him almost immediately. The court however insisted that the patient receive treatment or at least extensive observation.

The forensic psychiatrist in the prison

Difficult problems arise when psychiatrists work in prisons, particularly if they lack a clear contractual relationship with the institution and do not make their position clear to the patient (inmate). It might be tempting for such psychiatrists to align themselves with the administration and to ferret out possible riots, smuggling of contraband, or other illegal acts. Perverting the role of therapist in this manner is certainly improper. On the other hand, some psychiatrists tend to identify with the prisoner, align themselves not with, but against, the administration, and offer inmates a level of confidentiality which they cannot guarantee. In one such situation the warden, following a murder within his institution, attempted to obtain the psychiatrist's records so that he could get more information about the suspect. The psychiatrist believed incorrectly that he had a confidential relationship with the inmate and that the records were in his control. However, no psychiatrist employed in that institution had ever established such a contract with the warden, and the psychiatrist's records were turned over. Was the doctor irresponsible in not making a prior clarification of this issue and in believing that he could walk into a public institution and set his own ground rules? For instance, what should one do when an inmate in individual therapy reveals that he is currently involved in an escape plan? Is it ethical to report this to the prison authorities? The answer might depend on the psychiatrist's contract with the patient and with the administration. At the very least, it would be a difficult problem, particularly if the incipient escape or riot plan could cause injury to others.

Summary

Forensic psychiatry is not a field into which a psychiatrist should step without a good deal of forethought. It contains many ethical pitfalls.

The contract of the forensic psychiatrist is essentially not with the patient but with the latter's lawyer or the court. In fact, the 'patient' is not really a patient in the usual doctor–patient sense. This needs to be made clear to the examinee at the outset. Another house is being entered, not the house of medicine but that of law — with its different motives, goals, and rules of conduct. In medicine we communicate openly, in the law we may not. In medicine we listen to everything, and may discuss it with colleagues. In law, the attorney by whom we are employed may not want or allow us to do this. He may even wish us to omit information which he believes will harm his client; we may want to omit material which we feel is irrelevant. We may be tempted to say too much or too little, or in our zeal advance ideas and theories which have no foundation, or allow our personal bias to appear as professional opinion. These are all ethical problems and there are many more.

I have raised more questions than I have provided answers. Forensic psychiatry as a sub-specialty is in its infancy and is not always able to supply clear-cut ethical positions or guidelines. Hopefully experience and discussion will assist in the reduction of these difficult problems. I have undertaken to give my opinion when I have felt justified in doing so. Certainly the most important maxim for the psychiatrist is not to take advantage of the doctor–client relationship by encouraging the subject to talk without making it absolutely clear whom he represents and what use will be made of the information. The forensic psychiatrist has an opportunity to assist people in a way which is different from that of the therapist and to assist society through the law, but he is also in a position to do much harm. As George Moore once said: 'The difficulty in life is the choice.'

References

1. POLLACK, S.: Forensic psychiatry, a specialty. *American Academy of Psychiatry and the Law Bulletin* **II**: 1–6, 1974.
2. ROBITSCHER, J.: Isaac Ray lectures, 6 October George Washington University, Washington DC, 1977.
3. SZASZ, T.: *Psychiatric justice*. New York, Macmillan, 1975.
4. BAZELON, D.: The role of the psychiatrist in the criminal justice system. *American Academy of Psychiatry and the Law Bulletin* **VI**, 139–46, 1978.
5. ROBITSCHER, J.: *The powers of psychiatry*. Boston, Houghton Mifflin, 1980.
6. BAZELON, D.: The role of the psychiatrist in the criminal justice system. *American Academy of Psychiatry and the Law Bulletin* **VI**:145, 1978.
7. ROTH, L. N.: To respect persons, families and communities: some problems in ethics of mental health care. *Psychiatry Digest* **40**:17–26, 1979.
8. ZISKIN, J.: Speech before California District Attorney Association. *Psychiatric News* 5 May, 1978.
9. ZISKIN, J.: *Coping with psychiatric and psychological testimony*. Beverley Hills, Ca, Law and Psychology Press, 1970.

10. ENNIS, B. J. and LITWACH, T. R.: Psychiatry and the presumption of expertise: flipping coins in the courtroom. *California Law Review* **62**:693–752, 1974.
11. MENNINGER, K.: *Crime of punishment*. New York, Viking Press, 1966.
12. HALLECK, S. L.: *Psychiatry and the dilemmas of crime.*. Los Angeles, University of California, 1971.
13. HALPERN, A. L.: Use and abuse of psychiatry in competency examinations of criminal defendants. *Psychiatric Annals* **5**:4, 1975.
14. BAZELON, D.: The role of the psychiatrist in the criminal justice system. *American Academy of Psychiatry and the Law Bulletin* **VI**, 139, 1978.
15. BROOKS, A. D.: *Law, psychiatry, and the mental health system*. Boston, Little Brown, 1974, pp. 1011–16.
16. The principles of medical ethics with annotations especially applicable to psychiatry. *American journal of psychiatry* **130**:1057–64, 1973.
17. MOORE, R. A.: Rights for the dead. Guest editorial. *Psychiatric News* 21 March, 1980.
18. GOLDZBAND, M. G.: Personal communication, July 1980.
19. HOFFMAN, P. B.: Forensic evaluation of criminal cases: Confidential? Annual meeting of the American Psychiatric Association, May 1978, Atlanta.
20. GOLDZBAND, M. G.: Pre-arraignment psychiatric examinations and criminal responsibility — a personal Odyssey through the law and psychiatry west of the Pecos. *Journal of Psychiatry and Law* **4**:447–66, 1976.
21. GOLDZBAND, M. G.: Pre-arraignment psychiatric examinations and criminal responsibility — a personal Odyssey through the law and psychiatry west of the Pecos. *Journal of Psychiatry and Law* **4**:3, 456–7, 1976.
22. RAPPEPORT, J. R.: The psychiatrist as expert witness. *Medical World News* October 1976, pp. 18–25.
23. RAPPEPORT, J. R.: The role of the psychiatrist in the criminal justice system — the psychiatrist and criminal justice, in *Police investigation to prisoner rehabilitation*. Ed. Brady, J. P. and Brodie, H. K. Philadelphia, W. B. Saunders, 1978, pp. 918–32.
24. RAPPEPORT, J. R.: Forensic psychiatry, in *The psychiatric foundations of medicine*. Ed. Balis, G. U., Wurmser, L., McDabuek, E., and Grenell, R. G. Boston, Butterworth, 1978, pp. 301–24.
25. DIAMOND, BERNARD. Personal communication, July 1980.
26. *New York Times* 7 October 1977.
27. *American Medical News* 19 September 1977.
28. RADA, RICHARD T. (ed.): *Clinical aspects of the rapist*. New York, Grune and Stratton, 1978, p. 52.
29. SMITH V. ESTELLE 602 F 2d 694 at 697.
30. SMITH V. ESTELLE 602 F 2d 694 at 708.
31. GOLDZBAND, M. G.: *Custody cases and expert witnesses*. New York, Harcourt Brace Jovanovich, 1980.
32. THORNBERRY, T. P. and JACOBY, J. E.: *The criminally insane*. Chicago, University of Chicago Press, 1979.

15
Ethics and psychiatric research
John Wing

In the last chapter of his intellectual autobiography,[1] Karl Popper explains, paraphrasing Wolfgang Köhler, why few scientists care to write about values: 'The reason is simply that so much of the talk about values is hot air.' A value is involved every time a practical and immediate problem has to be solved or a decision made and there is no satisfactory substitute for rational consideration of the pros and cons of each issue. We evolve general ethical guidelines or principles (which differ, however, in different societies) in order to avoid having to think out the rights and wrongs of every possible alternative before taking everyday decisions, but they must always be open to challenge and to rational argument.

Many ethical theorists reject this commonsense approach to ethics. Comte, who created positivism, and Marx, who created dialectical materialism, are prime examples. They thought, though for quite different reasons, that they could forecast, far ahead of events, the way that human society would evolve. Once the predictions had been made, the task of the politician was to ensure a smooth transition towards the inevitable future. The criterion of morality, therefore, was whether an action was or was not likely to bring forward the golden age; the end justified the means.[2]

Plato, who was a historicist of rather a different kind, created a system of ethics that has been much admired, but he was able to propose the establishment of a correctional institution where those with atheistic views would be incarcerated for a period of five years in order to be given appropriate instruction. 'And when the time of their imprisonment has expired, if any of them be of sound mind let him be restored to sane company, but if not, and if he be condemned a second time, let him be punished with death.' The idea that the state should designate what is healthy and what is sick is part of what the author who has brought this platonic equation of insanity and dissent to our notice calls 'social psychiatry.'[3] Although this concept of social psychiatry is unrecognizable in Britain it is important for psychiatrists everywhere to understand the nature of the claims that are being made in its name; for example, that radical social reconstruction

I should like to thank Dr. F. Goodwin for his helpful comments on this chapter.

based on freeing the people from 'surplus repression' will solve the ills of western societies.[4] If such theories ever were seriously applied the outcome could not be guaranteed to be more democratic than in Plato's *Republic*. Another example of historicist morality applied to psychiatry is discussed in Chapter 18.

The authors in this volume are unlikely to espouse any of these ideologies. They will no doubt adopt a broadly liberal stance; regarding the rights of individuals (in this case, patients) as more important than the rights of agents who might be thought to be acting for the good of society and therefore, in the long run, for the good of the individuals who constitute society. Robert Neville has made an attempt to look at the recommendations of one such commission of enquiry[5] through the eyes of a modern equivalent of a seventeenth-century Puritan divine.[6] The exercise is not wholly convincing but the notion that each individual is flawed, and in order to achieve grace has to seek the common good rather than his own necessarily incomplete fulfilment, is indeed still latent in modern western societies. Such a sense of responsibility is shown by those who carry kidney donor cards and by those who regard it as their duty to take part in research projects if their reasonable scruples can be overcome. Perhaps this individual responsibility is insufficiently recognized in debates on the ethics of clinical and research practice.

This introduction may serve to remind the reader that the ethical aspects of research are no more controversial than the ethical aspects of any other subject. In particular, the ethics of clinical research depend almost completely on the ethics of clinical practice. Sir George Pickering once pointed out that every clinical decision involves an experiment. Certainly it ought to do so. Ethical problems are most likely to arise when treatment is based on theories which have been insufficiently tested in order to discover whether they have harmful consequences, or when the theories are virtually untestable because they are stated with insufficient clarity and detail. The scientific testing of diagnostic and therapeutic claims is therefore itself a moral imperative.

There is nowadays a fairly general acceptance of the view that new drugs should not be introduced without being tested. There is no similar consensus in respect of social treatments, most of which become firmly adopted before they have been thoroughly examined. The harm that may come from the application of misguided social theories, or the misapplication of sensible theories, is at least as great as any harm that can follow the prescription of a harmful drug or an unnecessary course of psychotherapy. In fact, it can be much greater, since harmful social practices can become institutionalized into the structure of a complete psychiatric service. The 'custodial era' in psychiatry, although it was not as black as it has sometimes been painted, nevertheless illustrates how the practices inherent in the concept of the 'total institution' can become generally and uncritically adopted, even though many of them were quite unnecessary and demonstrably harmful.

Medicine (or any other activity) would come to a full stop if every decision had to be monitored by an ethical committee. What then constitutes an experiment of sufficient substance to warrant such an opinion being obtained? Who is to judge when some item of practice ought to be referred to a committee? When does clinical practice become 'research'?

Before attempting to answer these questions, I will consider three main practical problems that ethical committees are always concerned about; the balance of good and harm to which a patient may be exposed, what constitutes informed consent, and confidentiality.

The balance of good and harm

The principle of least harm

The central ethical principle in clinical practice is that a doctor must not knowingly act against the interests of his patient and must take all reasonable steps to ensure that he does not do so unwittingly. The doctor has to decide, first of all, whether his expertise can be applied to any of the problems brought to him by the patient. If one of these problems does seem to be explicable in terms of some medical theory or theories ('diagnosis'), he then has to weigh the consequences of advising the patient to accept further investigation or treatment based on the predictions of that theory. This means balancing the advantages and the disadvantages of giving the advice against those of not giving it, in the light of knowledge that is rarely complete and may be conflicting. This uncertainty is particularly great in psychiatry; first, because disease theories are not as well developed as in other branches of medicine and secondly, because many of the problems brought by patients arise out of difficulties in everyday life to which disease theories have almost no relevance at all. It is the doctor's duty to be as well informed as possible. Some of the most reasonable criticisms of psychiatric practice have arisen because psychiatric expertise has been applied to people who were not mentally ill or because treatments (physical, psychological, and social) have been applied without the psychiatrist's being aware that they could have harmful effects. This has often been due to the fact that the necessary research has not been undertaken. The more the relevant theories have been subjected to rigorous tests, the better-informed the doctor can be and the less likely is he to cause unwitting harm.

Apart from the ethical obligation on any doctor to be as well equipped as possible for clinical practice, no special ethical issue is raised by accidental or unforeseeable damage and, in any case, there is provision through the courts for deciding issues of negligence. There are, however, circumstances in which the possibility of doing damage may be accepted because of the likelihood of a greater good. The amputation of a gangrenous foot is a case in point; by losing a foot the patient may save the rest of a limb. The fact that phenothiazine medication helps to prevent acute relapses in schizophrenia, at least in the short term, is so important to the welfare of patient and relatives that some uncertainty as to whether there will be harmful side-effects in the longer term is accepted (see Chapter 7).

It is at the growing points of clinical practice, where the balance of good and harm is not yet clear, that the most difficult decisions have to be made, and the advice of disinterested colleagues may be most helpful. Even here, as in the case of the first heart transplants, and the introduction of new forms of medication for schizophrenia and the manic and depressive disorders, the decision had to be made by physician and patient together, each trusting the other's judgement after a consideration of the risks and possible benefits.

Harm from research projects

The vast majority of research projects do not involve any probability of serious harm coming to those involved. The 1978 United States National Commission investigating what measures were needed to protect mentally disabled subjects of biomedical and behavioural research was persuaded that there was no risk at all in one-third of projects, and a 'very low' risk of only minimal stress or embarrassment, or minor medical complications (a bruise after taking blood, for example), in nearly all the rest. Fewer than five per cent of projects involving the mentally disabled presented more risk than this[5] My own experience of an ethical committee confirms this.

Although studies entailing little or no risk to the patient do require a consideration of the balance of good against harm (a project that will almost certainly do nobody any harm but is equally likely to do nobody any good is not worth undertaking) they do not raise profound ethical problems.

The ethics of clinical trials

This still leaves a number of awkward situations in which the possible harm from a given procedure comes closer to outweighing the benefit expected from it. In such circumstances there would appear to be an ethical duty to carry out a clinical trial. But a clinical trial itself, if it is to yield the maximum information, demands that the effects of receiving the treatment should be compared with the consequences of receiving the procedure previously accepted as the best, and the latter may also entail risks as well as possible benefits. Helmchen and Müller-Oerlinghausen call this dilemma the paradox of the clinical trial: 'First, it is unethical to use treatment the efficacy of which has not been examined scientifically; second, it is also unethical to examine the efficacy of treatment scientifically.'[7] In fact, no paradox is involved, only a complication in drawing up the balance between good and harm. But it is a complication that must always be considered, not only in research projects but whenever clinical practice is innovative rather than routine. The question of what good (or prevention of harm) may come to *other* patients than the specific individual under consideration for treatment is not only of legitimate but of obligatory, though secondary, concern to the doctor. The value of considering the ethical aspects of projects with an avowedly research aim is that such issues become explicit.

The British Medical Research Council, in an influential paper, specified the principles that should guide medical research workers setting up trials of treatments or methods of prevention which require control groups.[8] The value of such designs is that they speed up the acquisition of knowledge concerning the advantages and disadvantages of new methods. The more representative the group of patients selected for the trial, and the more random the allocation of patients to experimental or control groups, the more useful will be the information gained.

The research worker is concerned to ensure that the trial is conducted in accordance with strict scientific principles and it must therefore be considered whether this motivation (excellent in itself) is compatible with the overriding necessity to assess the balance of good and harm and inform the patient accordingly. It is not suggested that research workers will knowingly give inaccurate information in order to persuade patients to enter a trial but the possibility of unconscious bias cannot be discounted. Undoubtedly the safest procedure is that the patient's own clinician should not be involved in the research and that he should undertake the discussion necessary to decide consent. If this is not possible, as may be the case in small University departments, there will always be a clinician available who can undertake this important responsibility and who can be given authority to advise the patient where the balance of good and harm lies.

The issues involved in deciding whether and how to obtain 'true consent' will be discussed below but they are nowhere clearer than when procedures are involved that are not of direct benefit to the individual asked to take part in the project. The possibility or probability that an investigation will be of benefit to humanity or posterity is no defence in the event of legal proceedings. Nor can an individual consent to be harmed: 'The individual has rights that the law protects and nobody can infringe those rights for the public good.'[8]

Informed consent

What is informed consent?

There will be no disagreement with the general rule that people chosen to participate in research projects should be told frankly what the risks and benefits are likely to be and what the purpose of the research is. There are, however, many difficulties in the way of achieving completely informed consent.

First it is impossible for the clinician to tell the patient (or client) everything that is in his mind. He must select. Secondly, the patient can only rarely be as well informed as the clinician. Even when, in exceptional cases, the patient is himself a doctor, has taken a second opinion, looked up the textbooks, consulted the original papers, obtained the best statistics as to cure rates and side effects and so on, he will usually still need advice as to the best course of action. Most patients, of course, do not wish to go to such length. They simply want advice. Thirdly, even if it were feasible to spend a very long time with each patient, attempting to inform him of all the ins and outs influencing some particular recommendation it would often be undesirable to do so on ethical grounds, since the patient might well receive the impression that the clinician was unwilling to take responsibility and therefore come to doubt the value of the advice. Finally there is the difficult question of gauging how far the patient can understand an explanation of why a particular treatment or course of action is recommended rather than all the various alternatives available to the clinician. In the last resort, the matter is one of whether the patient can trust the clinician or not.

Must consent always be obtained?

Occasionally, telling patients that they are to take part in a trial may actually be contra-indicated. 'For example, to awaken patients with a possibly fatal illness to the existence of such doubts about effective treatment may not always be in their best interest; or suspicion may have arisen as to whether a particular treatment has any effect apart from suggestion and it may be necessary to introduce a placebo into part of the trial to determine this.'[8] An important example of the latter situation arises when a treatment has become generally adopted because it is believed, on the basis of its proved efficacy in ameliorating an acute disorder, that it has preventive value, even though this has *not* been demonstrated. It is precisely in such situations that the dangers of adverse reactions developing after long periods of administration are most apparent.

This was the problem, for example, with long-term maintenance medication with the phenothiazines. Was it justifiable to inform a patient, after he had been taking the medication for a long time, that it was uncertain whether it was effective and uncertain whether it was dangerous? The result might very well be to destroy his trust in a form of preventive medication that might be both effective and safe. The ethical problem can only be resolved by the clinician, in the light of his scientific knowledge and his acquaintance with the individual patient. In a recent trial of fluphenazine decanoate, the psychiatrists concerned decided that it was ethically correct to include certain of their patients without obtaining their informed consent.[9] A colleague objected to this trial (and indeed to all trials) on 'ethical' grounds but he was assuming that his personal faith in the drug's efficacy and safety ought to have been shared by the clinicians who allowed their patients to take part in the trial. The fact that his faith was not so shared is not a matter for ethics at all but for rational argument about evidence.[10]

This particular trial did show a superior preventative effect of drug over placebo in the short term and, taken together with other scientific data about the interaction between social and pharmacological treatments, it allows a much better informed decision to be made by psychiatrists in future. It does not, however, answer the question as to whether dangerous side-effects might develop in the longer term and thus some ethical doubt remains, in clinical practice, about the duration of therapy.

Consent by people whose judgement is impaired or not free

Obtaining informed consent presents special difficulties in the case of minors, mentally disabled people, prisoners, and others whose freedom of choice might be limited. Strictly speaking, in Britain, 'parents and guardians of children cannot give consent on the childrens' behalf to any procedures which are of no particular benefit to them and which might carry some risk of harm;[8] and the children themselves are not regarded as capable of giving such consent. Parents or guardians can assume this responsibility if no risk of injury is involved.

In the case of the mentally disabled (including the severely mentally retarded, the acutely disturbed, and the demented) whose judgement may be impaired, there is a similar obligation on clinicians and research workers to avoid any procedure which is not of direct benefit if there is a risk of harm. If there is only a minor risk (equivalent to those ordinarily met in everyday life or during ordinary clinical examination), and the patient is unable to give true consent, a relative or guardian can undertake the responsibility instead.

This relatively relaxed attitude, with major reliance on the trustworthiness of the relationship between researchers and mentally disabled research subjects appears to be more characteristic in Britain than in the United States, at least at the present time. In the United States these predominantly benevolent relationships are rapidly being replaced by contractual obligation embedded in a legal framework. This legalistic and protective direction of the United States research establishment may be a harbinger for other Western countries. It certainly tends to shift the emphasis away from individual ethical judgements by researchers.

The 1978 Report of the United States National Commission for the Protection of Human Subjects of Biomedical and Behavioral Research[5] is very much to the point. Proposed regulations based on this report and issued by the United States Department of Health, Education, and Welfare in 1978 were extremely detailed and specific. They provoked a storm of critical responses mostly, but not exclusively, from academic psychiatrists who objected to the seeming implication that research was intrinsically bad and to be tolerated only under stringent controls; they argued that the proposed regulations would hamper clinical research in psychiatry and thereby represented discrimination against the mentally ill as a class by denying them the fruit of new knowledge.[11]

The simple premise that the researcher is an ethical person who, within relatively wide limits, can be trusted to deal fairly with mentally disabled subjects thus is being superseded in the United States by the assumption that such research involves a contract between equals. An example of the complications engendered by this new state of affairs is the variety of permutations in the concept of informed consent. A sophisticated literature is evolving about such new and derivative concepts as proxy consent, consent by group process, and formal (by signature) versus oral consent.

Not only research with mentally disturbed subjects is becoming a problem in the United States. The position of prisoner as research subject is changing in the same direction. Increasingly stringent restrictions are being imposed on the freedom of the prisoner to volunteer for such a role. Thus, it is held that the prisoner cannot be promised a reduction of his sentence or any reward whatever for his participation, since the expectation of these rewards might interfere with his ability to understand the conditions of the experiment. This movement has developed such momentum that it is now being argued that there is an inherent incompatibility between the ability to give truly informed consent and the status of being a prisoner. Interestingly, opposition to these developments is appearing among prisoners themselves on the ethical grounds that they are being deprived of an opportunity to contribute to society.

Confidentiality

Confidentiality in modern clinical practice

A basic ethical principle in psychiatry is that the doctor should take all reasonable precautions to preserve the confidentiality of the information given to him by patients. Sometimes circumstances arise when this information cannot and should not be used only within the context of the personal psychiatrist–patient relationship. This creates a problem since the information is divulged in the first place only because the patient wants advice and there is an assumption on both sides that confidentiality will be maintained. The evidence given on behalf of the British Medical Association to a government Committee on Privacy [12] included the following statement: 'It is no longer practicable to look upon the single physician as the patient's sole confidant in any serious illness and it is assumed by public and profession alike that any contact with the complex medical machinery of today implies acquiescence in some degree of extended confidence.'

This concept of extended confidence is essential to a discussion of privacy. It is taken for granted that the immediate members of a clinical team in group practice, medical and non-medical, professional and clerical, must have access to confidential information and that they will not abuse this trust. In Britain, the doctor in charge of the team is responsible to the General Medical Council should any ethical lapse occur. But doctors and nurses talk to each other about their patients and often they have easy access to each other's medical records, without there necessarily being any clear-cut benefit to the patient apart from general medical education. It is common for the doctor, through his professional skill, to learn something about the patient which he is reluctant to share with him, for example the presence of a fatal illness. This dilemma has been much discussed both in the medical and lay press without any resolution other than that the doctor has to use his own judgement whether or not to tell the patient. The doctor sometimes intentionally and one-sidedly breaches his confidential relationship with his patients without there being a public and professional outcry. This is presumably because in these circumstances the interests of patients are best served by allowing the physician to exercise his clinical judgement.

Behind clinical medical practice there stands an implied bond of trust between the public and the medical profession, as well as the individual patient's confidence in his own doctor. It is assumed that the actions taken by the responsible doctor are intended to be beneficial and that no harm will result from them. These actions include the passing of confidential data to other people who, in turn, will act responsibly since they would not otherwise be given the information. It is well accepted in practice, by both parties, that specific permission cannot be sought every time confidential information is transferred[13] (See Chapter 12 for a somewhat different view).

Even if it were possible for a patient to give a blanket permission for all the acts of transfer of information from one doctor to another that are necessary in modern clinical practice, it would not protect the doctor from legal action if any harm should come from such a transfer. A patient cannot, in law, consent to be damaged. The question therefore, even in purely clinical practice, is not whether information can be transferred by the responsible doctor, or by a doctor standing in for him, without the explicit consent of the patient; the question is, under what circumstances should such transfers take place? The most likely source of a leak of information to unauthorized persons is a lack of security in the clinical records system. An attention to security at this level is probably as important as any other. However, public concern has mainly been aroused by the possibility of unauthorized access to medical information systems where there is a facility for computer linking. We are not concerned here with the administrative uses of such registers but the security issues are much the same as for research registers.

A statement by the British Medical Research Council points out:

> The systematic collection and analysis of medical information has always been an important requisite for those doctors, particularly medical officers of health, concerned with the study and control of the health of the whole population rather than the individual patient . . . The control of epidemics of infectious disease was achieved in part through the notification of its onset in individual patients by family doctors to the medical officers of health. Similarly, the control of non-infectious diseases may be assisted by the transfer of medical information between doctors. The origins of many of these non-infectious diseases may lie in early life, their evolution is slow and insidious, and the relation between cause and effect is often obscure and complex. The changing social habits and conditions of life in a congested urban community, together with changes in industrial processes, continually create new health hazards, such as the toxic hazards of food additives, combustion of fuel on a new scale or of a new type of environmental pollution. Advances in the production of new powerful therapeutic and prophylactic agents have created a need not only to assess their effectiveness, in comparison with existing drugs or forms of treatment, but also to maintain a continued watch for the development of adverse reactions.[14]

There are three main categories of use of medical data for research purposes: small research projects in which information is collected from medical records and associated documents such as death certificates; moderately-sized data-collection systems utilizing record linkage, such as on-going or *ad hoc* case registers, which are still under local medical control; and regional or national data collection systems which allow record linkage. The problems posed are somewhat different at each level but what all three have in common is that it is often impossible to gain the patient's informed consent for each act of transfer of data. Underlying the three categories lies a single dimension of increasing scale, complexity, and longevity of the system of data collection and storage. What the psychiatrist will be concerned with, therefore, is the likelihood of public benefits accruing from each transfer of information, balanced against the possibility of harm to the patient.

Small-scale research projects

In small-scale research projects the main problem is likely to be carelessness. Documents tend to be left lying around and information about identifiable patients might in this way become known to unauthorized people. However, few research workers or assistants are likely to be involved and there is usually one psychiatrist personally responsible for the project. The risks are much the same as those in ordinary clinical practice. The most famous recent case of breach of confidentiality was actually the result of a burglary at a physician's private office, so that it can hardly be argued that 'state' systems are uniquely vulnerable. Attention to security should be a part of all research projects. In particular, it it is rarely necessary for identifying data to be included on documents which contain confidential material. A name–number list is much more easily kept under secure conditions than a large set of bulky files. Larger-scale collaborative projects, in which information about identified individuals is collected in a number of medical centres, pose more complicated problems but the precautions taken locally are the same: the security of the name–number list, restriction of access to specified persons, supervision by a named doctor responsible for confidentiality, and licence by an ethical committee. It is best for data forwarded to a central office for collation to be identified by number only; it should not be necessary to hold names or other identifiers on a computer file.

Local case registers

Psychiatric case registers under local medical control have been developed for research purposes in several parts of Europe and the United States. It is necessary to collect identifying data, such as names and addresses, for two reasons. First, the name, address, date of birth, and sometimes other identifying items are needed to link records from different agencies or different occasions, so that cohort studies can be undertaken. Thus, for example, it is possible to make the vital distinction between person and event statistics (e.g. between one person being in hospital ten times and ten people being in hospital once), without which a wide range of scientific and administrative studies would be impossible. Secondly, the register can be used as a sampling frame. In general, registers in the United Kingdom do not place identifying data on the computer file and the whole operation is small enough to be under the direct control of one doctor authorized by an ethical committee. Medical information is transferred only under very restricted circumstances and only from one doctor to another. Identifying data are kept under conditions of strict security and all staff who have access are fully aware of their responsibility. If an approach to a patient on the register is desired, permission is sought from the responsible clinician and the patient's informed consent is obtained before any further inquiry is made.

These characteristics form the basis of recommendations made by the Royal College of Psychiatrists for ensuring confidentiality in medical information systems. These include the licensing of registers, the appointment of a named physician to be responsible for confidentiality, surveillance of each register by an ethical committee with non-medical as well as medical members including some who are expert in computer security, and the adoption of a strict code of practice dealing with the conditions under which identifying data may be stored, transferred, or published. A model code of practice has been recommended.[13]

National and regional registers

It is at national and regional registers that most recent criticism has been directed. This is not because any breach of confidentiality has in fact occurred. There has been no example of misuse of information supplied to the Mental Health Enquiry covering England and Wales during the 30 years of its operation. Names are not even given to *bona-fide* research workers; they must produce their own list of names which has been obtained by permission of local clinicians.

Without identifying information, it would be impossible even to produce statistics of first admissions to psychiatric hospitals, which are the raw data required both for epidemiological and administrative purposes. The fact that the names and addresses of patients are collected in a central computer file, together with sensitive information (e.g. religion, diagnosis, marital status) leads to fears that a corrupt regime, or a few corrupt officials, would be presented with the opportunity to misuse the system. A further argument, that a well-intentioned official would allow the data to be fed into other computer systems, or would make information on named individuals available to other government agencies, must be discounted. In view of the very specific regulations, no such transfer could be regarded as anything but sinister.

It is impossible to say that such a situation will never come about although it is certainly not with us at present. The Royal College of Psychiatrists therefore recommends that, as is already the case in Scotland, ethical responsibility for the Mental Health Enquiry should be transferred to a committee on which nominees from government are not in a majority and that there should be an independent chairman.[15]

Privacy regulations and the restriction of useful research

Precautions of this kind should not unduly restrict research but protective legislation is developing in some countries to such an extent that legitimate data-gathering activities are being hampered. 'For example, in Sweden, epidemiologists are complaining that their research has been rendered tedious, time-consuming and ineffective because of the regulations governing the establishment of information systems.'[16] It is extremely expensive to break the current computer security systems and, political corruption apart, there can be little incentive to do so in order to obtain the kind of information held in medical information systems.

Sir Richard Doll has given four examples of medical research that depended for their success 'on the maintenance of clinical records in hospitals, the existence of nosological indexes, and the willingness of doctors to provide access to their notes and to allow their patients to be followed up and, on occasions, interviewed. Sometimes they required access to industrial or other social records and very often to central registers of death or morbidity.' He points out that a proper concern over the possibility, for example, of linking records of treatment for venereal disease or psychiatric disorder with employment records, has led to a mistrust of all interchange of medical information, so that it is suggested that no such exchange should ever be made without the explicit consent of the patient.[17]

Doll quotes the statement by the British Medical Research Council: 'The Council considers that, subject to certain safeguards, medical information obtained about identified individual patients should continue to be made available without their explicit consent for the purposes of medical research.'[14] He sums up his own experience, which most research workers will endorse, as follows: 'the vast majority of people are glad to assist in medical research, even at the cost of some personal inconvenience.'

Lee Robins, a distinguished American medical sociologist, reviewed the value of long-term follow-up studies, which depend upon the ability to select unbiased samples and to obtain unbiased information about these samples throughout the period of follow-up. 'For many follow-up studies, the researcher needs access both to the subject himself and to records about him. Seeing the subject personally is valuable because the subject can provide information that has never been recorded, and he can alert the researcher to records about himself that would otherwise be missed. Record searches permit verifying the veracity of the subject's statements and also provide information he cannot supply.'[18] Robins's own research provides examples of how important such studies are in psychiatry but she points out that access to records has been severely curtailed by the United States Privacy Act of 1974 and the Family Educational Rights Act of 1974. A more recent report of the Privacy Protection Study Commission makes the same point.[19]

The recent report of the British Data Protection Committee is much more aware of the need to preserve a proper basis for useful research as well as to ensure that harm does not come to individuals. Its recommendations, while preserving reasonable safeguards, are unlikely seriously to curtail legitimate access to records.[20] It may be permissible to hope that public opinion will turn towards an appreciation of the value of research and a realization that preserving a base for research can be fully compatible with respect for human rights.

Committees on the ethics of research

The operation of ethical committees

'The object of ethical committees is to safeguard patients, healthy volunteers and the reputation of the profession and its institutions in matters of clinical research investigation.'[21] The report of a committee of the Royal College of Physicians suggested that such committees should be small, expert, contain a lay member, and be able to call upon specialist advice when needed. They should be responsible to the governing authority of the hospital or institute.

Grant-giving bodies such as the Medical Research Council in the United Kingdom and the National Institutes of Health and National Institute of Mental Health in the United States, require all proposals for research to be vetted by an ethical committee, and many such committees advise research workers to submit *all* their proposed projects, although this advice does not have the force of law. Some committees specify that the decision whether to submit is left to the senior member of staff concerned, with the proviso that there is a moral obligation to consult the Committee whenever there is the slightest doubt. A simple form is provided identifying the applicant, the responsible worker, and the sponsor, and including a brief description of the research and the ethical aspects involved.

Most ethical committees have now had several years of experience of considering the ethical problems raised by a wide variety of research proposals, most of which have been discussed in general terms earlier in this chapter. In my own experience, while there have been a few instances in which research workers thought a committee's recommendations too cautious, there has been no single case in which they were not accepted. Research workers have the opportunity to defend their proposals if they so wish and there is often a process of revision in order to devise a design and methodology acceptable to the committee. The lay member has had long experience of representing consumer interests and legal advice is available as required.

Most applications present few problems. A typical example would be the drawing of blood samples during the course of a depressive disorder in order to determine whether a chemical compound, hypothesized to be associated with severity, can in fact be found to vary appropriately in concentration. The applicant must explain why it is necessary to undertake the project. He must say how he proposes to explain it to patients, including telling them that it will not be helpful to their own treatment but may be useful in accumulating knowledge about the nature of the condition, that there can occasionally be some temporary bruising, and that they are free to take part or not, as they choose. The committee will consider whether the applicant has met its ethical criteria, asking, for example, whether patients are capable of giving informed consent in this instance. If so, they will decide whether the probable balance of good and harm is such that they can give their approval. If the procedure were a lumbar puncture rather than a venepuncture, the committee would take into account the somewhat greater risk involved but the principles they used would be the same.

After a time, an ethical committee becomes experienced in selecting problems that require more extended discussion because they have not previously arisen in its deliberations. When computerized tomography was introduced, for example, it was necessary for the particular indications and contraindications to be considered in detail. The balance of good and harm is different when the procedure is used as an aid in the assessment of dementia, as a means of investigating abnormality in alcoholism or schizophrenia, and as a method of studying cerebral pathology in, say, autistic children. In the last case, the possible addition to knowledge might not be considered worth the risk to the child, even if the parents were willing to give a fully informed consent.

Another kind of issue which requires detailed consideration during the early stages of a committee's existence is the use of 'normal volunteers' in research. In most instances, the ethical problems are similar to those arising in clinical research with patients but marginal questions do arise. For example, I have had experience of one application which sought permission to deliver a questionnaire concerning, among other things, attitudes to various sexual practices, through the letter-boxes of randomly selected houses in a certain geographical area, with a request that they should be completed and returned to the investigator in a stamped-addressed envelope. The committee's discussion turned on the problem of how far it was reasonable to expose people to such questions without obtaining their prior permission, as well as on the scientific value of this method of data-collection.

These examples, and others mentioned earlier in the chapter, indicate the way that ethical issues arise during the discussion of practical problems in research. An experienced committee develops an expertise which colleagues find impressive and which should, one hopes, reassure the public.

There is less of a consensus on the constitution and functions of ethical committees dealing with the special problems raised by computerized medical information systems. There seems no reason why ordinary ethical committees (or subcommittees of them) should not take on such duties. The only particular requirements are that those who supply information to the register should be represented and that a member of the committee should understand the problems of computer security. The Younger Committee has proposed a licensing authority for information systems and a central committee which can deal with issues not solved by other bodies.[20] The suggestion is still under consideration by the British Government.

Conclusion

I believe that the general answer to the set of questions I posed at the beginning of this chapter is that no line can be drawn between innovatory clinical practice in psychiatry and more formal research investigation. Whenever there is any doubt at all, it is the duty of the responsible psychiatrist to seek the advice of an ethical committee. An inescapable concomitant of this conclusion is that there are no ethical issues specific to clinical research. Every problem that arises in research — whether it involves the balance of good against harm, a decision to undertake a laboratory procedure or to give or withhold a treatment, or to pass information to some other person — also arises in everyday clinical work.

Several bodies have put forward lists of principles that can form a useful guide to individual psychiatrists and to members of ethical committees.[5,22] However, it is necessary to distinguish between the individual psychiatrist's own decision in any given case, which must be his own moral responsibility, and a set of ethical guidelines which may be laid down by a professional or lay body in order to help him take the decision. In the last resort, the trust of the public, individually and collectively, in the psychiatric profession will depend upon the cumulative effect of a myriad decisions of the first kind. A psychiatrist must be free to follow his conscience.

In my view, no matter what 'society' thinks about the necessity or otherwise for clinical trials, the freedom of an individual psychiatrist to decide whether or not to allow his own patients to be included in a trial, and whether or not 'fully informed consent' is feasible or necessary, must be preserved at all costs. We must be clear, however, that we are dealing with individual and not group ethics. The decision must be made in precisely the same way as it would have been if no clinical trial were involved. One psychiatrist may believe that the value of the treatment under test has already been sufficiently demonstrated and will therefore refuse to expose his patient to the risk of its withdrawal in a clinical trial. This decision must be respected but it cannot be imposed on other psychiatrists who think differently. Clearly, as Helmchen and Müller-Oerlinghausen point out,[7] this will introduce biases, but a variety of designs is available to take care of this problem and, in any case, an epidemiological approach always needs to be adopted in order to determine the limits within which the results can be generalized.[23]

Karl Popper's comment on personal responsibility for one's ethical decisions applies perfectly to the psychiatrist in his role as researcher: 'The responsibility for our ethical decisions is entirely ours and can be shifted on to nobody else; neither to God, nor to nature, nor to society, nor to history . . . Whatever authority we may accept, it is we who accept it. We only deceive ourselves if we do not realize this simple point.'[24]

References

1. POPPER, K.: *Unended quest: an intellectual autobiography.* Glasgow, Fontana/Collins, 1976, p. 193.
2. WING, J. K.: *Reasoning about madness.* London, Oxford University Press, 1978, p. 5.
3. SIMON, B.: *Mind and madness in ancient Greece: the classical roots of modern psychiatry.* Ithaca, Cornell University Press, 1978, p. 187.
4. MARCUSE, H.: *Negations: essays in critical theory.* Harmondsworth: Penguin, 1968.
5. National Commission for the Protection of Human Subjects of Biomedical and Behavioral Research. Report and Recommendations, Department of Health, Education, and Welfare, Publication No. (OS) 78–0006. Bethesda, 1978.

6. NEVILLE, R.: *On the national commission: a puritan critique of consensus ethics.* Hastings Center Report, April 1979, p. 22.
7. HELMCHEN, H., MÜLLER-OERLINGHAUSEN, B.: The inherent paradox of clinical trials in psychiatry. *Journal of Medical Ethics* **1**:168–73, 1975.
8. Medical Research Council: *Responsibility in investigations on human subjects* Report of the Medical Research Council for 1962–63. Cmnd. 2382.
9. HIRSCH, S. R., GAIND, R., ROHDE, P. D., *et al.*: Outpatient maintenance of chronic schizophrenic patients with long-acting fluphenazine. *British Medical Journal 1*:633–7, 1973.
10. WING, J. K.: The ethics of clinical trials. *Journal of Medical Ethics* **1**:174–5, 1975.
11. GOODWIN, F.: Personal communication, 8 August, 1980.
12. HOME OFFICE: *Computers and privacy.* Cmnd. 6353. London, HMSO, 1975.
13. BALDWIN, J. A., LEFF, J. P., and WING, J. K.: Confidentiality of psychiatric data in medical information systems. *British Journal of Psychiatry* **128**:417–27, 1976.
14. Medical Research Council: Responsibility in the use of medical information for research. *British Medical Journal* **1**:213–16, 1973.
15. Special Committee on Confidentiality and Medical Information Systems. Report. *Bulletin of the Royal College of Psychiatrists*, June 1979, p. 103.
16. VUORI, H.: Privacy, confidentiality and automated health information systems. *Journal of Medical Ethics* **3**:174–8, 1977.
17. DOLL, R.: Public benefit and personal privacy: The problems of medical investigation in the community. *Proceedings of the Royal Society of Medicine* **67**:1281–5, 1974.
18. ROBINS, L.: Privacy regulations and longitudinal studies. Paper read to American Association for the Advancement of Science, February 1978.
19. PRIVACY PROTECTION STUDY COMMISSION: *Personal privacy in an information society.* Washington DC, US Government Printing Office, 1977.
20. *Report of the Committee on Data Protection.* Cmnd. 7341. London: HMSO, 1978.
21. ROYAL COLLEGE OF PHYSICIANS, LONDON: *Supervision of the ethics of clinical research investigations in institutions.* July 1973.
22. AMERICAN COLLEGE OF NEUROPSYCHOPHARMACOLOGY: Statement of principles of ethical conduct for neuropsychopharmacologic research in human subjects, in *Legal and ethical issues in human research and treatment.* Ed. Gallant, D. M. and Force, R. New York, Spectrum Publications, 1978, Chapter 1.
23. LEFF, J. P.: Influence of selection of patients on results of clinical trials. *British Medical Journal* **iv**:156–8, 1973.
25. POPPER, K. R.: *The open society and its enemies.* Vol. 1. London: Routledge, 1945, p. 62 and note 18.

16

Training in psychiatric ethics

Robert Michels

THE recent growth of interest in the ethical aspects of psychiatry began with concerns about specific issues: involuntary confinement, the distinction between treatment of mental illness and social control of deviance, the right to treatment, least restrictive settings, confidentiality, informed consent, and so on.[1] Initially, attention was frequently directed to some real or alleged evil or abuse, and the discussion was conducted in a 'moral' (e.g. stamping out evil) rather than an 'ethical' framework. Since it seems unlikely that psychiatrists are inherently either more or less evil than other citizens, a discussion of their moral judgements leads to the question of how they come to be the way they are, what factors in their training or their socialization shape their ethical sensitivities and responses? A closely related theme is the role of ethics in psychiatric education; how should our knowledge about ethics influence the content and conduct of our training programmes? In view of this, it is interesting that there is little written about the teaching of ethics in psychiatry, and that both the profession and the public seem to prefer discussing the problems that psychiatrists face (and produce) rather than the method that seems most likely to alter their behaviour.

Can psychiatric ethics be taught?

There are several points of view about the teaching of ethics in psychiatry. Perhaps the oldest and the most widespread is that ethics cannot be taught. Proponents argue that certainly psychiatrists should be 'ethical' (by which they mean virtuous), but that the only way that this can be assured is to select ethical individuals and train them to become psychiatrists. The general structure of this argument is familiar to psychiatrists, since it is analogous to the view held by many physicians about the skills involved in the doctor–patient relationship. There are at least three counter-arguments that are important for our consideration. The first is that this position confuses ethics with morals. Ethics has to do with the way in which one thinks about and discusses moral problems and choices. A good man may not understand ethics, while a bad man might be quite sophisticated about it. Certainly we would like psychiatrists to be good people, but independent of this we would also like them to understand the ethical aspects of psychiatric issues.

Secondly, something may have a basis in temperament or talent or character and yet be enhanced or developed or refined through education. Musical skill, athletic ability, and the conduct of psychotherapy are all examples of this. It may be important to consider ethical capacities in selecting trainees, but also important to train them in ethics.

Finally, there are special problems that emerge in the consideration of the ethical aspects of psychiatry. Psychiatric ethics may be a branch of medical ethics or of general ethics, but it is a branch that has unique characteristics. There has been considerable effort devoted to the study and analysis of these issues, particularly in recent years, and it would be unfortunate if we expected each student of the field to explore these issues anew without access to the wisdom that has already been collected and formulated.

Teaching by modelling

A second view of the teaching of ethics in psychiatry is that it can be taught, but that the only appropriate way to do this is through modelling. This view would suggest that the critical problem is not selecting students, but rather selecting teachers. The importance of education through modelling and identification is a prominent theme in psychiatry in general, emphasized in psychodynamic, behaviourist, and developmental approaches to psychiatry. Some psychiatrists believe that most psychiatric education occurs through modelling, and almost all believe it to be important. Accepting this, it shifts or broadens our problem rather than solving it. We must consider how to teach the teachers as well as how to teach the students.

Teaching by cases

A third approach would see psychiatric ethics as an aspect of practical wisdom, taught by the case method in the discussion of specific clinical situations or practical decisions. Rounds, case conferences, and the supervision of specific treatments form the core of most psychiatric training programmes, and ethical aspects of the psychiatrist's work would be studied in the same way as psychodynamic or psychopharmacologic aspects. This has the virtue of bringing the teaching of psychiatric ethics into the pedagogic setting that has the trainee's greatest attention and emotional investment. The disadvantage is that ethical issues are often set aside because of the urgency of specific therapeutic problems, and there is a tendency to associate psychiatric ethics with unusual or 'tough' cases, rather than to recognize the universality of ethics as a framework for understanding professional functioning. Furthermore, this method of teaching focuses on issues related to specific patients, rather than those that emerge in consideration of broader questions of professional functioning. Ethical aspects of the relationship between the psychiatric profession and society, distribution of scarce resources, the role of the public in professional decisions, and similar matters will rarely be discussed in the context of specific cases, but they should be discussed in the course of psychiatric education. This is a general problem not unique to ethics. The same could be said about those aspects of psychopharmacology or psychodynamics or personality development that are part of the knowledge base of psychiatry. Finally, psychiatric educators who are excellent teachers of clinical psychiatry may not have the knowledge or interest required to teach about ethics, while moral philosophers who could enrich the experience of psychiatric trainees might not be competent or appropriate as general psychiatric supervisors. It would be unfortunate if the structure of the curriculum in psychiatric ethics precluded participation by those who were most competent to teach.

Teaching by seminars

A fourth approach to the teaching of ethics in psychiatry would see ethics as one of the themes of a core curriculum. A fundamental body of knowledge would be taught in seminars and courses, while applications to specific problems would appear in the discussion of ward rounds and supervision. This would provide exposure to the philosophical or theoretical aspects of ethics — theories of justice, concepts of right and duty, etc., the application of these principles to the major problems of psychiatry, and experience with evaluating decisions in concrete situations. This model may seem more comprehensive, and, therefore, more attractive than the others discussed above, but in fact, it is rarely if every employed, and tells us more about what might be done in the future than what is actually done in any programme today. In part, this reflects the relatively short period during which psychiatric ethics has seemed an appropriate part of psychiatric education; in part, the immense competition among an unusually wide range of subjects for time in the psychiatric curriculum.

When to Teach?

Teaching in medical school

Turning from how to teach psychiatric ethics to when the teaching should occur, we have the choice of pre-professional education, medical school, psychiatric training, or continuing education. The undergraduate period would seem to be the obvious time to develop a basis in the philosophical underpinnings of ethics, and there has been a growing interest in the subject in college curricula.[2] However, the pre-medical preparation of medical students is so heterogeneous that courses on medical ethics in medical schools, whether required or elective, have become customary.[3] These programmes have been reviewed extensively, and although the specific formats employed have varied, they seem to have found a firm place in the medical school curriculum. Their history is analogous in many ways to that of the teaching of psychiatry in medical schools. Everyone pays lip-service to their importance, but faculty and students both act as if the subject-matter is an adornment to the curriculum rather than an essential component of it.[4] Many believe that there is no real expertise in the area, and, therefore, no need for specially trained faculty. It is seen as part of the 'art' of medicine rather than the 'science', part of the humanistic tradition shared by all physicians. Although this attitude may present as enthusiasm for the new programme in ethics as a long missing and important part of the curriculum, it often conceals a subtle disparagement of the intellectual and scholarly basis of the field.

This similarity in the attitudes toward psychiatry and medical ethics on the part of the medical school community has led to certain strategic and political problems in introducing medical ethics into the medical school psychiatry curriculum. Most psychiatry teachers and departments are sensitive to and concerned about student attitudes toward their discipline, and are particularly eager to be seen as similar to other areas of the curriculum. This became increasingly true in American medical schools in the 1970s, as a backlash to the community psychiatry movement of the 1960s, reflecting the attempt to 'remedicalize' American psychiatry. One result has been an attempt to de-emphasize whatever is special or unique about psychiatry; its concern with social issues, its interest in subjective experience, those aspects of its practice that may not fit neatly into the narrowest definition of the medical model, and finally, its close links to medical humanism including medical ethics.

Teaching in psychiatric training programmes

The most natural setting for teaching the ethical aspects of psychiatry would seem to be during psychiatric training programmes. It is surprising that with one recent exception[5] there is almost nothing written about such teaching, and informal anecdotal communication suggests that relatively little occurs during training other than an occasional seminar or a brief elective course. This is in spite of the fact that a number of prominent psychiatric educators have a strong interest in ethical issues.

The relatively recent growth of interest in psychiatric ethics and the number of different subjects packed into psychiatric training make it important not to over-interpret the failure to develop these programmes. However, there are some special problems that emerge in including the teaching of ethics in psychiatric training that are worthy of consideration. First, a great deal of this training occurs in monstrously immoral social institutions, outdated, uncomfortable, inhumane, and reflecting the stigma and fear of mental illness as well as the political refusal to recognize and accept the inevitable costs if the mentally ill are regarded as full citizens and members of the community. The psychiatric trainee participating in these institutions — whether hospitals, community programmes, prisons, old people's homes, schools for the retarded, or the network of social services that usually fails to integrate them, feels the discomfort that has marked the entire profession's relation to the mental health system. There are several possible responses to this discomfort: guilt, anger at the profession, political activism, cynical nihilism, or withdrawal from involvement in mental health. However, whatever the specific form of the response, it is not usually a comfortable time to think about the basic ethical issues involved. Those who do become interested in such issues early in their training often tend to turn against the profession as a result. The pattern should be familiar to psychiatrists; the group tries to avoid and deny the painful aspects of their roles, and those who deviate from this group norm are likely to be rebellious in other respects and are also likely to be rejected by the group. Fortunately, the problem seems to be diminishing in recent years, with the growing interest and awareness of the profession in the social, political, and ethical significance of its work, and perhaps the beginning recognition that consideration of these is an essential component of a training programme.

A second problem in teaching ethics in psychiatric training programmes relates to the subject matter itself. Trainees, or at least those in 'dynamically' oriented programmes that focus attention on the inner psychological world of patients, are struggling to acquire a new paradigm, to think of behaviour as determined by mental forces, wishes, fears, conflicts, and so on. This requires a suspension of their more customary framework for regarding the same behaviour, the everyday common sense approach that includes a considerable amount of moral judgement. An important theme of psychodynamic psychiatric training is to learn to suspend moral judgements in areas where they would naturally be employed. At times this can lead to an unfortunate generalization outside of the clinical psychodynamic setting and a kind of amorality that seeks to understand all behaviour while judging nothing. Optimally, good psychodynamic training eventually leads to the recognition that in certain carefully specified clinical situations there are advantages to suspending moral judgements in order to create a field of inquiry that will make it possible to dissect the psychological determinants of behaviour, and indeed of morality itself. If not, the emotional atmosphere essential for the inquiry process cannot be established. The problem in training is that while a student is struggling to acquire a new paradigm, experiences that reinforce the old one may work against the immediate educational goal. In the jargon of the field, ethics may be used as a resistance against psychodynamics. It is not that ethics is inherently antagonistic or incompatible with a psychodynamic approach, only that they are different and that there may be interactions between them that have educational significance. In a sense, learning psychodynamics can be like learning a foreign language, and it may be useful to stop using one's native tongue for a while. This interaction can work in both directions, and just as learning a new language can enhance one's understanding of a familiar one, so these two different frameworks for considering human behaviour can each clarify and explicate the characteristics of the other.

Ethics in continuing education

Psychiatric education extends beyond the formal training programme and psychiatric ethics has an important role to play in continuing medical education. It has been a major theme of several recent psychiatric meetings, including the Plenary Session of the World Psychiatric Association in 1977, the American College of Psychiatrists in 1980, and the American Psychiatric Association in 1980. Seminars and symposia have received wide attention, such as the discussion of 'the psychiatrist as double agent', co-sponsored by the American Psychiatric Association and the Institute of Society, Ethics and the Life Sciences,[6] or the several conferences of the same Institute on ethical aspects of psychiatric treatment and research. There has also been a growing awareness of ethical issues in those psychiatrists who completed their formal training before these topics were included in educational programmes and now participate in postgraduate courses, although the appropriate way to introduce discussions of ethical problems into these curricula is not yet clear.[7]

What to teach?

The teaching of metaethics

The content of the curriculum in psychiatric ethics can be considered on three levels. First is the basic introduction to ethics, the philosophical basis of moral discourse, or metaethics. If a psychiatrist is to have more than opinions on right and wrong, if he is to understand the place of these views in the larger sphere of moral reasoning, the types of justification that are being used or being discarded, and the history of these views in general ethics; in short, if he is to have an ethical understanding of his moral positions, then he must have some education in metaethics. This is analogous to the need for training in basic biochemistry and pharmacology for the psychiatrist who will understand the drugs that he is prescribing, and even be prepared to understand those that have not yet been discovered.

Few psychiatrists are prepared to teach metaethics, and, if it is to be taken seriously, it requires the collaboration of philosophers, ethicists, or others with similar backgrounds. It can be taught as a distinct body of knowledge, with the advantage of emphasizing the inherent structure and relationships of the discipline itself, but the disadvantage of being given low priority by trainees who are preoccupied with more immediate and practical concerns. Alternatively, the meta-ethical dimensions of specific ethical issues can be explored in the context of discussing those specific issues. For example, a discussion of the relationship between individual autonomy, involuntary treatment, and the right to treatment in psychiatric settings can be used to explore the relationship between utilitarian and absolutist modes of ethical reasoning. This second approach reverses the advantages and disadvantages of the first; the material is organized in categories that 'feel' more relevant to the students, but at risk of diluting and fragmenting the critical issues in the underlying philosophical dialogue. There are practical problems that also must be considered; if qualified teachers are scarce, the first mode of presentation, a systematic review of ethical theory, requires less of their time, while the second format is more likely to encourage interaction between psychiatrists and professional philosophers.

The teaching of codes of ethics

The second level of the curriculum in psychiatric ethics would involve discussions of normative rules, standards, and codes of the profession, what psychiatrists and psychiatry ought to do, and why.[8,9,10†] This also could be taught either in a separate discussion or integrated with the teaching of specific issues in psychiatry. This level of ethics is closely related to issues of law, politics, and social policy, and their teaching can be co-ordinated in the curriculum. The teaching of rules of conduct can easily degenerate into moralistic sermons; a fate that is best prevented by serious efforts to expore professional codes or prescriptions in a metaethical framework, while at the same time

---

† See Appendix for codes of ethics relevant to psychiatrists.

considering their application to concrete situations and their practical consequences for society and for the profession.

The discussion of the codes and standards of the profession will also offer an opportunity to explore the nature of professions and their relationship to the general society.[11] Many of the recent controversies about psychiatric ethics have focused on this theme; issues of peer review, the psychiatrist as 'double agent',[6] and the role of the profession in responding to an individual member who breaches the professional code of ethics would all be examples.

The teaching of situational ethics

The third level of the curriculum in psychiatric ethics would be the consideration of a series of specific issues in the field. The list of potential subjects is long enough that any course would have to make selections. Possible subjects might include:

(1) the right to treatment;
(2) consent and involuntary treatment;
(3) invasive or irreversible treatments;
(4) institutions, total institutions, and deinstitutionalization;
(5) least restrictive settings and professional decisions;
(6) coercion and psychotherapy;
(7) prediction of dangerousness and the role of the psychiatrist in its prevention;
(8) children, the retarded, and the incompetent; guardianship and proxy;
(9) psychiatrist as agent of society and patient; the social and political abuse of psychiatry;
(10) behaviour control, social engineering, and deviance;
(11) responsibility and guilt;
(12) autonomy and competence; self-determination;
(13) performance enhancement, optimalization, and the psychopharmacology of hedonism;
(14) labelling and stigma;
(15) privacy and confidentiality;
(16) distributive justice and access to health services;
(17) resource allocation and the determination of priorities.

Each of these topics could be explored in terms of the values and choices they entail, the history of the profession's response, the arguments that have been presented on behalf of various positions that have been taken, the basic ethical issues that are implicit in these arguments, and the patterns of views on the entire array of topics that reflect more general ethical positions. Clearly, this detailed an analysis of all of these subjects would consume an inappropriate amount of time in a training curriculum, and selections would be required.

Goals and objectives

There is a range of possible goals in a teaching programme in psychiatric ethics, and although any specific curriculum is likely to pursue several goals at the same time, it is helpful to consider just what a curriculum is trying to do. Goals related to knowledge include understanding major systems of ethical reasoning and their similarities and differences, learning the terms and concepts used in ethical discourse, and learning the history of the contemporary ethical dilemmas in psychiatry with the positions and arguments that have developed around them. Goals related to attitudes include sensitizing the student to the ethical aspects of issues that might otherwise be seen as scientific or technical in nature, and acquainting him with the subtlety and complexity of ethical reasoning, often seen by those who are not familiar with it as little more than 'common sense'. The goals defined in terms of skill would include the student's ability to recognize ethical problems in psychiatry; to reason about them in a coherent, systematic, and useful way; and to understand the reasoning of others and participate with them in ethical discourse. Finally, the goals might include modifying the professional behaviour of the student so that it is informed and guided by his understanding of psychiatric ethics.

The selection of goals for a specific curriculum will be determined by the stage in the student's professional education, the time available, the setting, and the faculty. Generally, programmes that aim exclusively at modifying the student's behaviour in a specific direction without attending to knowledge and attitudes have little lasting impact, while those that focus on knowledge without attention to skill have difficulty involving more pragmatically oriented students.

Constructing curricula

Educational programmes are most successful if the students acquire knowledge that helps them to accomplish tasks in which they are currently engaged, and if they are given opportunities to apply the knowledge they are acquiring while they are acquiring it. When these principles are applied to the subject matter of psychiatric ethics, some general guidelines for constructing curricula emerge. One is that although lectures about ethical issues may impart information about terms, concepts, and the history of arguments and positions, the student will gain familiarity with moral reasoning only by participating more actively through dialogue and discussion. Secondly, although the 'classic' issues of psychiatric ethics should be explored, and the student has much to learn about them and from participating in discussions of them, a valuable dimension is added if the underlying themes and problems are traced in the student's current professional experience. For example, the 'double agent' issue of the psychiatrist's responsibility to his patient and to society is clearly articulated in the discussions of recent problems in Soviet psychiatry (see Chapter 18) or in the judicial decisions concerning the psychiatrist's obligation to warn potential victims of violent patients. However, the question will have additional meaning to the trainee who discusses it in terms, for example, of the psychotic patient currently receiving treatment who wants to return to an occupation involving public safety for which he is not yet competent, or the adolescent patient who is involved in sexual or drug-related behaviour that is not acceptable to family or society.

Psychiatric ethics involves intellectual areas in which psychiatrists have no special claim to expertise, and there are advantages to constructing programmes that will bring psychiatrists together with other mental health professionals, lawyers, sociologists, and philosophers, both in the student body and on the faculty. The broader meaning of one's routine daily decisions is experienced dramatically when seen through the eyes of an intelligent observer who has been socialized into a different perspective. For example, courses including psychiatric trainees and law students provide each of these groups with an opportunity to explore ethical questions in involuntary treatment or criminal responsibility that greatly enlarge the perspective of either group meeting alone.

Finally, like any other curriculum, attention to evaluation enriches the programme. Not only does it force the faculty to specify goals and objectives, all too often ignored when the subject matter is obviously relevant but necessarily vague and amorphous, but it also forces a dialogue between students and faculty about the goals. Students often approach programmes in psychiatric ethics with the assumption that the intent is to teach them what to do in difficult or special situations. A well constructed curriculum and evaluation procedure can convey that the goal is to help them to identify alternatives and analyse the ethical aspects of choices they face in their daily professional activities, to discuss these intelligently with their colleagues, and to clarify and, when appropriate, resolve differences and conflicts.

Summary

The recent interest in psychiatric ethics has not yet produced an interest in the teaching of psychiatric ethics, but this is likely to follow. Such teaching is more likely to occur in psychiatric and continuing education programmes than in pre-medical or medical school curricula. It should include discussion of metaethics or the basic principles of ethical reasoning, normative codes of professional conduct or the rules for psychiatrists facing choices, and the specific situations and problems that interest and trouble psychiatrists today.

References

1. REDLICH, F. and MOLLICA, R. F.: Overview: ethical issues in contemporary psychiatry. *Ameican Journal of Psychiatry* **133**:125–36, 1976.
2. *The teaching of bioethics*. Hastings-on-Hudson, New York, Institute of Society, Ethics, and the Life Sciences, 1976.
3. VEATCH, R. M. and SOLLITTO, S.: Medical ethics teaching: report of a national medical school survey. *Journal of the American Medical Associaiton* **235**:1030–3, 1976.
4. VEATCH, R. M., GAYLIN, W., and MORGAN, C. (ed.): *The teaching of medical ethics*. Hastings-on-Hudson, New York, Institute of Society, Ethics and the Life Sciences, 1973.
5. BLOCH, S.: Teaching of psychiatric ethics. *British Journal of Psychiatry* **136**:300–1, 1980.
6. *A conference on conflicting loyalties*. Hastings-on-Hudson, New York, Institute of Society, Ethics and the Life Sciences, Special Supplement, April, 1978.
7. JELLINEK, M. and PARMELEE, D.: Is there a role for medical ethics in postgraduate psychiatry courses? *American Journal of Psychiatry* **134**:1438–9, 1977.
8. MOORE, R. A.: Ethics in the practice of psychiatry — origins, functions, models, and enforcement. *American Journal of Psychiatry* **135**:157–63, 1978.
9. The principles of medical ethics with annotations especially applicable to psychiatry. *American Journal of Psychiatry* **130**:1057–64, 1973.
10. MICHELS, R.: The physician and medical education. *P & S quarterly* **19**:13–15, 1974.
11. MICHELS, R.: Professional ethics and social value. *International Review of Psychoanalysis* **3**:377–84, 1976.

17

The responsibility of the psychiatrist to his society

Paul Chodoff

THIS chapter will be concerned with the responsibilities of individual psychiatrists and the profession of psychiatry to society as a whole and the ethical issues arising therefrom. These responsibilities are: of citizenship; of being accountable to the public and its representatives; and of fostering an equitable distribution of psychiatric services throughout the entire socio-economic range of the society.

The responsibilities of citizenship

The psychiatrist, like any good citizen, can be expected to comport himself in a useful and decent manner in the general society; he should share his special knowledge with the public; and he should make his voice heard in the public discussion and determination of issues of legitimate interest to psychiatry. The psychiatrist also has the responsibility to his society to establish, maintain, and adhere to standards of professional integrity.

Although the above precepts can be taken as self-evident, other issues arise which are not so obvious. For instance, does his responsibility to his society also require that, like other well educated citizens occupying favoured positions, the psychiatrist ought to devote time and effort to an informed participation in the affairs of his community and country? Some psychiatrists, particularly among those who practice in the psychoanalytic mode, may feel that this decision involves an ethical question since their duties as a citizen in this regard may conflict with their belief that any activity which exposes them to public scrutiny will compromise transference relationships and thus interfere with their ability to provide optimal treatment for their patients. The conflict here is a familiar one within the utilitarian tradition of resolving moral issues, and its solution, at least as far as its ethical aspects are concerned, will depend on the individual psychiatrist's perception of the consequences of his behaviour to the community at large and to his patients. Some help in resolving this issue, as is true for a number of issues within psychiatry, could be provided by a factual demonstration of how treatment is affected when the psychiatrist comes to the patient's attention in a public rather than in a private, psychotherapeutic role.

Does an ethical issue arise when psychiatrists are asked by legitimate organs of the media or public information to comment on a subject thought to be within the area of psychiatric expertise? Asking psychiatrists questions about a wide gamut of subjects is common practice, possibly reflecting a popular belief in the seer-like qualities of the profession, a belief, one should remember, representing only one side of a popular ambivalence towards the psychiatrist, who also may be seen at times as a bombastic simpleton. Questions may range from the political misuse of psychiatry or the mental health of world leaders to the psychology of changing styles of dress. Psychiatrists confronted with such questions may get out of their depth. Intoxicated by the illusion of omnipotence which is an occupational hazard of the profession,[1] they may find themselves succumbing to the temptation to believe that their special training makes them experts on everything under the sun. They may have a problem in drawing the line between really having something to say of benefit to the public and gazing into a crystal ball which is just as clouded as anyone else's. Instances of such misuse of their professional reputations by psychiatrists unfortunately are not rare. A particularly heinous example occurred in the United States in 1964 when a number of psychiatrists expressed negative opinions about the mental health of Barry Goldwater, then a candidate for Presidency of the United States. They were swayed, it appears, by their adverse view of Mr Goldwater's political beliefs rather than by evidence about his emotional stability. Other examples of such misuse, also unfortunately rather popular at present, are certain psychobiographies undertaken by psychiatrists or written with their aid which dissect public figures in painful and embarrassing ways on the basis of little or no direct data.

Another ethical consideration for a psychiatrist is his responsibility when he holds an opinion contrary to that generally held by his colleagues or which has been put forward officially by the organization which represents him. If his self-interest and professional advancement are in conflict with his beliefs it may be difficult for him to act in accordance with the latter. Such a conflict is of course familiar to all of us and though it may be difficult to act honestly, serious ethical considerations may not be involved. However, there will be other instances when the issue is more complex and ambiguous and the psychiatrist may have to acknowledge that his dissent, especially if stated very strongly, can harm his profession and, in addition, might confuse the public. The psychiatrist needs to weigh such considerations carefully. As an ethical matter, however, it is clear that he ought not to allow himself to be influenced by self-serving motivations to align himself with a position which is not his. To act simply as an 'apparatchik' is never ethically proper and psychiatrists particularly need to be aware of rationalizations which enable them to ignore their true beliefs.

Thus far, I have dealt with situations which pose ethical problems because legitimate societal requirements need to be weighed against personal and professional goals. More serious ethical delemmas may arise when the opposite situation obtains — when there is a need to balance the canons of professional integrity against certain doubtful or problematical demands of society. It is a hallmark of the psychiatric profession that in a number of areas (e.g. involuntary hospitalization, the insanity defence) its practitioners operate at an interface between the rights of the individual and the requirements of society. The psychiatrist is particularly vulnerable to pressure from governmental and cultural sources and instances will inevitably arise when these come into conflict with professional convictions. On such occasions, a difficult ethical issue is whether genuine responsibility to society is discharged better by adhering to professional standards or by obeying the dictates of law and custom.

Threats to personal integrity posed by state or social expectations will vary depending on the prevalent cultural norms and on the nature of the relationship between government and citizens. As can be seen by the perversions of psychiatry which have occurred and still occur in the Soviet Union, adverse state pressures are likely to be more serious in totalitarian than in democratic countries. Because of the relatively open nature and individualistic rather than state orientation of western society, it is improbable that the professional integrity of western psychiatrists will run the risk of being thus compromised; this does not mean that more subtle ethical problems of this type do not occur. Psychiatrists employed by and therefore dependent on government, may submit to state pressure. Thus state or public hospital psychiatrists may accede without protest to inadequate standards of care or may detain patients for too long or, what is more likely today, for too short a time in response to outside forces rather than the patients' best interests. Factors other than patients' real needs may guide the treatment decisions of military or prison psychiatrists. Although private practitioners are less susceptible to government influence, they, like their colleagues everywhere, no matter what the setting, operate within a cultural context which produces a pervasive though sometimes unnoticed bias in their judgements. Resulting ethical issues include the dilemma faced by the psychiatrist who is asked to legitimize a request for an abortion on the grounds of a non-existent or tenuous suicidal tendency or to write a certificate for a draft deferment during wartime because of an equally non-existent mental illness. In both instances, the psychiatrist may have strong beliefs in favour of abortion on demand or in opposition to the war. As in the case of state pressure on institutional psychiatrists, the serious question to be faced is whether this hypothetical psychiatrist is acting ethically when he ignores the standards of his profession even for what he considers a good cause.

The responsibility to be accountable

I turn now to a discussion of the responsibility of psychiatrists to be accountable to the public and its representatives. Accountability is defined as 'liability to give account of an answer for the discharge of duties and conduct; usually accountable for acting' in the *Oxford English Dictionary*. This means that like anyone else engaging in activities which are sanctioned by society and which involve a certain degree of power, psychiatrists must be able to provide responsive answers to questions about the scope, legitimacy, and effectiveness of what they do, and must provide machinery to redress errors or wrongs.

The concept of accountability has descended a long historical path since philosophers first debated whether kings and lords could be controlled and held responsible for their actions.[2] By accepting his rule, did the people thereby abrogate their right to any accounting for the power which they had turned over to the ruler? This is what Hobbes thought and it is a doctrine also manifested as the divine right of kings: the king was accountable only to God, while the sole resource of the people was to petition the former and pray to the latter. An opinion contrary to this absolutist view held that the monarch was a representative of the people, from whom he received his power and to whom he was accountable. In modern societies, of course, the latter theory has achieved primacy to such an extent that even in totalitarian regimes it is paid lip-service by dictators. The world now being in a relatively short supply of monarchs, the present application of this ancient debate is that anyone wielding significant power must account for it. Thus, in the United States, Britain, and other democracies, those who hold the reins of government must explain and justify their actions to their constituents. This requirement holds not only for politicians; it is also true in varying degrees for educators, business leaders, researchers, managers of athletic teams, and so on; this equation of power–responsibility–accountability can also be applied to psychiatrists and to organized psychiatry. Jonas Robitscher[3] has gone so far as to assert that the psychiatrist in the United States has become the most important non-governmental decision-maker in modern life, disposing of more power than most state officials. Robitscher views this state of affairs with alarm. He believes that psychiatric power is not subject to public scrutiny, enlightening review, constitution limitations, and it may not be responsive to personal protest. In short, he sees the psychiatrist as operating in relative immunity from the necessity to account for himself. Without taking so apocalyptic a view, I believe we must acknowledge that the psychiatrist exerts a significant influence in many areas of public life as well as in the lives of his patients and that the possibility must be taken seriously that he is insufficiently responsible to the public in accounting for his power. If this statement is true, a number of important ethical implications follow.

Before considering ethical aspects of the need to account for psychiatric power, it is necessary to discuss a derivative and special use of the term accountability which has been prevalent in recent years, particularly in the United States. In this sense accountability refers specifically to the relationships between psychiatrists and third-party fiscal agents,[4] usually insurance companies, either of the commercial or doctor sponsored variety, which provide a substantial proportion of the payment for many psychiatric services. Problems arising in this connection merge into similar but not identical ones in connection with government programmes like Medicare and Medicaid in the United States and National Health Insurance in Britain. As medical insurance (including psychiatry to varying degrees) has become increasingly important to the United States, its requirements for accountability have been complemented by those of the burgeoning consumer movement — which holds that the purveyor of any goods or services must be accountable to the public or its representatives for the operations for which he is paid. This includes the psychiatrist. These two influences have induced a considerable ferment among American psychiatrists and have also been responsible for a variety of conflicts with ethical dimensions. The most urgent one is between the value inherent in the concept of accountability and the value of confidentiality in the relationship between psychiatrist and patient.

An article of faith most fervently held by psychiatrists is that their profession is unique in being able to offer its patients the assurance that any information revealed in the course of the therapeutic encounter will be inviolate. This assurance is compromised by the introduction into the patient–psychiatrist relationship of a non-involved third party which requires diagnostic and other information as protection against over-utilization, fraud, abuse, and misuse of the services their subscribers are paying for. Without a reasonable amount of relevant data, third-party agents are handicapped in their efforts rationally to plan and to protect their operations. They need to do this to insulate their subscribers from crippling expenses and to maintain a competitive position in the health insurance market. Thus, we have the ingredients of a classic dilemma. The psychiatrist wants to promise his patient confidentiality but the latter may require insurance help to continue treatment. Though the conflict is a complex one involving economic, therapeutic, and other aspects, certainly it also contains an important ethical dimension. On the one hand, the psychiatrist needs to be alert to the real danger that disclosures to third parties will compromise his therapeutic efforts. This can happen in two ways. First, the patient may fear that sensitive personal material will become available to outsiders in employer personnel offices or in vast and impersonal insurance networks. This fear may hamper the patient's ability to communicate with his psychiatrist or even to undertake treatment at all.[5] Secondly, the psychiatrist will have to decide whether to disclose to his patient the information he is transmitting to the insurance company. In either case, damage to the therapeutic relationship may ensue through transference complications or the implications of the diagnosis. The psychiatrist's resistance to disclosing diagnostic information to insurance companies for the above reasons is reinforced by his belief, which has some justification, that they treat him differently by seeking more information about the patient and his treatment plan than they do for other medical specialities. Finally, as citizens living in an increasingly interdependent and technological society, psychiatrists share the general revulsion at the spectre of Big Brother brooding over and monitoring their every activity, even the most private. For all the above reasons, the psychiatrist is determined to protect at all costs the confidentiality of his relationship with his patient and to resist the efforts of third parties to extract clinical data.

But there is another side to this conflict. The possibility exists that some of the concern about breaches of confidentiality is excessive and is fuelled by other factors, perhaps more covert than obvious. For one, even if confidentiality must be partially compromised, we need bear in mind the counter-balancing social value of extensive third-party coverage. Since these benefits increase the availability of needed psychiatric services to a wider socio-economic range of the community, it is in the interest both of the public and psychiatrists that third-party operations succeed. Then, it is not clear that the fear of damaging disclosure of confidential personal material is justified by the evidence. On the one hand allegations about unauthorized disclosure have been made before United States congressional committees of the Privacy Protection Study Commission.[6] On the other, in the case of the extensive psychiatric programme of Blue Shield and Blue Cross in Washington DC, under the Federal Employees Benefit

Program, so far as can be ascertained, there have been no authenti-
cated cases in which psychiatric information has been improperly
disseminated.[7]

Although certainly not the general opinion among American
psychiatrists, it has even been suggested that patient–psychiatrist
confidentiality is of more concern to the latter than to the former.[8]
Preoccupation with confidentiality may serve almost as a shibboleth
for some psychiatrists, particularly those with a psychoanalytic
orientation who appear to offer the strongest opposition to the
transmission of diagnostic and other material to insurance companies.
An obvious reason is the importance to them of transference issues.
However, another, more covert factor, must also be considered: a
significant number of patients who consult these psychotherapeutic
psychiatrists present with significant psychopathology and serious
problems about living but their disorders do not fit medical diagnostic
criteria very readily. Thus, psychiatrists who treat these patients may
feel uneasy and even defensive about the whole diagnostic process.
They may fear that their difficulty in conforming to this aspect of the
medical model will jeopardize the insurance coverage of their patients
or limit the amount of treatment authorized.

Although certainly important, the ethical conflict between the
confidentiality of the psychiatrist–patient relationship and the need
for accountability to fiscal third parties is not the only one engendered by this change in the method of payment for psychiatric
services.

It is also unfortunately true that misuse and abuse of psychiatric
services and even outright fraud are more likely to occur when
payment is made by third parties, not only insurance companies but
also government programmes (such as Medicaid and Medicare in the
United States), than in the traditional two party, out-of-pocket
method.[9] Dishonest or questionable practices may be initiated by the
patient alone (charging two insurance companies for the same
service) or may result from collusion between patient and psychiatrist. In addition to being obviously unethical, it is hard to
conceive that a treatment which relies on an assumption of uncom-
promising honesty could be carried out successfully in such a corrupt
atmosphere.

Most of the questionable practices occurring within the context of
third-party payment are the responsibility of psychiatrists alone.
These malfeasances include billing for services more extensive than
those provided or for services not rendered at all, or for multiple
services to members of a family either not rendered or rendered in a
casual fashion. Psychiatrists, as physicians, may retain all or a portion
of the charges for services actually performed by other mental health

professionals, who themselves are not eligible for insurance reimbursement. Behaviour of this kind is simply dishonest. There are, however, other practices in which the issues are somewhat more complex and less clear cut, such as charging a patient's family for time spent with them in discussing the patient's case, or increasing the number of group members for group therapy beyond the usually accepted standards. A question posing real ethical conflict is whether patients in psychotherapy or psychoanalysis should be regularly charged for missed appointments.[10] Here the difference between the two-party and three-party systems of payment is clear. In the former when a patient is properly informed of his therapist's rule in this regard and accepts it, there seems little reason for cavil. Is this also true when a substantial portion of the payment is coming not from the patient himself but from insurance funds? Some psychiatrists argue that the source of payment makes no difference, that their arrangement is entirely with their patients and they deny any direct role in the patient's relationship with the third party. On the other hand, it can be claimed that the public or subscriber source of the funds does make a difference and an ethical issue is involved, especially since it is more likely that missed sessions will be more frequent if the patients do not have to pay for them out of their own pockets.

I now turn to a consideration of accountability in the broader sense previously alluded to — the need to be accountable to the public for the powers of psychiatrists and the claims which they assert. This power is manifested in many ways; in important decisions involving the lives of patients and their families; in involuntary commitment procedures; in judicial decisions imputing responsibility for criminal behaviour; in methods of treatment sometimes administered against the patient's will and which have far reaching and sometimes troubling effects; in research activities involving human behaviour; in ventures involving national and international politics; and finally, and very important, in the application of diagnostic labels which may profoundly affect the lives of the people to whom they have been affixed. Ethical issues involving this power and its applications are the subject of many of the chapters of this book. Here I emphasize the responsibility of the individual psychiatrist and of the profession to provide channels of communication and monitoring agencies to assure the public that they are in effective control of their activities and are effectively policing their ranks. The public needs to know that it will be protected from unacceptable practices ranging from the improper to the illegal. These potential misprisions cover a wide range in accordance with the diverse nature of psychiatric activity. Already discussed in connection with third-party accountability are a number of acts of deception and collusion for financial gain. It needs to be said, however, that legitimate treatment modalities in the profession may also be abused, misused, or over-utilized in instances where payment is made in the traditional manner and not with the aid of third parties.

Internal policing measures are particulary necessary when a psychiatrist appears to be practising with improper or insufficient credentials or under the handicap of incapacitating physical or mental illness. Also requiring vigilant attention are those unhappy occasions when there is reason to believe that overt sexual relations have taken place between psychiatrist and patient.

What are the responsibilities of psychiatrists and of the profession when confronted with situations of the kind described above? It is unlikely that the individual psychiatrist can carry out corrective measures himself but he can be expected to report them to the appropriate channels within the profession. In many instances this expectation is more easily noted than carried out; a psychiatrist faced with such an unpleasant duty is likely to suppress his knowledge. Professional solidarity, uncertainty about the facts and motives both friendly and humanitarian towards the involved practitioner may impede action. Here too, as in the case of the need to divulge information to third parties, the psychiatrist may find himself in conflict between confidentiality and the duty to protect both the public and the good name of the profession.[11] What is he to do, for example, when he learns that an admired and esteemed colleague has developed such a failing of powers through aging as no longer to be competent in treating patients? Similarly, what of the colleague who has developed a severe alcohol or drug problem? Or one who has become mentally ill (as for instance with an incapacitating depression)? Equally or possibly even more difficult is the position of a psychiatrist who hears from a female patient allegations that a previous therapist has been sexually involved with her. In such a case the psychiatrist has, of course, an obligation to satisfy himself that the accusation is legitimate and credible and not generated by the patient's fantasy or by her covert or unconscious motives. Even when so assured, it is still difficult to undertake the ethical course of reporting the behaviour to responsible authorities.

In all of these instances, any action taken should be the result of due consideration of all factors involved not the least of which are the wishes of the patient, and the effects of such disclosure on his or her welfare. As experts in the multifarious ways in which human beings disguise their behaviour and deceive themselves about their motives, psychiatrists need to be alert to the possibility that they are avoiding responsible action because it is difficult and painful.

What about the response of organized psychiatry to complaints of the kind described above when brought to official attention by psychiatrists or other sources? The usual procedure is to refer the complaints to ethics or peer review committees. These operate in different but overlapping areas but share the functions of fact finding and making judgements within the limits of their powers. In the United States they consist entirely of physician psychiatrists affiliated with the organizations which sponsor the committees. This fact has led to the charge[12] that they are nothing more than company unions engaged in charades and that in fact the profession of psychiatry (like any profession) is incapable of policing itself. Critics maintain that in the interests of justice to the public it is essential that non-professional representatives also take part in deliberations about the derelictions and misdeeds of psychiatrists. In reply, spokesmen for the psychiatric profession stress the disruptive effects on the review process of uninformed outsiders and they adduce evidence that such committees, composed as they are, can function effectively.[13] The questions raised by the opponents of regulation of professionals by professionals must however be taken seriously. As with other issues discussed in this chapter, the true merit of the argument made by defenders of this practice must be weighed against the possibility of self-serving rationalization.

If the purpose of accountability is to maintain public confidence in psychiatry as a service-providing institution then it is not enough to ensure that an equitable balance be established between the provision of necessary information to fiscal agents and the protection of the confidentiality of the therapeutic relationship. It is not enough that internal monitoring mechanisms are available to weed out unaccredited or incompetent psychiatrists or to check the few who engage in acts of moral turpitude. Accountability in the broad sense also obliges the profession to be clear about what it is, what it does, its capabilities, and its limits, and to make a reasonable amount of this information available to the interested public.

The profession of psychiatry is not in agreement about these matters of definition. As a matter of fact, that psychiatry is currently involved in an identity crisis is widely accepted and is a frequent source of comment and discussion. To some extent this crisis is inherent in the nature of the profession, a reflection of the reality that psychiatrists must maintain as best they can an uneasy balance with one foot in biological medicine and the other in social concerns. This characteristic has been compounded by real differences within the ranks of psychiatrists. Conflicts of direction and interest exist and are accentuated by the impact of rapidly changing customs and values. The new third-party methods of payment for psychiatric services at least in the United States has been one factor among many in inducing cracks in whatever facade of unanimity was previously maintained by the profession.[4]

Questions about the scope and function of psychiatry which remain unsolved and confuse the public include the following: to what extent is a psychiatrist a physician and to what extent a 'mental health professional'? Is there a schism developing between the 'doctors' among psychiatrists and the 'therapists'? Is a medical education necessary to undertake a primarily psychotherapeutic career? Should psychoanalysis be a psychiatric subspecialty or a separate discipline? Is there justification for the hierarchical order in which the physician-psychiatrist claims dominance over social workers, psychologists, etc. in psychiatric hospitals and clinics and in receiving third-party reimbursement?

Whom should the psychiatrist treat? Should his patients include only individuals suffering from significant mental illness or at least those whose disorder conforms to a reasonable definition of the medical model? What definition of that model should psychiatrists accept? To what extent should the psychiatrist devote himself to the treatment of the 'worried well' — people suffering from discomfort or distress which is not strictly medical — or to attempts to enhance human potential?

How effective are psychiatric treatments? Although this question can be asked of all forms of psychiatric treatment including drugs and somatic methods, it is most urgent with regard to the psychotherapies. What are the reasons for the paucity of reliable outcome studies on psychotherapy? Are such studies feasible at all or is the very attempt to undertake them destructive of the more subtle goals of such treatment? Can third-party or government payment be justified for psychotherapeutic methods which have not been proven effective in accordance with the usual scientific criteria?

Does psychiatry have anything to offer in the care and cure of society or should it confine itself to individual patients? [14] Are attempts to relieve broad social problems evidence of hubris or are they politics disguised as psychiatry? On the other hand, do objections to such efforts reflect a rigid, sterile, and non-humanistic attitude in psychiatrists simply opposed to social change?

Answers to questions such as these are not easily forthcoming. To some extent the manifestations of ferment in a profession responding vigorously to the need to change, they contain economic, scientific, clinical, and political elements. However, it is clear that ethical considerations also apply to some of these questions and to the more general one which asks whether psychiatry is justified in keeping these matters to itself rather than exposing its disarray to public scrutiny.

To be of help in the resolution of the ethical component of these questions, psychiatrists must be able to do more than convey injunctions against fraudulent or exploitative actions or merely supply a code of professional etiquette.[15] A grounding in a theory of values is also required. I suggest that as Freud based the analytic relationship on the love of truth precluding sham or deceit, this same value should guide and inform psychiatric ethics.[16]

Distributive justice

I conclude this chapter with some remarks about distributive justice, by which I refer to the responsibility of psychiatrists to promote an equitable distribution of services throughout the society wherein they dwell and practise their profession. The failure to achieve this goal is a serious problem for all western countries as can be illustrated by a brief description of relevant aspects of the American psychiatric scene.

In the United States at present psychiatric resources are far from being shared out equally; disparities exist at many levels.[17] There is a great difference between the quality of mental health care received by poor people and the middle and upper socio-economic classes (and this difference is compounded by social and ethnic distinctions). The poor have inadequate contact with skilled professionals able to recognize early signs of mental illness. When they enter into a mental health care system, they lack the financial resources or the insurance coverage which would make available to them expert attention and well equipped and well staffed hospitals. The disparity between American state psychiatric hospitals and their private counterparts is staggering — a disgrace to any fair minded observer. The community mental health system and the extension of insurance coverage to the indigent through Medicaid have attempted to correct some of the discrepancies but, for various reasons, what has been accomplished has been only marginal. An important ethical issue arises from the fact that physicians undertaking training in psychiatry are much more inclined to prefer a career in private practice than in public institutions. By making this choice they elect to spend their time treating relatively few patients many of them not seriously ill rather than the chronically ill and often hospitalized schizophrenics, alcoholics, and drug addicts who make up the bulk of the psychiatric population in the United States.[14] As a result of what might almost be termed an abdication of professional responsibility, state hospitals and public facilities are often staffed by foreign medical graduates whose inevitably serious deficiencies in communication impair their ability to help their patients. If we accept that it is a responsibility of psychiatrists to distribute their services fairly, how can we reconcile ourselves to the large proportion each of whom treats a mere 'handful' of patients?

One way in which these inequities are manifested is in the difference in treatment goals[18] for the economically disadvantaged and for the better off. Ambitious attempts to produce significant character changes in middle-class patients can be compared with the aim of merely returning those from the lower class to a previous level of functioning. Reasons having to do with levels of intelligence, sophistication, and psychological-mindedness are given for the difference, and to some extent they have merit. But again, as has so often been pointed out in this chapter, we may be rationalizing rather than reasoning. The support given by the United States government to Health Maintenance Organizations which provide only short-term psychotherapy because it is less expensive rather than also making available long-term and more intensive treatment when indicated[19] may be taken as a example of this trend.

The unequal allocation of psychiatric services between the two worlds of the rich and poor is not the only example of a failure of distributive justice in this regard. Certain geographical areas of the United States are favoured over others, dwellers in the suburbs over those in urban ghettos and the moderately disturbed over the severely ill. A present form of inequality which will inevitably become even more apparent with the changing age distribution of the population is the inadequacy of the care afforded the elderly as compared with younger patients. Tancredi and Slaby[17] state, 'although persons 65 years of age and over are more than 10 per cent of the U.S. population and are known to have a higher incidence of mental health problems than other age groups, they constitute less than 4 per cent of all patients seen in private practice or community mental health centers'.

These inequalities are reflected in the fact that budgetary allotments at various governmental levels are insufficient to meet mental health care needs. Within the mental health budget itself, there is inadequate provision for care of the chronically ill and for psychiatric research.

This maldistribution of psychiatric care has complex roots. To some extent, it is inherent in the structure of a capitalist society — all the more reason why these problems and their ethical implications should not be ignored by psychiatrists who enjoy the bounty of such a society. Individual psychiatrists need to bear them in mind both in career planning and in assessing political choices. The profession as a whole, including psychiatrists in private practice, should participate more actively than at present in the formulation of public goals[20] which would improve the distribution of psychiatric services. Efforts in this direction would constitute a form of advocacy for the mentally ill — certainly an important role for psychiatrists and a significant element in their responsibility to society. Adopting a position which favours extension and equalization of mental health care might however confront some practitioners with an ethical conflict since their levelling efforts could divert third-party and government money from the reimbursement of their middle class patients to the care of the disadvantaged and chronically ill. The pertinent question is whether it can be justified to provide money for the moderately distressed when the disabled are being short-changed? Another ethical question involves the implications of expending resources to care for badly damaged patients who need the care right now, rather than allocating them preventively to improve the mental health of others from similar backgrounds so that they might stand a better chance to avoid serious mental illness.

If psychiatrists accept that it is their responsibility to ameliorate the unequal distribution of their services, they are also accepting, implicitly perhaps, that mental health, like health care in general, is a right of citizens rather than an 'optimal consumer good'.[21] But if this assumption is made explicit, then psychiatrists must go further. If society is asking the profession to help it to achieve mental health, then psychiatrists must define what they mean by the concept itself— is mental health freedom from disease or is it a state of self-actualization? The differing implications of these two interpretations are vast, particularly with regard to the role of psychotherapy. Whether this modality can be considered a significant therapeutic instrument against serious mental illness is an important factor in determining the amount of support it should receive from public sources. As indicated earlier in this chapter, psychiatry has not as yet provided a firm answer to this question; it is its ethical duty to do so if possible or to acknowledge that it cannot.

Whatever definition of mental health ultimately is accepted, financial and budgetary considerations, of course, must be taken into account in making public provision for it. This immediately raises the question of the extent to which it is ethically proper to use cost–benefit considerations to decide how to spend public money for psychiatric services. In absolutist terms, they should not be overriding but in the practical universe, where such decisions are made, a morally utilitarian stance is the best that can be hoped for. In attempting to ensure that the field of mental health care is treated fairly financially, it would be difficult for the psychiatrist to insist that every mental health problem be dealt with financially in equal fashion. To do so might expose him to the charge either of Utopianism or self-interest.

Obviously, if priorities were not set, the health budget of a nation would be astronomical. Although important in the United States, this problem is particularly pertinent for a national health service such as that in Britain where government constantly has to make difficult choices concerning the allocation of resources. For instance, cuts in public expenditure have recently threatened the existence of some intensive psychotherapy units. It was implied that because they were said to provide concentrated service to too few clients they were a luxury the nation could not afford.

The need to decide what sums will be allotted for various psychiatric services also brings different programmes into competition — how much, for instance, for research v. actual treatment programme or for treatment v. prevention. If all citizens are entitled to mental health care as a right, political, practical, and ethical considerations like these will be numerous and troublesome, and it will be incumbent on psychiatrists involved in the process to set priorities firmly and to be clear about the ethical ground on which they operate.

References

1. MARMOR, J.: The feeling of superiority: an occupational hazard in the practice of psychotherapy. *American Journal of Psychiatry* **110**:370–6, 1953–4.
2. SIBLEY, MILFORD Q.: *Political ideas and ideologies.* New York, Harper and Row, 1970.
3. ROBITSCHER, JONAS: *The powers of psychiatry.* New York, Houghton-Mifflin, 1980.
4. CHODOFF, PAUL: Psychiatry and the fiscal third party. *American Journal of Psychiatry* **135**:497–510, 1978.
5. BEIGLER, J. S.: Privacy and confidentiality. Paper presented to the American College of Psychiatrists, San Antonio, Texas, 7 Feb., 1980. (In press.)
6. LINNOWES, D. F. (Chairman): *Personal privacy in an information society.* Report of the Privacy Protection Study Commission, Washington DC, US Government Printing Office, July, 1977.
7. ADLAND, M.: Personal Communication, July, 1979.
8. MODLIN, HERBERT C.: How private is privacy? *Psychiatry Digest* **30**,13–17, 1969.
9. TOWERY, O. B. and SHARFSTEIN, STEVEN S.: Fraud and abuse in psychiatric practice. *American Journal of Psychiatry* **135**:92–4, 1978.
10. CHODOFF, PAUL: The effect of third party payment on the practice of psychotherapy. *American Journal of Psychiatry* **129**:540–5, 1972.
11. DOYLE, BRIAN B.: Psychiatric illness in physicians: confidentiality v. responsibility. Presented at a special session on 'The impaired physician', Annual Meeting of the American Psychiatric Association, Atlanta, 10 May, 1978.
12. FRIEDSON, ELIOT: *Profession of medicine.* New York, Dodd, Meade, 1972.
13. CHODOFF P., and SANTORA, P. J.: Psychiatric peer review: the Washington DC experience, 1972–1975. *American Journal of Psychiatry* **134**:121–5, 1977.
14. KLERMAN, G. L.: The limits of mental health. Presented at Staff College, National Institute of Mental Health, 13 June, 1979.
15. MURRAY, G. B.: Ethics at the crossroads. *Psychiatric Annals* **9**:21–8, 1979.
16. FREUD, S.: *Analysis terminable and interminable.* Standard Edition Vol. 23. London, Hogarth Press, 1978, pp. 211–53.
17. TANCREDI, L. R. and SLABY, A. E.: Ethical policy in mental health care. New York, Prodist/Heinemann, 1977.
18. MICHELS, R.: The responsibility of psychiatry to society. Presented at Annual Meeting, American College of Psychiatrists, San Antonio, Texas, 8 Feb., 1980.

19. Group for the Advancement of Psychiatry: *The effects of the method of payment on mental health care practice*, Report 95, New York, 1975.
20. SOMERS, A. R.: Accountability, public policy and psychiatry. *American Journal of Psychiatry* **134**:959–65, 1977.
21. LEVINE, C.: Ethics and health cost containment. Report from a Hastings Center Conference, *Hastings Center Report* **9**:10–17, 1979.

18

The political misuse of psychiatry in the Soviet Union

Sidney Bloch

That psychiatry is bedevilled by complex ethical problems is abundantly clear from the mushrooming literature on the subject in recent years, and from the other contributions to this book. The vast majority of psychiatrists strive to practise their profession as ethically as they can, guided chiefly by the principle that they do all in their power to serve the interests and needs of the patient. Unfortunately, these interests and needs are sometimes neglected, or even intentionally ignored. Here, we need to distinguish between poor practice — the inept or inconsiderate actions and attitudes of psychiatrists who, because of inadequate training or poor working conditions or disturbed personal functioning, cause patients to suffer rather than to benefit — and misuse of psychiatric theory and treatment for purposes other than medical.

In this chapter I am concerned with psychiatry's improper use, and then, with a quite specific form of misuse: the suppression of political and other forms of dissent through their designation as mental illness. Although there is evidence that such abuse has occurred in a number of countries, the most notable example of it is in the Soviet Union. The Soviet case can also serve to illustrate most pertinently the ethical complexity of the psychiatrist's position wherever he works. I hope this chapter will therefore enable the reader to reflect on how the many thorny issues raised by other contributors to this book are involved in the political abuse of psychiatry as it currently occurs in the Soviet Union.

The features of the abuse, having been decribed in detail by several observers, are today well known (see for example refs 1–9) and it would serve little purpose to recount them here. My concern rather is with the *underlying causes of the abuse — how is it possible that Soviet psychiatry has been exploited as a punitive weapon of the state?* To answer this question we will need to consider (1) the role of the professional

I am indebted to Peter Reddaway, Senior Lecturer in Political Science at the London School of Economics, for his collaboration in much of the research on which this chapter is based, research which found fuller expression in our joint book *Russia's political hospitals* (*Psychiatric terror* in the US).[4] He also made helpful critical comments on the draft of this chapter.

generally, and the psychiatrist specifically, in a totalitarian state; (2) the features of the Soviet system in which, on the one hand, deviance is abhorred and suspected, and on the other, conformism is valued; and (3) the effects of these attitudes on the definition and treatment of psychiatric illness.

Before embarking on a consideration of the causes of Soviet psychiatric abuse, it would be well to sketch out the facts. The abuse can be summarized thus: since the late 1950s a small, but nevertheless significant, proportion of dissenters in the Soviet Union have been diagnosed, although mentally well, as suffering from such serious psychiatric conditions as schizophrenia and paranoid personality disorder. As a result of their 'illness', they have been detained involuntarily in ordinary or prison psychiatric hospitals for periods ranging from weeks to many years. While in hospital some have been given tranquillizing and other drugs for which they have no need; the purpose rather has been to use medication as a form of social control.†

All have experienced the severe trauma of being placed alongside genuinely ill patients; the fear of not knowing when, and indeed whether, they would ever be released; and some the indignity of being pressed to recant their dissenting views, often held with considerable conviction and over many years, in order to signify their 'recovery' and expedite their release.

Those detained in this way have been loosely termed dissenters or dissidents; they share the characteristic that they have deviated in some way from social norms and conventions laid down, and regarded as obligatory by the Soviet state. The dissenters fall into five main groups:

1. *Advocates of human rights and democratization.* They have, through various peaceful and legal means, called on the regime to respect citizens' rights as accorded in the Soviet Constitution and to permit democratic processes to operate.
2. *Nationalists.* Those dissenters who have protested about the lack of rights of ethnic groups, e.g. the Crimean Tatars, the Ukrainians, the Estonians, the Lithuanians, and appealed for the granting of political and economic autonomy to each of the Soviet Union's 15 national republics, again in accordance with the Constitution.

---

† The well known case of the Ukranian mathematician, Leonid Plyushch[9,11] shows dramatically the severely deleterious effects that psychotropic drugs can have when they are used to punish a person or to control his undesirable 'political behaviour'. Klerman and Schechter in their contribution (see Chapter 7) on the ethical aspects of drug treatment, have considered the potential application of medication for non-medical purposes more generally, while McGarry and Chodoff (see Chapter 11) have examined the issue of the patient's right to refuse treatment. It would seem that in the case of dissenters detained in psychiatric hospitals, this right has not been respected by the treating psychiatrist. Neither has informed consent been a feature of the physician–patient relationship.

3. *Would-be emigrants.* Those who have applied, or tried physically, to leave the Soviet Union.
4. *Religious believers.* People belonging to a variety of religious groups, who have been detained solely because of their religious convictions; they wish to practise their religion freely and to see an end to the state's domination and restriction of the church.
5. *Citizens inconvenient to the State.* A more amorphous group, comprising those who are inconvenient to Party or state officials because of their obdurate complaints about bureaucratic excesses and abuses.

The repression of representatives of these dissenter groups by 'political psychiatry' has been only one of several state strategies — the mental hospital has joined the labour camp, the prison, and exile as means of social control and punishment. Why have the authorities resorted to psychiatry when the alternatives available are well established and more than adequate? The psychiatric gambit has certain attractive features (though now also one unattractive one, since the huge and continuing wave of protest and opposition to psychiatric abuse, both in the Soviet Union and abroad, has led to much unfavourable publicity and embarrassment for the Soviet regime). With the dawn of détente during the Krushchev era, the Government sought to portray the Soviet Union as a state which respected the rule of law and where the arbitrariness and excesses of the Stalin period no longer applied. Political trials in which the defendant could proclaim his innocence and highlight the abuses of the legal system had to be avoided. Psychiatry was a convenient ally: by declaring the defendant ill and, therefore, not responsible, the trial became a mere formality, with no opportunity for the dissenter — who was deemed too disturbed to attend the proceedings — to defend himself. Once declared not responsible and placed in a mental hospital, the dissenter's release could result — in many cases — only from his recantation, that is, an admission that his 'dissenting behaviour' was a product of a diseased mind, and with his promise not to 'relapse' into such behaviour after his discharge. Along with the indignity and distress of recantation came other unpleasant experiences mentioned earlier: in some respects these were even more tormenting than those suffered in prison or labour camp. One other key advantage of the psychiatric option has been the opportunity it provides to the regime to discredit ideas which it regards as heterodox and dangerous; such 'crazy' ideas are, therefore, not worth consideration. The human rights campaign of figures like a Red Army Major — General (Pyotr Grigorenko)[10] or a Marxist academic (Leonid Plyushch) [11] are especially threatening in so far as they suggest serious 'internal' flaws in the system. Such criticism cannot be brooked and must be quashed as the rantings of the insane. Potential critics can be deterred from expressing their views publicly.

Hitherto I have referred to a system of psychiatric misuse which is inspired and manipulated by the state. In the Soviet context this means the Communist Party – State. I have not commented on how the psychiatrist fits into the picture. Clearly the state authorities could not execute 'political psychiatry' without the collaboration and connivance of the practising psychiatrist. We can now turn to the question posed at the outset: *how has Soviet psychiatry been deflected from its ethical course?* Although the explanation is neither straightforward nor clear-cut, I would like to offer an analysis based on evidence from several different sources, including the testimony of dissenters who have been dealt with psychiatrically; the reports of Soviet psychiatrists who have spoken out against the abuse; the attitudes expressed by the Soviet psychiatric establishment in its defence of the profession against allegations of unethical character;[12] the voluminous documentation that has reached the west over the past decade, in particular, smuggled-out copies of actual case reports of dissenters[13]; and the observations by social scientists of the dominant role of the state and Party in the supposedly autonomous profession of psychiatry throughout most of the post-Revolutionary period.

The psychiatrist in the Soviet system

The most appropriate first step in our analysis is a consideration of the relationship between the psychiatrist and the Soviet state. In a totalitarian system of government such as that of the Soviet Union, the interlocked state and Party are supreme: every aspect of life is subordinate to them and no one and nothing escapes their tenacious grip and control. And so it is with a profession like psychiatry. Whether the individual psychiatrist wishes it or not, he is faced with the reality that he is not a member of an independent profession and that his actions are guided by political overlords. This position is to be contrasted with the psychiatric profession in Western states. There, governments, through legislation, also exert some control of psychiatrists' activities. For example, in England the 1959 Mental Health Act governs the way in which psychiatrists can and cannot deprive a person of his liberty while a statutory body, the General Medical Council, has the power to strip a psychiatrist of his right to practise if he is found to have acted unethically. Similarly, in the United States, the professional activities of the psychiatrist must be carried out within a framework of limiting laws. But in both countries these forms of control do not prevent the psychiatrist from practising his profession according to his own clinical and ethical judgements.

True, there are other subtle social and political pressures that face the psychiatrist, and against which he needs to be vigilant. However, he is in a much stronger position than his Soviet colleague to fend off the pressures (see Chapter 4).

This is because the Soviet situation differs in several crucial respects. Probably the most significant is the *omnipresence of political control and ideology*. This begins in the psychiatrist's professional life whilst he is still a medical student. Political studies — Marxism–Leninism, political economy, dialectical materialism, historical materialism, history of the Communist Party, and scientific atheism are the subjects involved — occupy a quarter of his curriculum. The medical teacher is enjoined to assume a special responsibility to inculcate the proper political attitudes. He 'must present himself as an agitator and propagandist of Bolshevik ideology in all that he discusses . . . a clinical lecture must constantly refer to the classics of Marxism–Leninism; there must also be references to our philosophical literature for the purpose of correctly explaining pure medical questions to students' [p. 75].[14]

The medical student may harbour private views about these political studies but he cannot fail to recognize the importance attached to them by the state. Later, he will be reminded of their relevance by comments like the following, which appeared in *Medical Worker*, the organ of the Ministry of Health: 'In order to be a working representative of the physician's noble profession, it is necessary not only to have an excellent professional education, but also to be well acquainted with the principles of Marxism–Leninism' [p. 33].[15] The medical student, therefore, graduates with two interwoven qualifications — medical and political. The oath he then takes strengthens this medico-political link since, in addition to the customary patient-directed ethical promises he also declares, 'That I will in all my actions be *guided by the principles of communist morality*, ever to bear in mind the high calling of the Soviet physician and of *my responsibility to the people and the Soviet State*'.[16] The 'principles of communist morality' are not elaborated upon but the mere inclusion of such a phrase in the oath, coupled with the statement about the doctor's responsibility to the people and state, introduces a political tone into what should, ideally, be a document exclusively concerned with the care and welfare of patients.

That a hefty dose of political studies is included in the medical course and that the physician's oath contains political elements are not surprising in the light of the dominance of ideology in the Soviet Union, a dominance which stems from Stalin's view of the place of profession in Soviet society. This view is clearly seen in Stalin's attitude to professional qualifications:

There is one branch of science which Bolsheviks in all branches of science are in duty bound to know, that is the Marxist–Leninist science of society . . . a Leninist cannot just be a specialist in his favourite science; he must also be a political and social worker, keenly interested in the destinies of his country, acquainted with the laws of social development, capable of applying these laws, and striving to be an actual participant in the political guidance of the country [p. 74].[14]

Stalin's emphasis on political qualifications has always been associated in the first place with Party membership, with its attendant loyalties, acceptance of Party policy and a preparedness to obey directives. Generally, professionals who occupy positions of power, such as heads of institutions or senior officials in government bodies, are Party members. This pattern holds for the medical profession too and doctors who are members of the Party — one in five — tend to occupy posts of influence and authority in medical institutions and in the Ministry of Health [p. 126].[14] We can assume that in this regard the speciality of psychiatry is no different from the rest of medicine.

There is good reason for the concentration of Party members in the top echelons, since their presence there enables the regime to monitor the working of the system and to manipulate it. The implementation of Party policy through its 'loyal' membership is virtually guaranteed; not to comply with directives is hazardous and promptly results in demotion or worse. It can be readily seen that the psychiatrist in a senior position is obliged to function as 'double agent', on the one hand he is duty bound to the Party and on the other his allegiance is supposedly to his patients and psychiatric colleagues (see Chapter 4). Lest the impression be gained that senior psychiatrists glide into their positions, there is reason to believe that many of them join the Party in the first place for careerist reasons, in order to fulfil personal ambitions. And, even for those whose professional integrity might have been intact at the outset, the need, for career purposes, to subordinate themselves to the political and ideological demands of the regime leads inexorably to its erosion.

This decline in integrity has been well described by Dr Yury Novikov, a young Moscow psychiatrist, who defected to the West in 1977.[17] In a series of illuminating articles, he uses his own case to illustrate his 'slide' into potentially unprofessional conduct. He concluded that defection was his only option to avoid becoming corrupt. As a promising forensic psychiatrist on the staff of The Serbsky Institute for Forensic Psychiatry (incidentally the chief locus of psychiatric abuse), he became the protégé of its Director, Professor G. Morozov (a central figure in political psychiatry). Novikov was clearly being groomed to become a very senior psychiatrist at the Serbsky. This process entailed a role for Novikov in the manipulation of visiting western psychiatrists in order to convince them that hospitalized dissenters were mentally ill. He also turned a blind eye to the diagnosis of political dissenters as disturbed, (which he knew to be occurring, although he was hardly involved himself) so as not to disturb his privileged status.

The structure of the Soviet health service certainly contributes to the erosion of a physician's integrity. The Ministry of Health is the sole employer of psychiatrists (apart from military, and prison psychiatrists who are under the Ministry of the Interior) and for professional advancement and promotion they are limited to the institutions controlled by the Ministry. And control it is. Following the 1917 Revolution, the model of local government, the zemstvo — which had existed for fifty years and which had exercised some control over medical services — was entirely revamped and replaced by a tightly directed, pyramidal, central government model. The newly formed Federal Ministry of Health assumed, and has maintained since, a dominant role in the setting and implementation of all aspects of health policy. Although each of the Soviet Republics has its own Health Ministry, all major decisions emanate from Moscow. The Federal Minister of Health, therefore, enjoys enormous power. This includes the determination of psychiatric policy, for which the responsible subordinate is the Chief Psychiatrist. The latter is an extremely influential figure, since all decisions regarding the practice of psychiatry must meet with his approval. Both officials, in turn, are advised by the Institute of Psychiatry, a branch of the prestigious Academy of Medical Sciences. This body was originally set up to advise the Minister of Health. The Director of the Institute of Psychiatry wields considerable power and plays a key role, with the Serbsky's chief, in shaping virtually every facet of psychiatry including clinical practice, training, and research (it is significant that the current Director, Professor Andrei Snezhnevsky; the Deputy Director, Dr Ruben Nadzharov; a senior member, Dr Marat Vartanyan; and an ex-Chief Psychiatrist, Dr Zoya Serebryakova; have all been involved in one way or another in the psychiatric repression of dissent.)

Concentration of power and influence in the hands of a minute group and the rigid hierarchical system go hand-in-glove with the disproportionate number of Communist Party members who occupy top positions. By these means control can be efficiently exercised and any unorthodoxy among rank and file psychiatrists checked. Rank and file psychiatrists as a result must submit to official policies and have little freedom to initiate or experiment. No wonder that clinical innovation in Soviet psychiatry tends to be slow and uncommon.

The best illustration of this system of tight control is the virtual domination of diagnostic theory by Professor Snezhnevsky. To appreciate his monopoly we need to return to 1950. In that year a battle was waged at a special joint session of the Academy of Medical Sciences and the Academy of Sciences between the advocates and opponents of the thesis that Pavlovian theory was central to psychiatric practice. Snezhnevsky, at that time a senior academic and Chief of the Serbsky Institute, successfully led the pro-Pavlov forces. His achievement was another step in a rapidly developing career which included his appointment at the relatively young age of twenty-eight as head of a psychiatric hospital. Ten years later, in 1938, he had become a Deputy Director of the prestigious Gannushkin Institute. Snezhnevsky, it appeared, was an ambitious man talented as a psychiatrist and astute as a politician. Thus, in the intense ideological turmoil that characterized the 1950 conference, having confirmed his readiness to serve the political machine, he was the obvious person to promote the 'Party' line. The conference took place in the context of an extensive purge in science, the rise of dogma, strong anti-semitism and the repudiation of opponents to Pavlov. Pavlovian ideas were approved as the only right approach and the entire psychiatric profession was remoulded to fit the new dogma. Anti-Pavlovian psychiatrists were removed from any important jobs they held and forced into retirement or transferred to lesser assignments.

Snezhnevsky's triumph led to his progressive elevation to supreme power: he was soon appointed to the chair of psychiatry at the Central Post-Graduate Medical Institute in Moscow and in 1962 reached the acme of his career when he was admitted to full membership of the esteemed Academy of Medical Sciences, a rare honour for a psychiatrist. He also took over the directorship of the Institute of Psychiatry.

In the course of Snezhnevsky's rise to power he fought a second battle, this time over the concept of schizophrenia. This campaign, and Snezhnevsky's ultimate victory, illustrate further the immense power of the Soviet psychiatric establishment and it's capacity to curb critics and independently minded psychiatrists. Soon after the adoption of the Pavlovian doctrine, Snezhnevsky began to promote his theories on schizophrenia. We shall turn to these later. For the moment, suffice it to say, his views amounted to a broadening of the concept of schizophrenia sufficient to encompass even relatively minor behavioural change as evidence of the condition. His theories were vehemently rejected by other schools of psychiatry, particularly those based in Leningrad and Kiev. Opposition, however, gradually declined — some critical psychiatrists died, others were demoted — and Snezhnevsky, with official support, and in command of the Institute of Psychiatry and also of the country's only psychiatric journal, gained almost complete control. This control has, with the odd abortive revolt, remained intact.

It is perhaps too facile to suggest that Snezhnevsky is, in effect, a Party 'apparatchik'. But the centralization of professional power, the dominance of the Party and the pervasiveness of ideology all point to the politicization of psychiatry and to Snezhnevsky's career as an example. It would appear that a requisite for advancement is 'political-mindedness', a quality obviously demonstrated by Professor Snezhnevsky.

One might reasonably ponder over the value of waging these battles for professional power. What has driven Snezhnevsky (and his colleagues) to battle over several years for complete power? His motives, undoubtedly complex and manifold, have probably been a blend of the following. First, an ideological motive, its strength difficult to assess, may apply: namely, a conviction that the Party is supreme and its interests paramount; the psychiatrist, like any other loyal citizen, recognizes that the Party knows best and that it must be respected. Secondly, careerist ambition — the knowledge early on in a person like Snezhnevsky, that like all other professions in the Soviet Union, psychiatry was hierarchical in nature with much power wielded from the top made it clear to him the means whereby personal ambitiousness could be satisfied. Thirdly, the rewards that result from loyalty to the Party and adherence to its directives are substantial and varied. For example, only a minuscule group of Soviet psychiatrists receive permission to attend foreign conferences. Inevitably the same psychiatric notables arrive no matter whether the subject of the meeting is schizophrenia or psychosomatic disorders or genetics or social psychiatry. One might infer that all expertise in Soviet psychiatry is limited to a handful of psychiatrists, but it soon becomes obvious that repeated opportunities for international travel are granted only to the small coteries of 'trusted' psychiatrists who occupy top administrative or hospital positions, and rarely to anyone else.

The rewards are also ample at a material level and include salaries about three times those of ordinary psychiatrists, access to special stores selling luxury goods at moderate prices, the possibility of owning a country cottage, and the opportunity to holiday at special sanatoria or abroad. The reward system remains intact so long as the recipient satisfies the donor by acting loyally to the Party and obeying its directives. It is obvious that a psychiatrist who wishes to receive these rewards is vulnerable to manipulation by his political masters, and that the way is greased for his entry into the role of double agent: the Party –State on the one hand and the patient on the other.

The problem of multiple allegiance affects any psychiatrist, as discussed by David Mechanic in his chapter (see Chapter 4) on the social context of psychiatric practice. As he puts it: 'When psychiatrists work for organizations other than the patient, they have, by definition, a split loyalty.' And he cites the most dramatic example of this as the psychiatrist who serves as state bureaucrat in a totalitarian society. This as we have seen earlier in this chapter, is precisely the situation that obtains in the Soviet Union, and that enables psychiatry to perform the function of social control at the state's bidding.

How does this pattern link up with the political misuse of psychiatry? Peter Reddaway and I[4] have suggested elsewhere that Soviet psychiatrists can be categorized into three groups *vis-à-vis* their involvement in, and attitudes to, the misuse. The *core* group of psychiatrists is probably no more than several dozen in number. They tend to occupy senior hospital or administrative positions and have participated in the assessment of moderately or well known dissenters, or at least been consulted in some way about them. Particularly noteworthy in this group are Professor Georgy Morozov, the head of The Serbsky Institute, Professor Nadzharov, the Deputy Director of the Institute of Psychiatry, Drs. Margarita Taltse and Yakov Landau, senior forensic psychiatrists at the Serbsky, and Professor Snezhnevsky himself. The second group consists of *average* psychiatrists — the vast majority of the profession who, after they have become aware of the abuse (it only began to become common knowledge in the 1970s) have tried to steer clear of any dealings with 'the complicated cases' of political patients. Motivated by fear and a strong need to conform they have gone along with the system probably using denial and rationalization to avoid their entrapment in ethical dilemmas. The third group comprises a very small number of *dissenting psychiatrists*, who have openly criticized some of their colleagues for perpetrating the non-medical use of psychiatry. Some of them, like Dr Semyon Gluzman, have been punished severely for their criticism, whereas others — Dr Yury Novikov, Dr Marina Voikhanskaya, Dr Boris Zoubok, Dr Avtandil Papiashvili, Dr Alexander Voloshanovich among them — have emigrated to the West and there expressed their condemnation of the Soviet practices. Dr Voloshanovich, for instance, has stated in a letter to the president of The American Psychiatric Association that, 'while working as a psychiatrist in a hospital, and later as a consultant with the Working Commission to Investigate the Use of Psychiatry for Political Purposes I have become convinced that the indictment brought in against Soviet psychiatrists is substantiated, and the abuse of psychiatry for punitive goals does exist in the country indeed. In all the cases I am aware of, psychiatrists are definitely responsible for the abuses.'[18] Dr Voloshanovich is a particularly interesting member of the dissenting group in that he served, until his emigration in 1980, as psychiatric consultant to the Moscow-based Working Commission, a small body, composed of human rights activists seeking to publicize political psychiatry and bring it to an end. In his consultant capacity, he undertook a remarkable task: to assess and prepare reports on dissenters who had been previously hospitalized and on others who had reason to fear that they might become the victims of psychiatric abuse. Their motive for submitting to psychiatric examination was simple — they hoped that a clean bill of mental health, publicized widely both in the Soviet Union and abroad, might deter the authorities from applying the psychiatric gambit to them (and perhaps to others) in future.

Another form of dissent is appearing among Soviet psychiatrists — the indirect challenge to the Snezhnevsky school, through the publication of books and journal articles. A striking example of this development is the research paper by Dr Etely Kazanetz, published in a western psychiatric journal in 1979.[19] Dr Kazanetz, a psychiatrist at the Serbsky Institute, takes issue with Snezhnevsky's diagnostic schema and argues that it leads to an excessive use of schizophrenia as a diagnosis and consequently to undesirable labelling effects on the patient of the schizophrenic diagnosis itself. It is especially significant that Kazantetz has openly criticized Snezhnevsky's hegemony. But he has since paid for this by being dismissed from the Serbsky Institute.

The attitudes of psychiatrists are probably more complex than the above classification suggests. With the school of Professor Snezhnevsky so solidly entrenched over the last twenty years or so, it is more than likely that a younger generation of psychiatrists, who have known no other diagnostic system than that of Snezhnevsky, have been influenced by his doctrine. Thus, they could be sincere in viewing dissent in a serious light and the boundaries of mental illness as much broader than their western counterparts. They could well be influenced by senior colleagues such as Professor N. Timofeyev who has maintained that: 'dissent is a different way of thinking . . . a way of thinking which is in disagreement with that of other people. It can be of various origins . . . it may also be determined by a disease of the brain in which the morbid process develops very slowly (sluggish form of schizophrenia) so that its other manifestations remain imperceptible . . . diagnostic difficulties increase if the subject relates in a formally correct way to the environment.'[20]

This does not rule out that the psychiatrists' own intrinsic conformity and their reluctance to 'rock the boat' lest they jeopardize their careers have also, no doubt, affected their professional attitudes to dissenters. The tragic fact is that the average Soviet psychiatrist is not encouraged to think about ethical issues for himself; and even with personal or second-hand knowledge of unethical conduct among his colleagues, he is likely to avoid the whole issue of his profession's accountability to the public (see Chapters 16 and 17).

We now turn to a more detailed consideration of Snezhnevsky's theories to note their place in the overall picture of psychiatric abuse.

The Soviet attitude to mental illness

The labelling of political and other modes of dissent in the Soviet Union as severe mental illness appears to be a recent phenomenon, closely linked with the theories espoused and promoted by the Snezhnevsky school. But the general intolerance of dissent has always been a hallmark of Soviet society, and indeed of the Tsarist era too. The authoritarian nature of both Soviet and Tsarist rule have been concerned that dissent always spelled danger and threat.

However, a society's concern about unorthodox ideas and behaviour amid its members appears to be universal, although certainly varying widely in degree. The essence of this anxiety is summarized impressively by the British sociologist, Kathleen Jones, when she comments:

without the stigmatization of some acts and some people as 'abnormal' or 'anti-social', there would be no idea of the normal, no rules to govern social behaviour . . . it follows that people whose behaviour is labelled as schizophrenic, criminal, inadequate or otherwise anti-social provide the yardstick by which acceptable conduct is measured. Society is making use of them for its own ends, the orthodox depend on the unorthodox to define their own orthodoxy; but the labels tend to be attached to people haphazardly. Behaviour which is seen as psychiatric disturbance in one society may be regarded as criminal in another, and simply tolerated in a third.[21]

Since the 1917 Revolution unorthodoxy has been labelled both as a criminal offence and a psychiatric illness, undoubtedly with the main goal of defusing its potential to shake the rather fragile equilibirum of Soviet society. The threshold for deviance from conventionally accepted norms has been low, and the level of conformity high. Conformity became deeply entrenched in Soviet citizens for good reason: during Stalin's Great Terror it was a means to survival. Any demonstration of independent thinking could bring Stalin's repressive machine into action, with death or long-term imprisonment the result. A wide range of behaviour — social practices like homosexuality, certain attitudes to religion, particular styles in personal appearance, a love of certain music, art, or literature, and the like — is still readily viewed as deviant in the Soviet Union and the person who exhibits it labelled as 'different' and therefore suspect. Moreover, in a society where the collective is a central feature, and the group takes priority, the individual cannot afford to act idiosyncratically or unconventionally. Rather, he must adhere to the collective and its norms.

Thus deviance, troubling and unwelcome to the average, strongly conformist, Soviet citizen (and this includes most psychiatrists) can be explained away as stemming from a disturbed mind. Bukovsky and Gluzman portray this attitude vividly in their famous *Manual on psychiatry for dissenters*,[22] when they advise the dissenter liable to a psychiatric interview to reply thus:

Unless your studies or your profession require it, you show no interest (and never have) in philosophical problems (for there is a term 'metaphysical intoxication') in psychiatry, parapsychology, or mathematics ... do not display any interest in modern art and especially any understanding of it [p. 109].

In sum, act the complete conformist!

The tendency to label deviant behaviour as illness has escalated considerably with the advent of Snezhnevsky's diagnostic scheme. Earlier we noted his triumph in the medico-ideological upheaval of 1950. In the subsequent two decades he achieved another victory in the successful dissemination of his theories on schizophrenia. As chief psychiatric adviser to the Minister of Health, Director of the Institute of Psychiatry, and therefore the architect of training and research throughout the profession, and editor of the only psychiatric journal in the Soviet Union, he was powerfully placed to emasculate all opposition to his theories. The ascendancy of his school probably constitutes the most significant milestone in Soviet psychiatry since the Second World War, in terms of reshaping the diagnostic practice of an entire profession, and of facilitating the exploitation of psychiatry for political purposes.

Let us turn then to Snezhnevsky's diagnostic approach† which has had such profound effects on Soviet psychiatry. Its most radical element is the prominence given to schizophrenia. This condition is considered to be basically genetic in origin and to produce ineluctable personality deterioration. Thus the diagnosis has very serious import. Once a patient is diagnosed as schizophrenic he is regarded as a life-long victim of the illness and this is true even if he does not show features of it. The Snezhnevsky school postulates the existence of three forms of schizophrenia: continuous, shift-like, and periodic, with sub-types in each form. In the continuous form the patient's course is progressively downhill and no remission occurs thus differentiating it from the periodic form where attacks of the illness are followed by remission and the shift-like form which is a cross between the

† Walter Reich in his chapter (see Chapter 5) on 'Psychiatric diagnosis as an ethical problem' provides additional details on the Snezhnevsky schema. He also shows convincingly in his discussion of the 'power of diagnostic theory to shape psychiatric vision' that diagnosis is a social act, affected by what the psychiatrist views as the society's norms; and how easily — particularly in the absence of competing theories of diagnosis — illness categories can become reified. His observations are most cogent in our consideration of the Snezhnevsky school of psychiatry and its approach to dissent.

continuous and the periodic. Sub-types of the continuous form — rapid or malignant, moderate and sluggish or mild — are distinguishable by the rate of progression of the illness. In all sub-types the onset may be so gradual that the disease is not at all obvious — so-called 'seeming normality', of which more later. The early behavioural changes are often subtle, for example, the patient tends to withdraw, lose interest, and become apathetic. Thereafter follow the 'positive' and obviously psychotic features such as delusions and hallucinations.

The mild, sluggish variety is all important to our purposes in so far as it reflects a broadening of the schizophrenic concept so extensive as to allow even the mildest and subtlest behavioural change to be readily labelled as one of the most severe psychiatric conditions. And it is also sluggish schizophrenia which is the diagnosis accorded dissenters who have been the victims of political psychiatry. Typical of this form of schizophrenia is its slow, insidious development and a picture of 'pseudo-neurotic' symptoms, which may be obsessional, hysterical, or hypochondriacal. Other clinical manifestations include psychopathic or paranoid symptoms. The patient showing paranoid symptoms tends to be middle aged. Although he often retains insight into his illness he overvalues his own importance and may develop unrealistic plans for reforming society or for inventions of extraordinary significance.

The Snezhnevsky school and dissent

'Delusional reformism', 'overestimation of the personality', and 'poor adaptation to society' are some of the criteria regularly encountered in the diagnostic reports of dissenters. Two alternative possibilities exist: (1) do these 'patients' genuinely exhibit reformist ideas which are unrealistic, irrational, grandiose, and extraordinary; and (2) have Snezhnevsky and his colleagues — following 'official pressure' — intentionally widened the schizophrenic net so as to entrap political and other dissenters? The widening of the criteria for schizophrenia is indisputable (it was shown clearly in the 1972 International Study on Schizophrenia[23] conducted by the World Health Organization); but Snezhnevsky could well aver that, based on his extensive clinical research (the study of thousands of cases at the Institute of Psychiatry), milder forms of the psychosis occur. That other Soviet schools of psychiatry and most western psychiatrists fail to subscribe to his views is neither here nor there. The concept of schizophrenia has, since its creation by Kraepelin, attracted much controversy over the extent of its boundaries, the primary criteria required for the use of the label, its cause and its treatment — indeed, every facet of this illness remains cluttered with uncertainties. With no objective yardstick to confirm the presence or absence of schizophrenia in a patient, the Snezhnevsky view of how the concept should be applied is arguably as valid as any other. In any event, most psychiatrists would subscribe to the notion that the belief tenaciously held by a person that he, and only he, has exceptional plans to reshape society or the world, may point to a psychotic disorder. Certainly in my own clinical practice I have had occasion to treat patients who were utterly convinced that they possessed extraordinary powers or wisdom, and that others should listen to their 'message'. The patient as Christ, prophet, or other exalted personage is familiar to most clinicians. But, the question remains, do contemporary Soviet dissenters belong in this group? The voluminous evidence indicates that they do not. While not an easy matter for research, sufficient examples exist of prominent Soviet dissenters once labelled as schizophrenic who have enjoyed normal mental health since their emigration to the west. The Soviet psychiatric establishment's retort that such 'patients' were actively treated while in the Soviet Union and are now enjoying a remission lacks credibility. Is it mere coincidence that Zhores Medvedev, Pyotr Grigorenko,[24] Vladimir Bukovsky, Leonid Plyushch, Natalya Gorbanevskaya, Ilya Rips, Alexander Volpin, and many others have remained 'free of relapse' for periods of up to a decade?

One approach to the issue is to examine closely the criteria used by Soviet diagnosticians. Peter Reddaway and I have done this in detail in *Russia's political hospitals*[4] and the reader is referred to the accounts in Chapters 5 and 6. Our study led us to the following conclusion: that even within the context of Snezhnevsky's model of schizophrenia 'the application of a diagnosis to dissenters is unwarranted, at least as regards those whose detailed case histories were sent to the west by Bukovsky' [p. 251]. Let us consider some of the key criteria used to make the diagnosis in these dissenters. Commonly used phrases are 'paranoid delusion of reforming society or of reorganizing the state or of revising Marxism-Leninism'. In fact, dissenters have acted in ways which in a western democratic society would be regarded as completely normal and reasonable, that is, they have protested about the state's neglect of basic rights as set out in the Constitution; they have called for a separation of church and state so as to permit a person to practise his religion freely according to his own conviction; they have criticized legitimately the severe restrictions imposed by the regime on scientists; they have appealed for the abolition of cults of personality amongst the Soviet leadership; and so on.

Such views have usually been expressed through letters and telegrams, and, rarely, peaceful demonstrations. Furthermore, dissenters have fought for the promotion of human rights within an international framework. This is epitomized in the explicit support given to the most prominent member of the Soviet movement, Dr Andrei Sakharov, (so far not dealt with by political psychiatry but always a potential target and the object of repeated official rumours that he is mentally ill) by President Carter and many other distinguished figures in the west who have recognized the justice and validity of various forms of Soviet dissent. If the Russian diagnostic system is valid, many of them would presumably find themselves tagged with a label of sluggish schizophrenia!

Another criterion used in the psychiatric case reports of dissenters is 'over-estimation of the personality' — usually a companion criterion to 'paranoid delusions of reformism'. Grandiosity certainly suggests a serious psychiatric condition but the concept, it would seem, has been distorted and perverted in the case of dissenters, who are aware of the task they have undertaken. They do not believe that their actions will automatically bear fruit or that the regime will necessarily heed their protests, and none are messianic in their messages. They recognize the frustrating, and above all, hazardous nature of their struggle. The passage into dissident territory is fraught with danger — demotion or loss of job, expulsion from the Party, mental hospitalization, internment in a prison or labour camp, exile — the penalties are obvious and well known. Yet, the dissenter considers the risk worth taking because of the importance of his objectives. He is not out to prove his courage but rather, he is convinced, justifiably, that he has the right, granted by his country's Constitution, to express his views about the state's lack of respect for that very right and for many other rights.

'Poor social adjustment' is another presumptive symptom of schizophrenia in dissenters' diagnostic reports. Social adjustment is regarded, reasonably, as an indicator of mental health. An inadequate adjustment may well suggest the presence of a psychiatric condition. Ironically, the Soviet citizen who assumes a dissenting role is, in a way, maladjusted to his social environment. He does deviate from the social conventions so characteristic of his totalitarian society — complete conformity stemming from a fear of the state's retaliation against unorthodoxy and lifelong social conditioning. The dissenter unlike the 'loyal' citizen proclaims his independence and autonomy, since his actions sheer him away from the compliant and subservient collective. He does not, however, withdraw from society. On the contrary, he is much concerned with its welfare and ultimate fate. Moreover, dissent is not an exclusive pre-occupation: he may work as a mathematician, artist, labourer, engineer, physicist, or doctor; and he may have achieved much success in his career; for example, Grigorenko as a Red Army Major-General, Medvedev as a biologist, Plyushch as a mathematician, Rafalsky as a headmaster, Ponamaryov as a research engineer (it should be noted that many dissenters have been fired from their positions as part of the state's policy of harrassment, and been prevented from continuing to work in their professions).

Perhaps we can now return to the questions we posed earlier. First, are the reformist ideas of dissenter 'patients' really delusional and do they show other symptoms of illness? The evidence from case reports smuggled out of the Soviet Union and from clinical assessments of dissenters made by western psychiatrists is persuasive. It would appear that the behaviour of dissenters is distorted in such a way as to fulfil the criteria for schizophrenia set down by the Snezhnevsky school. While these criteria are in, and of, themselves not unreasonable, when cut to fit the dissenter the fit simply does not match. As for the second question, evidence that the Snezhnevsky school's extension of the schizophrenic concept resulted from 'official pressure' or was originally engineered to provide a psychiatric weapon against the growing tide of dissent in the 1960s remains equivocal. In any event, the diffuse and extremely broad boundary of the diagnosis has paved the way for a subtle collusion between a political authority, determined to stamp out the ogre of dissent from its midst by any available means, and a compliant psychiatric establishment, quite willing to apply the newly established diagnosis of mild schizophrenia to dissenters. The most likely pattern therefore probably amounts to mostly implicit pressure by the state on psychiatrists to use their theories to place deviance and dissent within the orbit of mental illness. Snezhnevsky and his colleagues have managed to satisfy their political masters by developing and applying their comprehensively developed diagnostic package.

Interestingly in the wake of international publicity about Soviet political psychiatry and protest against it from both professional and lay sources, in the Soviet Union and in the west — this diagnostic scheme has come to contain other ingredients. The most striking additional to the Soviet psychiatric lexicon is 'seeming normality', a concept promulgated by twenty-one leading Soviet physicians in a letter defending their country's psychiatric profession.[25] The signatories adamantly refuted allegations that Soviet psychiatry was corrupt and argued that:

There is a small number of mental cases whose disease, as a result of a mental derangement, paranoia, and other psycho-pathological symptoms, can lead them to anti-social actions which fall in the category of those that are prohibited by law, such as disturbance of public order, dissemination of slander, manifestation of aggressive intentions, etc. It is noteworthy that they can do this after preliminary preparations, with 'a cunningly calculated plan of action' . . . To the people around them such mental cases do not create the impression of being obviously 'insane'. Most often, these are people suffering from schizophrenia or a paranoid pathological development of the personality. Such cases are known well both by Soviet and foreign psychiatrists.

The seeming normality of such sick persons when they commit socially dangerous actions is used by anti-Soviet propaganda for slanderous contentions that these persons are not suffering from a mental disorder.

The trial of Natalya Gorbanevskaya illustrates the use to which this concept has been put. The expert psychiatric witness, in defence of his diagnosis of sluggish schizophrenia, argued that well-defined clinical features of psychosis, such as delusions and hallucinations, did not have to be characteristically present for the diagnosis. Moreover, this form of schizophrenia did not require clear symptoms but was present 'from the theoretical point of view' [p. 140].[4] Professor Lunts seemed to be saying that a condition like schizophrenia could exist theoretically but not clinically in a patient — a diagnosis of mental illness in the absence of any features of mental illness! Or, as Dr Martynenko put it in the case of the dissenter Olga Iofe: 'The presence of this form of schizophrenia does not presuppose changes in the personality noticeable to others [p. 250].[4] Via 'seeming normality', schizophrenia becomes an Orwellian and forbidding creature — a giant amoeba which swallows up anything that lies across its path.

The Russian writer Chekhov, in his story *Ward number six*, portrays a chilling situation in which the boundaries of psychiatric illness became so utterly diffuse and blurred that the distinction between normality and abnormality evaporates. The Snezhnevsky doctrine brings us uncomfortably close to fiction.

Conclusion

The political misuse of psychiatry in the Soviet Union is unquestionably a flagrant example of unethical practice, but obviously it is not the only example. The euthanasia programme of Nazi psychiatrists, for example — responsible for the death of thousands of mentally disabled and handicapped patients[26] — constitutes one of the most unsavoury chapters in twentieth-century psychiatry. It could be argued that the current, inequitable distribution of mental health care to the poor members of some western societies, especially the United States — as described by Paul Chodoff in Chapter 17 — is another case of gross unethical conduct.

The Soviet case, however, is of extraordinary significance for psychiatrists because it demonstrates, in bold relief, the myriad vulnerabilities to which their profession is subject and how enormously complex are the ethical dilemmas which face them in their practice. Many of these vulnerabilities and dilemmas have been dealt with in earlier chapters of this book, where more often than not questions have been posed, rather than solutions offered. This is, it seems to me, how it should be. The Soviet abuse very much preoccupies the profession today; tomorrow a variety of other ethical problems will no doubt present themselves. Remedies for these future problems will prove as elusive and demanding as for those we grapple with now. What we as a profession can, and should strive for are two interrelated goals: to commit ourselves to the continuing task of facing the ethical dimensions of our work, and to try to clarify as clearly as possible the nature of these ethical dimensions. Should we succeed in reaching these two goals, the chance of an unethical system of practice like the Soviet one may decline; happily, even vanish.

References

1. FIRESIDE, H.: *Soviet psychoprisons*. New York, Norton, 1979.
2. NEKIPELOV, V.: *Institute of fools: notes from the Serbsky*. London, Gollancz, 1980.
3. LADER, M.: *Psychiatry on trial*. Harmondsworth, Penguin, 1977.
4. BLOCH S. and REDDAWAY, P.: *Russia's political hospitals. the abuse of psychiatry in the Soviet Union*. London, Gollancz, 1977. (In US *Psychiatric terror: how Soviet psychiatry is used to suppress dissent*. New York, Basic Books, 1977.)
5. MEDVEDEV Z and MEDVEDEV, R.: *A question of madness*. London, Macmillan, 1971.
6. PODRABINEK, A.: *Punitive medicine*. Ann Arbor, Karoma, 1980.
7. GORBANEVSKYA, N.: *Red Square at noon*. London, Deutsch, 1972.
8. BUKOVSKY, V.: *To build a castle: my life as a dissenter*. London, Deutsch, 1978.
9. PLYUSHCH, L.: *History's carnival..* London, Collins and Harvill Press, 1979.
10. GRIGORENKO, P.: *The Grigorenko papers*. London, Hurst, 1976
11. KHODOROVICH, T. (ed.): *The case of Leonid Plyushch*. London, Hurst, 1976.
12. See for example *The Guardian*, 29 September 1973; *British Medical Journal*, 10 August 1974.
13. Much of the material has been published in *The Chronicle of Current Events*, a journal produced in typescript every two to four months by an anonymous group of human rights activists, and published in English by Amnesty International, London.
14. Quoted in Field, M.G.: *Doctor and patient in Soviet Russia*. Cambridge, Mass., Harvard University Press, 1957.
15. Quoted in Field, M. G.: *Soviet socialized medicine: an introduction*. New York, Free Press, 1967.
16. Survey, No. 81, p. 114, 1971. Translation of Soviet Physician's Oath originally published in *Meditsinskaya Gazeta* , 20 April, 1971. (See Appendix for complete text.)
17. NOVIKOV, J.: Kronzeuge Gegen den KGB. *Der Stern*, 22 March–26 April, 1978.
18. *Psychiatric News*, 7 December, 1979.
19. KAZANETZ, E.: Differentiating exogenous psychiatric illness from schizophrenia. *Archives of General Psychiatry* **36**:740–5, 1979.
20. TIMOFEYEV, I. N.: Deontological aspects of diagnosing schizophrenia. *Zhurnal Nevropat. i Psikhiatrii* **74**:1065–9, 1974.
21. JONES, K.: Society looks at the psychiatrist. *British Journal of Psychiatry* **132**:321–32, 1978.
22. BUKOVSKY, V. and GLUZMAN, S.: A manual on psychiatry for dissidents. Appendix 1 in *Soviet psychoprisons* by Fireside, H. New York, Norton, 1979.
23. *The international pilot study of schizophrenia*. Vol. 1. Geneva, World Health Organization, 1973.

24. REICH, W.: Grigorenko gets a second opinion. *New York Times Magazine* 13 May 1979. Dr Reich summarizes the results of a comprehensive psychiatric examination carried out by Drs A. Stone, L. C. Kolb, and himself, as well as the results of psychological and neurological testing.
25. *The Guardian*, 29 September, 1973.
26. MITSCHERLIK, A. and MIELKE, F.: *The death doctors*. London, Elek, 1962, Chapter 10.

Appendix
Codes of ethics

CODES for the ethical guidance of physicians have been promulgated over many centuries and in many different countries. In this appendix we offer a selection which we believe are relevant to the psychiatrist. Included are the hallowed Hippocratic Oath and the most recent code — the revised Principles of Medical Ethics of the American Medical Association (1980). Also included is the well-known Declaration of Geneva (1948) of the World Medical Association and, because of its relevance to the chapter on the political misuse of psychiatry in the Soviet Union, the Oath of Soviet Physicians (1971).

Two codes for the ethical conduct of biomedical research in general are provided — the World Medical Association's Declaration of Helsinki (1975) and the Principles of Experimental Research on Human Beings of the British Medical Association (1963).

It is of interest that there are few specific codes of ethics for psychiatrists. We are aware of only two of them — The Principles of Medical Ethics with Annotations Especially Applicable to Psychiatry of the American Psychiatric Association (1978) and the World Psychiatric Association's Declaration of Hawaii (1977).

The Hippocratic Oath

I swear by Apollo Physician and Asclepius and Hygieia and Panaceia and all the gods and goddesses, making them my witnesses, that I will fulfil according to my ability and judgment this oath and this covenant:

To hold him who has taught me this art as equal to my parents and to live my life in partnership with him, and if he is in need of money to give him a share of mine, and to regard his offspring as equal to my brothers in male lineage and to teach them this art — if they desire to learn it — without fee and covenant; to give a share of precepts and oral instruction and all the other learning to my sons and to the sons of him who has instructed me and to pupils who have signed the covenant and have taken an oath according to the medical law, but to no one else.

I will apply dietetic measures for the benefit of the sick according to my ability and judgment; I will keep them from harm and injustice.

I will neither give a deadly drug to anybody if asked for it, nor will I make a suggestion to this effect. Similarly I will not give to a woman an abortive remedy. In purity and holiness I will guard my life and my art.

I will not use the knife, not even on sufferers from stone, but will withdraw in favor of such men as are engaged in this work.

Whatever houses I may visit, I will come for the benefit of the sick, remaining free of all intentional injustice, of all mischief and in particular of sexual relations with both female and male persons, be they free or slaves.

What I may see or hear in the course of the treatment or even outside of the treatment in regard to the life of men, which on no account one must spread abroad, I will keep to myself holding such things shameful to be spoken about.

If I fulfil this oath and do not violate it, may it be granted to me to enjoy life and art, being honored with fame among all men for all time to come; if I transgress it and swear falsely, may the opposite of all this be my lot.

[Reprinted by permission from *Ancient Medicine*: Selected Papers of Ludwig Edelstein edited by Oswei Temkin and C. Temkin, Baltimore: Johns Hopkins University Press, 1967.]

The Declaration of Geneva

Physician's Oath

At the time of being admitted as a member of the medical profession:

I solemnly pledge myself to consecrate my life to the service of humanity;

I will give to my teachers the respect and gratitude which is their due;

I will practise my profession with conscience and dignity; the health of my patient will be my first consideration;

I will maintain by all the means in my power, the honor and the noble traditions of the medical profession; my colleagues will be my brothers;

I will not permit considerations of religion, nationality, race, party politics or social standing to intervene between my duty and my patient;

I will maintain the utmost respect for human life from the time of conception, even under threat, I will not use my medical knowledge contrary to the laws of humanity;

I make these promises solemnly, freely and upon my honor.

[Adopted by the General Assembly of the World Medical Association, Geneva, 1948, amended 1968. Reprinted by permission.]

The Physician's Oath of the Soviet Union

Having attained the high calling of physician and entering medical practice I solemnly swear:

to devote all my knowledge and strength to the preservation and improvement of the health of man, to the curing and prevention of diseases, to work conscientiously wherever the interests of society demand;

to be ever ready to render medical aid, to be attentive and thoughtful of the patient, to maintain medical confidence;

constantly to perfect my medical knowledge and physician's skills, to further by my work the development of medical science and practice;

to turn, if the patient's interests demand it, for advice to my professional colleagues and that I myself will never refuse advice and help to them;

to preserve and further the noble traditions of our native medicine, that I will in all my actions be guided by the principles of communist morality, ever to bear in mind the high calling of the Soviet physician, and of my responsibility to the people and the Soviet state.

I swear that I will be faithful to this oath throughout the rest of my life.

[Originally published in *Meditsinskaya Gazeta*, 20 April 1971. English translation in *Survey* No. 4 (81) Autumn 1971, p. 114. Reprinted by permission.]

Principles of Medical Ethics of the American Medical Association

Preamble: the medical profession has long subscribed to a body of ethical statements developed primarily for the benefit of the patient. As a member of this profession, a physician must recognize responsibility not only to patients, but also to society, to other health professionals, and to self. The following Principles adopted by the American Medical Association are not laws, but standards of conduct which define the essentials of honorable behaviour for the physician.

I. A physician shall be dedicated to providing competent medical service with compassion and respect for human dignity.

II. A physician shall deal honestly with patients and colleagues, and strive to expose those physicans deficient in character or competence, or who engage in fraud or deception.

III. A physician shall respect the law and also recognize a responsibility to seek changes in those requirements which are contrary to the best interests of the patient.

IV. A physician shall respect the rights of patients, of colleagues,

344 Psychiatric Ethics

and of other health professionals, and shall safeguard patient confidences within the constraints of the law.

V. A physician shall continue to study, apply and advance scientific knowledge, make relevant information available to patients, colleagues, and the public, obtain consultation, and use the talents of other health professionals when indicated.

VI. A physician shall, in the provision of appropriate patient care, except in emergencies, be free to choose whom to serve, with whom to associate, and the environment in which to provide medical services.

VII. A physician shall recognize a responsibility to participate in activities contributing to an improved community.
[Adopted by the American Medical Association, Chicago, 1980. Reprinted by permission.]

The Declaration of Helsinki

Introduction

It is the mission of the medical doctor to safeguard the health of the people. His or her knowledge and conscience are dedicated to the fulfilment of this mission.

The Declaration of Geneva of the World Medical Association binds the doctor with the words, "The health of my patient will be my first consideration," and the International Code of Medical Ethics declares that, "Any act or advice which could weaken physical or mental resistance of a human being may be used only in his interest."

The purpose of biomedical research involving human subjects must be to improve diagnostic, therapeutic and prophylactic procedures and the understanding of the aetiology and pathogenesis of disease.

In current medical practice most diagnostic, therapeutic or prophylactic procedures involve hazards. This applies *a fortiori* to biomedical research.

Medical progress is based on research which ultimately must rest in part on experimentation involving human subjects.

In the field of biomedical research a fundamental distinction must be recognized between medical research in which the aim is essentially diagnostic or therapeutic for a patient, and medical research, the essential object of which is purely scientific and without direct diagnostic or therapeutic value to the person subjected to the research.

Special caution must be exercised in the conduct of research which may affect the environment, and the welfare of animals used for research must be respected.

Because it is essential that the results of laboratory experiments be applied to human beings to further scientific knowledge and to help suffering humanity, The World Medical Association has prepared the following recommendations as a guide to every doctor in biomedical research involving human subjects. They should be kept under review in the future. It must be stressed that the standards as drafted are only a guide to physicians all over the world. Doctors are not relieved from criminal, civil and ethical responsibilities under the laws of their own countries.

1. Basic principles

1. Biomedical research involving human subjects must conform to generally accepted scientific principles and should be based on adequately performed laboratory and animal experimentation and on a thorough knowledge of the scientific literature.

2. The design and performance of each experimental procedure involving human subjects should be clearly formulated in an experimental protocol which should be transmitted to a specially appointed independent committee for consideration, comment and guidance.

3. Biomedical research involving human subjects should be conducted only by scientifically qualified persons and under the supervision of a clinically competent medical person. The responsibility for the human subject must always rest with a medically qualified person and never rest on the subject of the research, even though the subject has given his or her consent.

4. Biomedical research involving human subjects cannot legitimately be carried out unless the importance of the objective is in proportion to the inherent risk to the subject.

5. Every biomedical research project involving human subjects should be preceded by careful assessment of predictable risks in comparison with foreseeable benefits to the subject or to others. Concern for the interests of the subject must always prevail over the interests of science and society.

6. The right of the research subject to safeguard his or her integrity must always be respected. Every precaution should be taken to respect the privacy of the subject and to minimize the impact of the study on the subject's physical and mental integrity and on the personality of the subject.

7. Doctors should abstain from engaging in research projects involving human subjects unless they are satisfied that the hazards involved are believed to be predictable. Doctors should cease any investigation if the hazards are found to outweigh the potential benefits.

8. In publication of the results of his or her research, the doctor is obliged to preserve the accuracy of the results. Reports of experimentation not in accordance with the principles laid down in this Declaration should not be accepted for publication.

9. In any research on human beings, each potential subject must be adequately informed of the aims, methods, anticipated benefits and potential hazards of the study and the discomfort it may entail. He or she should be informed that he or she is at liberty to abstain from participation in the study and that he or she is free to withdraw his or her consent to participation at any time. The doctor should then obtain the subject's freely-given informed consent, preferably in writing.

10. When obtaining informed consent for the research project the doctor should be particularly cautious if the subject is in a dependent relationship to him or her or may consent under duress. In that case the informed consent should be obtained by a doctor who is not engaged in the investigation and who is completely independent of this official relationship.

11. In case of legal incompetence, informed consent should be obtained from the legal guardian in accordance with national legislation. Where physical or mental incapacity makes it impossible to obtain informed consent, or when the subject is a minor, permission from the responsible relative replaces that of the subject in accordance with national legislation.

12. The research protocol should always contain a statement of the ethical considerations involved and should indicate that the principles enunciated in the present Declaration are complied with.

11. Medical research combined with professional care (clinical research)

1. In the treatment of the sick person, the doctor must be free to use a new diagnostic and therapeutic measure, if in his or her judgement it offers hope of saving life, reestablishing health or alleviating suffering.

2. The potential benefits, hazards and discomfort of a new method should be weighed against the advantages of the best current diagnostic and therapeutic methods.

3. In any medical study, every patient — including those of a control group, if any — should be assured of the best proven diagnostic and therapeutic method.

4. The refusal of the patient to participate in a study must never interfere with the doctor–patient relationship.

5. If the doctor considers it essential not to obtain informed consent, the specific reasons for this proposal should be stated in the experimental protocol for transmission to the independent committee.

6. The doctor can combine medical research with professional care, the objective being the acquisition of new medical knowledge, only to the extent that medical research is justified by its potential diagnostic or therapeutic value for the patient.

III. Non-therapeutic biomedical research involving human subjects (non-clinical biomedical research)

1. In the purely scientific application of medical research carried out on a human being, it is the duty of the doctor to remain the protector of the life and health of that person on whom biomedical research is being carried out.

2. The subjects should be volunteers — either healthy persons or patients for whom the experimental design is not related to the patient's illness.

3. The investigator or the investigating team should discontinue the research if in his/her or their judgement it may, if continued, be harmful to the individual.

4. In research on man, the interest of science and society should never take precedence over considerations related to the well-being of the subject.

[Adopted by the General Assembly of the World Medical Association, Helsinki 1964; revised Tokyo 1975. Reprinted by permission.]

Principles of Experimental Research on Human Beings

1. New drugs or other therapy should not be prescribed unless prior investigation as to the possible effects upon the human body has been fully adequate.

2. Before a new drug is used in treatment, the clinician should ensure that the distributors of the drug are reputable and the claims made for the products include reference to independent evidence of its effects.

3. No new technique or investigation shall be undertaken on a patient unless it is strictly necessary for the treatment of the patient, or, alternatively, that following a full explanation the doctor has obtained the patient's free and valid consent to his actions, preferably in writing.

4. A doctor wholly engaged in clinical research must be at special pains to remember the responsibility to the individual patient when his experimental work is conducted through the medium of a consultant who has clinical responsibility for the patient.

5. The patient must never take second place to a research project nor should he be given any such impression. Before embarking upon any research the doctor should ask himself these questions:
   (a) Does the patient know what it is I propose to do?
   (b) Have I explained fully and honestly to him the risks I am asking him to run?
   (c) Am I satisfied that his consent has been freely given and is legally valid?

(d) Is this procedure one which I would not hesitate to advise, or in which I would readily acquiesce, if it were to be undertaken upon my own wife or children?

[Adopted by the British Medical Association, 1963. Reprinted by permission.]

The Declaration of Hawaii

EVER since the dawn of culture ethics has been an essential part of the healing art. Conflicting loyalties for physicians in contemporary society, the delicate nature of the therapist–patient relationship, and the possibility of abuses of psychiatric concepts, knowledge and technology in actions contrary to the laws of humanity, all make high ethical standards more necessary than ever for those practising the art and science of psychiatry.

As a practitioner of medicine and a member of society, the psychiatrist has to consider the ethical implications specific to psychiatry as well as the ethical demands on all physicians and the societal duties of every man and woman.

A keen conscience and personal judgement is essential for ethical behaviour. Nevertheless, to clarify the profession's ethical implications and to guide individual psychiatrists and help form their consciences, written rules are needed.

Therefore, the General Assembly of the World Psychiatric Association has laid down the following ethical guidelines for psychiatrists all over the world.

1. The aim of psychiatry is to promote health and personal autonomy and growth. To the best of his or her ability, consistent with accepted scientific and ethical principles, the psychiatrist shall serve the best interests of the patient and be also concerned for the common good and a just allocation of health resources.

To fulfil these aims requires continuous research and continual education of health care personnel, patients and the public.

2. Every patient must be offered the best therapy available and be treated with the solicitude and respect due to the dignity of all human beings and to their autonomy over their own lives and health.

The psychiatrist is responsible for treatment given by the staff members and owes them qualified supervision and education. Whenever there is a need, or whenever a reasonable request is forthcoming from the patient, the psychiatrist should seek the help or the opinion of a more experienced colleague.

3. A therapeutic relationship between patient and psychiatrist is founded on mutual agreement. It requires trust, confidentiality, openness, co-operation and mutual responsibility. Such a relationship

may not be possible to establish with some severely ill patients. In that case, as in the treatment of children contact should be established with a person close to the patient and acceptable for him or her.

If and when a relationship is established for purposes other than therapeutic, such as in forensic psychiatry, its nature must be thoroughly explained to the person concerned.

4. The psychiatrist should inform the patient of the nature of the condition, of the proposed diagnostic and therapeutic procedures, including possible alternatives, and of the prognosis. This information must be offered in a considerate way and the patient be given the opportunity to choose between appropriate and available methods.

5. No procedure must be performed or treatment given against or independent of a patient's own will, unless the patient lacks capacity to express his or her own wishes or, owing to psychiatric illness, cannot see what is in his or her best interest or, for the same reason, is a severe threat to others.

In these cases compulsory treatment may or should be given, provided that it is done in the patient's best interests and over a reasonable period of time, a retroactive informed consent can be presumed and, whenever possible, consent has been obtained from someone close to the patient.

6. As soon as the above conditions for compulsory treatment no longer apply the patient must be released, unless he or she voluntarily consents to further treatment.

Whenever there is compulsory treatment or detention there must be an independent and neutral body of appeal for regular inquiry into these cases. Every patient must be informed of its existence and be permitted to appeal to it, personally or through a representative, without interference by the hospital staff or by anyone else.

7. The psychiatrist must never use the possibilities of the profession for maltreatment of individuals or groups, and should be concerned never to let inappropriate personal desires, feelings or prejudices interfere with the treatment.

The psychiatrist must not participate in compulsory psychiatric treatment in the absence of psychiatric illness. If the patient or some third party demands actions contrary to scientific or ethical principles the psychiatrist must refuse to co-operate. When, for any reason, either the wishes or the best interests of the patient cannot be promoted he or she must be so informed.

8. Whatever the psychiatrist has been told by the patient, or has noted during examination or treatment, must be kept confidential unless the patient releases the psychiatrist from professional secrecy, or else vital common values or the patient's best interest makes

disclosure imperative. In these cases, however, the patient must be immediately informed of the breach of secrecy.

9. To increase and propagate psychiatric knowledge and skill requires participation of the patients. Informed consent must, however, be obtained before presenting a patient to a class and, if possible, also when a case history is published, and all reasonable measures be taken to preserve the anonymity and to safeguard the personal reputation of the subject.

In clinical research, as in therapy, every subject must be offered the best available treatment. His or her participation must be voluntary, after full information has been given of the aims, procedures, risks and inconveniences of the project, and there must always be a reasonable relationship between calculated risks or inconveniences and the benefit of the study.

For children and other patients who cannot themselves give informed consent this should be obtained from someone close to them.

10. Every patient or research subject is free to withdraw for any reason at any time from any voluntary treatment and from any teaching or research programme in which he or she participates. This withdrawal, as well as any refusal to enter a programme, must never influence the psychiatrist's efforts to help the patient or subject.

The psychiatrist should stop all therapeutic, teaching or research programmes that may evolve contrary to the principles of this Declaration.

[Adopted by the General Assembly of the World Psychiatric Association, Honolulu, 1977. Reprinted by permission.]

Principles of Medical Ethics with Annotations Especially Applicable to Psychiatry of the American Psychiatric Association

Preamble

These principles are intended to aid physicians individually and collectively in maintaining a high level of ethical conduct. They are not laws but standards by which a physician may determine the propriety of his conduct in his relationship with patients, with colleagues, with members of allied professions, and with the public.

Section 1

The principal objective of the medical profession is to render service to humanity with full respect for the dignity of man. Physicians should merit the confidence of patients entrusted to their care, rendering to each a full measure of service and devotion.

1. The patient may place his/her trust in his/her psychiatrist knowing that the psychiatrist's ethics and professional responsibilities preclude him/her from gratifying his/her own needs by exploiting the patient. This becomes particularly important because of the essentially private, highly personal, and sometimes intensely emotional nature of the relationship established with the psychiatrist.

2. The requirement that the physician "conduct himself with propriety in his profession and in all the actions of his life" is especially important in the case of the psychiatrist because the patient tends to model his/her behaviour after that of his/her therapist by identification. Further, the necessary intensity of the therapeutic relationship may tend to activate sexual and other needs and fantasies on the part of both patient and therapist, while weakening the objectivity necessary for control. Sexual activity with a patient is unethical.

3. The psychiatrist should diligently guard against exploiting information furnished by the patient and should not use the unique position of power afforded him/her by the psychotherapeutic situation to influence the patient in any way not directly relevant to the treatment goals.

4. Physicians generally agree that the doctor-patient relationship is such a vital factor in effective treatment of the patient that preservation of optimal conditions for development of a sound working relationship between a doctor and his/her patient should take precedence over all other considerations. Professional courtesy may lead to

poor psychiatric care for physicians and their families because of embarrassment over the lack of a complete give-and-take contract.

Section 2

Physicians should strive continually to improve medical knowledge and skill, and should make available to their patients and colleagues the benefits of their professional attainments.

1. Psychiatrists are responsible for their own continuing education and should be mindful of the fact that theirs must be a lifetime of learning.

Section 3

A physician should practice a method of healing founded on a scientific basis and he should not voluntarily associate professionally with anyone who violates this principle.

Section 4

The medical profession should safeguard the public and itself against physicians deficient in moral character or professional competence. Physicians should observe all laws, uphold the dignity and honour of the profession and accept its self-imposed disciplines. They should expose, without hesitation, illegal or unethical conduct of fellow members of the profession.

1. It would seem self-evident that a psychiatrist who is a law-breaker might be ethically unsuited to practice his/her profession. When such illegal activities bear directly upon his/her practice, this would obviously be the case. However, in other instances, illegal activities such as those concerning the right to protest social injustices might not bear on either the image of the psychiatrist or the ability of the specific psychiatrist to treat his/her patient ethically and well. While no committee or board could offer prior assurance that any illegal activity would not be considered unethical, it is conceivable that an individual could violate a law without being guilty of professionally unethical behaviour. Physicians lose no right of citizenship on entry into the profession of medicine.

2. A psychiatrist who regularly practices outside his/her area of professional competence should be considered unethical. Determination of professional competence should be made by peer review boards or other appropriate bodies.

3. Special consideration should be given to those psychiatrists who, because of mental illness, jeopardize the welfare of their patients and their own reputations and practices. It is ethical, even encouraged, for another psychiatrist to intercede in such situations.

4. When a member has been found to have behaved unethically by the American Psychiatric Association or one of its constituent district

branches, there should not be automatic reporting to the local authorities responsible for medical licensure, but the decision to report should be decided upon the merits of the case.

5. Where not specifically prohibited by local laws governing medical practice, the practice of acupuncture by a psychiatrist is not unethical *per se*. The psychiatrist should have professional competence in the use of acupuncture (see Section 4, Annotation 2). Or, if he/she is supervising the use of acupuncture by non-medical individuals, he/she should provide proper medical supervision (see Section 6, Annotations 4 and 5).

Section 5

A physician may choose whom he will serve. In an emergency, however, he should render service to the best of his ability. Having undertaken the care of a patient, he may not neglect him; and unless he has been discharged he may discontinue his services only after giving adequate notice. He should not solicit patients.

1. A psychiatrist should not be a party to any type of policy that excludes, segregates, or demeans the dignity of any patient because of ethnic origin, race, sex, creed, age, or socioeconomic status.

2. What constitutes unethical advertising, in an attempt to solicit patients, varies in different parts of the country. Local guidance should be sought from the county or state medical society. Questions that should be asked include: to whom are materials distributed, when and what is distributed, and the form in which it is distributed.

Section 6

A physician should not dispose of his services under terms or conditions which tend to interfere with or impair the free and complete exercise of his medical judgment and skill or tend to cause a deterioration of the quality of medical care.

1. Contract practice as applied to medicine means the practice of medicine under an agreement between a physician or a group of physicians, as principals or agents, and a corporation, organization, political subdivision, or individual whereby partial or full medical services are provided for a group or class of individuals on the basis of a fee schedule, for a salary, or for a fixed rate per capita.

2. Contract practice *per se* is not unethical. Contract practice is unethical if it permits features or conditions that are declared unethical in these *Principles of Medical Ethics* or if the contract or any of its provisions causes deterioration of the quality of the medical services rendered.

3. The ethical question is not the contract itself but whether or not the physician is free of unnecessary nonmedical interference. The ultimate issue is his/her freedom to offer good quality medical care.

4. In relationships between psychiatrists and practicing licensed psychologists, the physician should not delegate to the psychologist or, in fact, to any nonmedical person any matter requiring the exercise of professional medical judgment.

5. When the psychiatrist assumes a collaborative or supervisory role with another mental health worker, he/she must expend sufficient time to assure that proper care is given. It is contrary to the interests of the patient and to patient care if he/she allows himself/herself to be used as a figurehead.

6. In the practice of his/her specialty, the psychiatrist consults, associates, collaborates, or integrates his/her work with that of many professionals, including psychologists, psychometricians, social workers, alcoholism counselors, marriage counselors, public health nurses, etc. Furthermore, the nature of modern psychiatric practice extends his/her contacts to such people as teachers, juvenile and adult probation officers, attorneys, welfare workers, agency volunteers, and neighborhood aides. In referring patients for treatment, counseling, or rehabilitation to any of these practitioners, the psychiatrist should ensure that the allied professional or para-professional with whom he/she is dealing is a recognized member of his/her own discipline and is competent to carry out the therapeutic task required. The psychiatrist should have the same attitude towards members of the medical profession to whom he/she refers patients. Whenever he/she has reason to doubt the training, skill, or ethical qualifications of the allied professional, the psychiatrist should not refer cases to him/her.

7. Also, he/she should neither lend the endorsement of the psychiatric specialty nor refer patients to persons, groups, or treatment programs with which he/she is not familiar, especially if their work is based only on dogma and authority and not on scientific validation and replication.

8. In accord with the requirements of law and accepted medical practice, it is ethical for a physician to submit his/her work to peer review and to the ultimate authority of the medical staff executive body and the hospital administration and its governing body.

9. In case of dispute, the ethical psychiatrist has the following steps available;

a. Seek appeal from the medical staff decision to a joint conference committee, including members of the medical staff executive committee and the executive committee of the governing board. At this appeal the ethical psychiatrist could request that outside opinions be considered.

b. Appeal to the governing body itself.

c. Appeal to state agencies regulating licensure of hospitals if, in the particular state, they concern themselves with matters of professional competency and quality of care.

d. Attempt to educate colleagues through development of research projects and data and presentations at professional meetings and in professional journals.

e. Seek redress in local courts, perhaps through an enjoining injunction against the governing body.

f. Public education as carried out by an ethical psychiatrist would not utilize appeals based solely upon emotion, but would be presented in a professional way and without any potential exploitation of patients through testimonials.

10. When involved in funded research, the ethical psychiatrist will advise human subjects of the funding source, retain his or her freedom to reveal data and results, and follow all appropriate and current guidelines relative to human subject protection.

Section 7

In the practice of medicine a physician should limit the source of his professional income to medical services actually rendered by him, or under his supervision, to his patients. His fee should be commensurate with the services rendered and the patient's ability to pay. He should neither pay nor receive a commission for referral of patients. Drugs, remedies or appliances may be dispensed or supplied by the physician provided it is in the best interests of the patient.

1. The psychiatrist may also receive income from administration, teaching, research, education, and consultation.

2. Charging for a missed appointment or for one not cancelled 24 hours in advance need not, in itself, be considered unethical if a patient is fully advised that the physician will make such a charge. The practice, however, should be resorted to infrequently and always with the utmost consideration of the patient and his circumstances.

3. Psychiatric services, like all medical services, are dispensed in the context of a contractual arrangement between the patient and the treating physician. The provisions of the contractual arrangement, which are binding on the physician as well as on the patient, should be explicitly established.

4 It is ethical for the psychiatrist to make a charge for a missed appointment when this falls within the terms of the specific contractual agreement with the patient.

5. An arrangement in which a psychiatrist provides supervision or administration to other physicians or non-medical persons for a percentage of their fees or gross income is not acceptable; this would constitute fee-splitting. In a team of practitioners, or a multidisciplinary team, it is ethical for the psychiatrist to receive income for

administration, research, education or consultation. This should be based upon a mutually agreed upon and set fee or salary, open to renegotiation when a change in the time demand occurs.

Section 8

A physician should seek consultation upon request; in doubtful or difficult cases; or whenever it appears that the quality of the medical service may be enhanced thereby.

1. The psychiatrist should agree to the request of a patient for consultation or to such a request from the family of an incompetent or minor patient. The psychiatrist may suggest possible consultants, but the patient or family should be given free choice of the consultant. If the psychiatrist disapproves of the professional qualifications of the consultant or if there is a difference of opinion that the primary therapist cannot resolve he/she may, after suitable notice, withdraw from the case. If this disagreement occurs within an institution or agency framework, the differences should be resolved by the mediation or arbitration of higher professional authority within the institution or agency.

Section 9

A physician may not reveal the confidences entrusted to him in the course of medical attendance, or the deficiencies he may observe in the character of patients, unless he is required to do so by law or unless it becomes necessary in order to protect the welfare of the individual or the community.

1. Psychiatric records, including even the identification of a person as a patient, must be protected with extreme care. Confidentiality is essential to psychiatric treatment. This is based in part on the special nature of psychiatric therapy as well as on the traditional ethical relationship between physician and patient. Growing concern regarding the civil rights of patients and the possible adverse effects of computerization, duplication equipment, and data banks makes the dissemination of confidential information an increasing hazard. Because of the sensitive and private nature of the information with which the psychiatrist deals, he/she must be circumspect in the information that he/she chooses to disclose to others about a patient. The welfare of the patient must be a continuing consideration.

2. A psychiatrist may release confidential information only with the authorization of the patient or under proper legal compulsion. The continuing duty of the psychiatrist to protect the patient includes fully apprising him/her of the connotations of waiving the privilege of privacy. This may become an issue when the patient is being investigated by a government agency, is applying for a position, or is involved in legal action. The same principles apply to the release of

information concerning treatment to medical departments of government agencies, business organizations, labor unions, and insurance companies. Information gained in confidence about patients seen in student health services should not be released without the student's explicit permission.

3. Clinical and other materials used in teaching and writing must be adequately disguised in order to preserve the anonymity of the individuals involved.

4. The ethical responsibility of maintaining confidentiality holds equally for the consultations in which the patient may not have been present and in which the consultee was not a physician. In such instances, the physician consultant should alert the consultee to his/her duty of confidentiality.

5. Ethically the psychiatrist may disclose only that information which is immediately relevant to a given situation. He/she should avoid offering speculation as fact. Sensitive information such as an individual's sexual orientation or fantasy material is usually unnecessary.

6. Psychiatrists are often asked to examine individuals for security purposes, to determine suitability for various jobs, and to determine legal competence. The psychiatrist must fully describe the nature and purpose and lack of confidentiality of the examination to the examinee at the beginning of the examination.

7. Psychiatrists at times may find it necessary, in order to protect the patient or the community from imminent danger, to reveal confidential information disclosed by the patient.

8. Careful judgement must be exercised by the psychiatrist in order to include, when appropriate, the parents or guardian in the treatment of a minor. At the same time the psychiatrist must assure the minor proper confidentiality.

9. When the psychiatrist is ordered by the court to reveal the confidences entrusted to him/her by patients he/she may comply or he/she may ethically hold the right to dissent within the framework of the law. When the psychiatrist is in doubt, the right of the patient to confidentiality and, by extension, to unimpaired treatment, should be given priority. The psychiatrist should reserve the right to raise the question of adequate need for disclosure. In the event that the necessity for legal disclosure is demonstrated by the court, the psychiatrist may request the right to disclosure of only that information which is relevant to the legal question at hand.

10. With regard for the person's dignity and privacy and with truly informed consent, it is ethical to present a patient to a scientific gathering, if the confidentiality of the presentation is understood and accepted by the audience. It is ethical to present a patient or former

patient to a public gathering or to thenews media only if that patient is fully informed of enduring loss of confidentiality, is competent, and consents in writing without coercion.

Section 10

The honored ideals of the medical profession imply that the responsibilities of the physician extend not only to the individual, but also to society where these responsibilities deserve his interest and participation in activities which have the purpose of improving both the health and the well-being of the individual and the community.

1. Psychiatrists should foster the cooperation of those legitimately concerned with the medical, psychological, social, and legal aspects of mental health and illness. Psychiatrists are encouraged to service society by advising and consulting with the executive, legislative, and judiciary branches of the government. A psychiatrist should clarify whether he/she speaks as an individual or as a representative of an organization. Furthermore, psychiatrists should avoid cloaking their public statements with the authority of the profession (e.g., "Psychiatrists know that . . .").

2. Psychiatrists may interpret and share with the public their expertise in the various psychosocial issues that may affect mental health and illness. Psychiatrists should always be mindful of their separate roles as dedicated citizens and as experts in psychological medicine.

3. On occasion psychiatrists are asked for an opinion about an individual who is in the light of public attention, or who has disclosed information about himself through public media. It is unethical for a psychiatrist to offer a professional opinion unless he/she has conducted an examination and has been granted proper authorization for such a statement.

4. The psychiatrist may only permit his/her certification to be used for the involuntary treatment of any person following his/her personal examination of that person. To do so, he/she must find that the person, because of mental illness, cannot form a judgement as to what is in his/her own best interests and without which treatment substantial impairment is likely to occur to the person or others.

[Adopted by the American Psychiatric Association, 1973, revised 1978. Reprinted by permission.]

Index